COMPUTED TOMOGRAPHY IN THE EVALUATION OF TRAUMA

SECOND EDITION

COMPUTED TOMOGRAPHY IN THE EVALUATION OF TRAUMA

SECOND EDITION

edited by
Michael P. Federle, M.D.

Professor of Radiology,
University of California
San Francisco
Chief, Department of Radiology
San Francisco General Hospital
San Francisco, California

Michael Brant-Zawadzki, M.D.

Associate Professor of Radiology
University of California
San Francisco, California

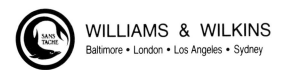

WILLIAMS & WILKINS
Baltimore • London • Los Angeles • Sydney

Editor: George Stamathis
Associate Editor: Victoria M. Vaughn
Copy Editor: Deborah K. Tourtlotte
Design: Bert Smith
Illustration Planning: Wayne Hubbel
Production: Anne G. Seitz

*First Edition, 1982

Library of Congress Cataloging-in-Publication Data

Main entry under title:
Computed tomography in the evaluation of trauma.

  Includes bibliographies and index.
  1. Wounds and injuries—Diagnosis. 2. Tomography. I. Federle, Michael
P. II. Brant-Zawadzki, Michael. [DNLM: 1. Tomography, X-Ray Computed—atlases.
2. Wounds and Injuries—diagnosis—atlases. WO 517 C738]
RD93.7.C65 1986   617'.1   85-16930
ISBN 0-683-03102-3

Printed at the Waverly Press, Inc.
            86 87 88 89 90   10 9 8 7 6 5 4 3 2 1

To our wives, Lynne and Toria,
for their patience and support.

Foreword

Since the first edition of this book 4 years ago, computed tomography has been established as the most important tool in the diagnostic imaging workup of many traumatic conditions. It has replaced many other radiographic and imaging procedures almost completely and has even replaced diagnostic peritoneal lavage for abdominal trauma. Since publication of the first edition we have found increasing uses for CT in evaluation of complex maxillofacial, spine, and chest injuries. We have now had the opportunity to study virtually all types of traumatic injuries to the abdominal and retroperitoneal organs and have even more confidence in the accuracy and utility of CT of abdominal trauma.

This new edition continues the practical presentation of the extensive experience the authors have at San Francisco General Hospital. This experience is invaluable and highlights the importance of the trauma team where the radiologist, surgeon, and other physicians have but one goal in mind: to return a functioning person back into society following a critical injury. The radiologist is a crucial component of this team, in both the preoperative and postoperative periods. While the technologic advances made in computed tomography are important, the ability and availability of the radiologists are essential to successful application of CT in trauma. I must emphasize that it is the experience that comes from countless patients, long nights, and dedication to their profession that makes this book and its contents so valuable. It has been a real pleasure to work with the authors over the past few years as this exciting diagnostic tool has developed and received a wide application to patient care.

Donald D. Trunkey, M.D.
Professor of Surgery
University of California, San Francisco
Chief of Surgery
San Francisco General Hospital

Preface to the Second Edition

As the second edition of *Computed Tomography in the Evaluation of Trauma* goes to press, it is gratifying to review the advances that have been made in the 4 years since the first edition was published. In the preface to the first edition we noted the cautious optimism shared by ourselves and our surgical colleagues as we accumulated experience and shared our findings with the few other investigators who were extensively using CT in the trauma setting at that time. Since that time, there have been dozens of publications attesting to the clinical impact of CT in trauma and the cautious optimism has been replaced by genuine enthusiasm and confidence. Our confidence is based on experience with thousands of additional cases that now include examples of virtually every type of traumatic injury to the cranium, face, larynx, chest, abdomen, and pelvis. This has allowed us to replace anecdotal accounts of interesting examples of traumatic injuries with comprehensive discussions of the sensitivity, specificity, and clinical impact of CT in specific organ systems and clinical settings.

Another major impetus in producing this second edition has been the further sophistication of CT equipment that is now in wide distribution. New hardware and software adaptations allow faster scan times, fewer artifacts, three-dimensional reconstruction of complex anatomic units, and higher resolution thin sections. These technologic advances have unquestionably resulted in better definition of pathologic lesions and more confident diagnoses, particularly in children and agitated or uncooperative adult patients.

We again acknowledge with pride the cooperation and support of all our clinical colleagues, both house staff and faculty, with particular gratitude to Don Trunkey, M.D., Professor and Chief of Surgery, and Jack McAninch, Chief of Urology, for their continued support and interest, allowing us to further advance the uses of CT in trauma, and for "spreading the gospel" to surgeons throughout this country and abroad.

We also gratefully acknowledge the excellent secretarial assistance of Carol Moreno, whose energy, enthusiasm, and efficiency were instrumental in getting this manuscript to press.

Finally, we thank the many editors and assistants at Williams & Wilkins, particularly George Stamathis, for encouraging the production of this second edition and for steering the project through to completion.

Michael P. Federle, M.D.
Michael Brant-Zawadzki, M.D.

Preface to the First Edition

This book represents the culmination of more than 2 years of active investigation of the role of computed tomography in trauma. We began with cautious optimism, having few references to cite or others with whom to compare experiences. New ways of looking at anatomy had to be learned, and criteria had to be established for dealing with a wealth of new information. Our surgical colleagues exhibited the same guarded enthusiasm, and their support made further progress and refinement possible. Being included in the "trauma team" in the form of consultations, conferences, and even in the operating room has been a source of satisfaction and joy to us, and has forced us continually to check the validity and usefulness of our observations.

In presenting this material we fully realize that we make some rather provocative claims as to the value of CT and its role relative to other more established imaging tests. We do so not out of a proprietary interest in CT for its own sake, as the authors and editors are actively engaged in all other facets of radiology and ultrasonography. Nor do we regard this material as "work-in-progress," merely an interesting new technique to be added to the already bewildering array of available studies. Rather, we hope to present material which, while new and challenging, represents the current standard in radiology proven in daily practice at this institution. We hope that our audience includes not only radiologists but all physicians whose increased knowledge of this powerful new tool will permit better care of the traumatized patient.

It is with pride that we acknowledge the cooperation and support of all our clinical colleagues, both housestaff and faculty, with particular gratitude to the following physicians: Don Trunkey and Richard Crass, General Surgery; Larry Pitts, Chief of Neurosurgery; Lee Rowe, former Chief of Otolaryngology; Jack McAninch, Chief of Urology; and Peter Trafton, Department of Orthopedics.

We also gratefully acknowledge the excellent secretarial assistance of Nicky Casciani and Shirley Soucie whose work was often overtime, always cheerful, and amazingly efficient.

Finally, we thank those devoted professionals at Williams & Wilkins, particularly Alice Reid, for steering this project through from its inception.

Michael P. Federle, M.D.
Michael Brant-Zawadzki, M.D.

Contributors

Michael Brant-Zawadzki, M.D.
Associate Professor of Radiology
University of California, San Francisco
San Francisco, California

Robert DeLaPaz, M.D.
Associate Professor of Radiology
Stanford University Medical Center
Stanford, California

Michael P. Federle, M.D.
Professor of Radiology
University of California, San Francisco
Chief of Radiology
San Francisco General Hospital
San Francisco, California

Philip C. Goodman, M.D.
Associate Professor of Radiology
University of California, San Francisco
San Francisco General Hospital
San Francisco, California

Betsy A. Holland, M.D.
Assistant Professor of Radiology
University of California, San Francisco
San Francisco General Hospital
San Francisco, California

R. Brooke Jeffrey, M.D.
Associate Professor of Radiology
University of California, San Francisco
San Francisco General Hospital
San Francisco, California

Hideyo Minagi, M.D.
Professor of Radiology
University of California, San Francisco
San Francisco General Hospital
San Francisco, California

Lawrence H. Pitts, M.D.
Associate Professor of Neurosurgery
University of California, San Francisco
San Francisco General Hospital
San Francisco, California

Lee D. Rowe, M.D.
Clinical Associate Professor of Radiology
University of Pennsylvania
Philadelphia, Pennsylvania

Contents

Chapter 1

The Role of CT in Evaluation of Head Trauma

BETSY A. HOLLAND, M.D.
MICHAEL BRANT-ZAWADZKI, M.D.
LAWRENCE H. PITTS, M.D.

INTRODUCTION

The introduction and development of computed tomography coincided with a growing awareness of the staggering problem caused by head trauma in our society. Accidents are the leading cause of death in the United States in persons from the ages of 1 to 45. A recent national survey found that more than 420,000 hospital admissions were prompted by head injury in a single year. Over 40,000 of these patients spent 3 or more weeks in a hospital. The overall cost associated with the care of these patients was estimated to be $3.9 billion (1980 dollars). The financial burden is overshadowed by the considerable emotional and social consequences of severe head injury, especially when one recognizes the fact that most of the patients affected are in their first three decades of life (1). Mortality and permanent neurologic and psychologic disability in severely head-injured patients have remained unacceptably high in recent years, despite the great strides made by modern neurosurgical techniques and intensive care therapy.

Given this context, the application of computed tomography to the early diagnosis of the head-injured patient offered great promise. The ability to diagnose intracranial hematoma and brain damage quickly with CT has revolutionized the radiographic approach in this setting. However, due to the complex pathophysiology of the brain produced by trauma, the beneficial impact of CT on the management and outcome of these patients has been difficult to demonstrate. Thus, although rapid and accurate information regarding the brain's status following trauma is readily available with the use of CT, such early insight does not always positively influence the prognosis of the severely traumatized patient. The purpose of this chapter is to review the utility of computed tomography in the diagnosis of brain injury, while giving the practicing radiologist a broad outline of the pathophysiologic complexity and therapeutic dilemmas which the managing clinician must face while caring for these patients.

Advantages of CT

Despite the major advantages of magnetic resonance imaging (MRI) in the evaluation of many brain insults, CT scanning remains the modality of choice in the initial evaluation of patients with acute head trauma for a variety of reasons. First, a diagnostic study can be performed in less than 20 minutes following a patient's admission to the emergency room. Life support equipment (such as respirators, ECG monitors, etc.) is not a major constraint in CT scanning, unlike in MRI. CT's sensitivity to soft tissue contrast differences allows an accuracy approaching 100% in the diagnosis of acute intra- and extracerebral collections of blood (2). MRI has difficulty in characterizing a focus of brain damage as hemorrhagic for the first day or two of the insult. Such rapid diagnosis of intracranial hematoma is vital, since delayed treatment of intracranial hematoma has been found to be one of the preventable factors contributing to the death of head injury patients (3). Before the introduction of CT, surgeons relied on immediate intracranial exploration in those traumatized patients with signs of incipient herniation presumed due to intracranial blood collections. Yet one study reported that in nearly half (48%) of such patients, a mass sufficiently large to allow its removal was not found at emergency surgical exploration (4). The inference one can draw from this study is that initial CT scanning of these patients prior to surgical intervention is useful, especially when such a study can be obtained rapidly.

In addition to detecting intracranial blood, CT can detect contusion, pneumocephalus, and radiodense foreign bodies reliably. The secondary effects of trauma—such as edema, ischemia and infarction, brain shift, and hydrocephalus—can likewise be assessed. Skull fractures, especially when displaced, are also depicted.

1

The noninvasive nature of CT is another major virtue, because it allows serial scanning without risk and permits monitoring of the patient's course and the effects of various therapeutic regimens. Late follow-up studies can detect chronic sequelae of trauma, such as communicating hydrocephalus, focal and/or diffuse cerebral atrophy, and porencephaly.

Technique

Routinely, a slice thickness of 10 mm suffices for detection of any lesion which would significantly alter therapy. Although one could argue that three or four selected slices through the brain are sufficient to evaluate the need for emergency surgical exploration, modern equipment allowing rapid-sequence scanning provides contiguous slices from the lower cerebellum through the cerebral convexities without significant loss of time, even in the most emergent setting. Because extravasated blood has a relatively high protein concentration, it attenuates X-rays more than surrounding brain and acts as an inherent contrast medium. Therefore, acute CT scanning in head trauma rarely requires infusion of intravenous contrast for diagnostic purposes.

A technical point of importance worth emphasizing is that blood appears white on the routine (narrow) window settings used for brain scanning due to the concentration of protein constituents in an acute hematoma. Therefore, shallow blood collections layered against the bony calvarium do not stand out easily unless the window width is expanded to show the inherent attenuation differences between blood and bone (Fig. 1.1A, B). Occasionally, image reformations in the sagittal and/or coronal planes may aid in the detection of blood collections which are distributed along the convexities in such a way as to make them difficult to detect on axial sections (Fig. 1.1C).

Contrast infusion may occasionally aid in detecting acute abnormalities, such as continued bleeding (Fig. 1.2). It is also useful in delineating post-traumatic vascular lesions such as cavernous-carotid fistula (Fig. 1.3) and traumatic aneurysm (Fig. 1.4). The use of contrast in follow-up scans of head trauma patients may show ring enhancement of the resolving hematoma (Fig. 1.5). It is also useful in the detection of isodense subdural blood collection (Fig. 1.6).

Nondisplaced skull fractures may be difficult to see due to partial-volume problems inherent to thick CT slices; thus thin slices or even specific bone detail reconstruction algorithms are helpful in their detection, especially at the skull base (Fig. 1.7).

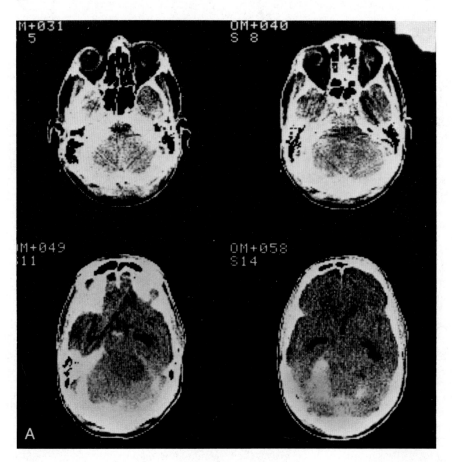

Figure 1.1.   Forty-year-old male, comatose after fall from a cliff.
A. Selected axial CT sections in the posterior fossa, photographed at routine gray scale settings, show blood lateral to the incisura (*lower right*) with effacement of the quadrigeminal plate and superior cerebellar cisterns. Early dilatation of the temporal horns is also seen, indicating obstructive hydrocephalus. The lower row slices show effacement of the paramesencephalic cisterns, and the fourth ventricle is not seen.

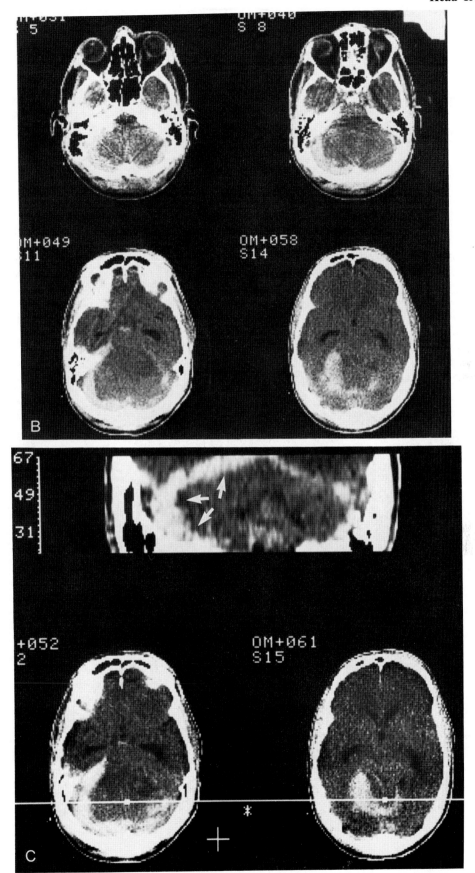

Figure 1.1.
B. Widening the gray scale settings allowed differentiation of the subdural collection extending from underneath the tent into the subdural space of the posterior fossa, along the cerebellopontine angle cisterns.
C. A coronal reconstruction delineates the blood in the subdural space surrounding the right cerebellar hemisphere (*arrows*).

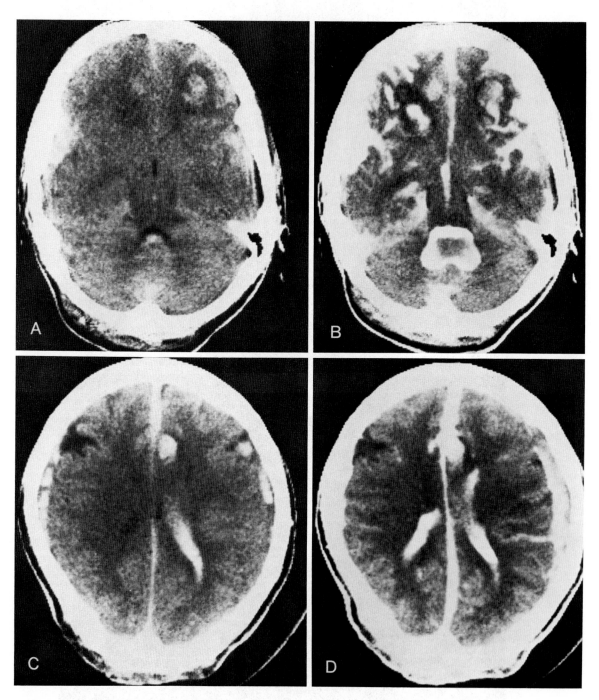

Figure 1.2.   This elderly woman became comatose after being hit by a trolley car.
A, B. Noncontrast CT slices showed extra-axial, parenchymal, and intraventricular blood.
C, D. Following contrast infusion, progressive extravasation of contrast-enhanced blood is seen at the same levels, most noted in the ventricles, the subdural space, and around the brain stem.

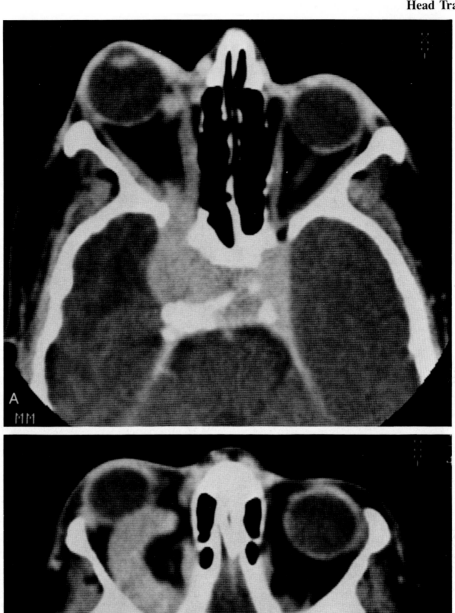

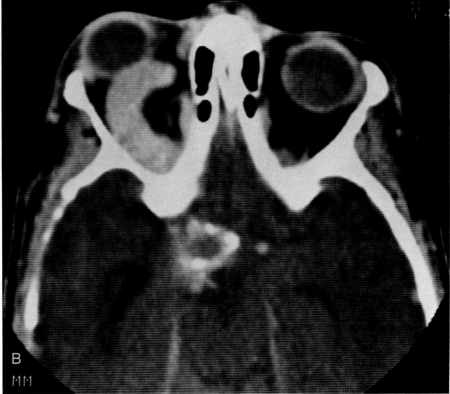

Figure 1.3.   Pulsatile exophthalmos developed shortly after trauma in this young female.
A, B. A contrast-enhanced CT scan showed an abnormal vascular structure expanding the right cavernous sinus, with marked expansion of the superior ophthalmic vein seen on the higher cut.

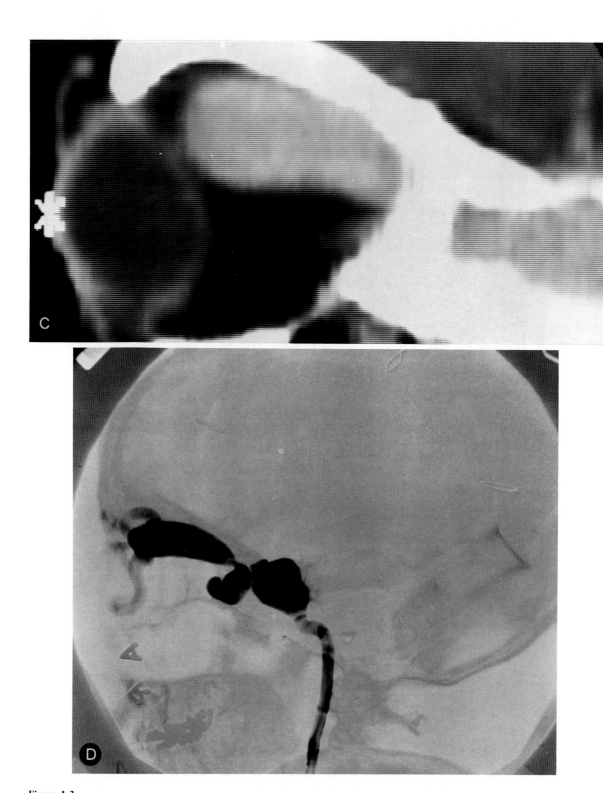

Figure 1.3.
C. Image reformation in the orbit's sagittal plane delineated the grossly hypertrophied ophthalmic vein, presumed due to a cavernous carotid fistula.
D. Angiography verified this impression.

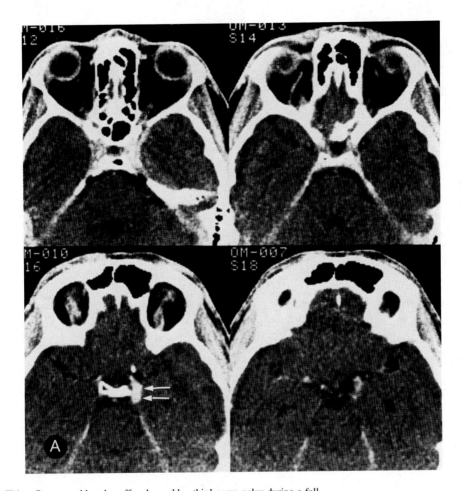

Figure 1.4.   Thirty-five-year-old male suffered a sudden third nerve palsy during a fall.
A. Sequential thin-section CT scans following contrast infusion depicted an abnormal vascular density in the posterior suprasellar cistern on the left (*arrows*).

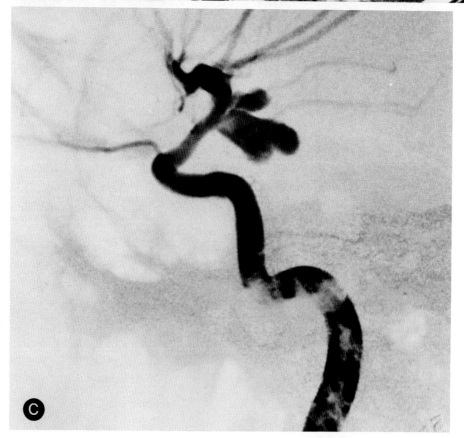

Figure 1.4.
B. Image reformation in the coronal plane suggested a bilobed aneurysm (*arrows*).
C. Two aneurysms off the internal carotid were documented with angiography.

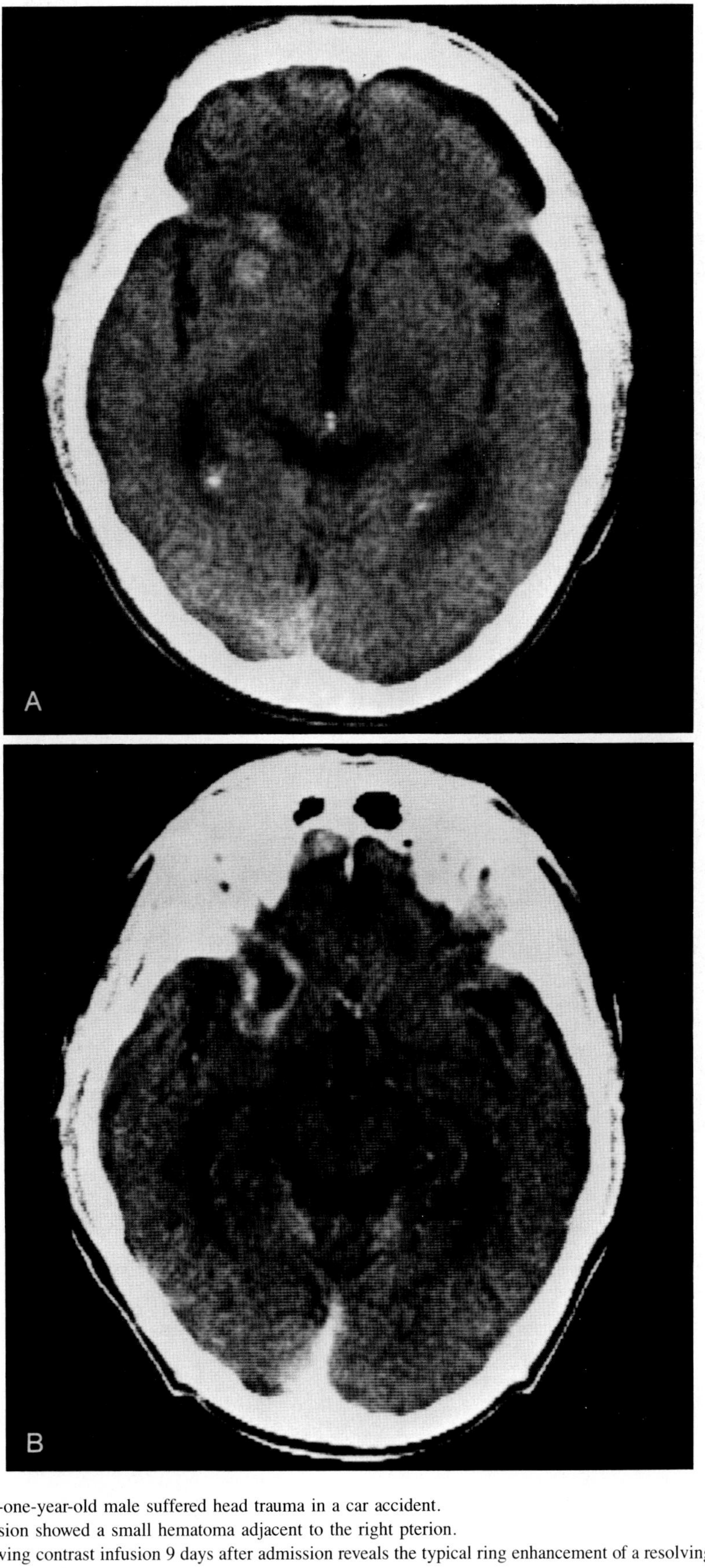

Figure 1.5. Seventy-one-year-old male suffered head trauma in a car accident.
A. CT scan on admission showed a small hematoma adjacent to the right pterion.
B. Repeat study following contrast infusion 9 days after admission reveals the typical ring enhancement of a resolving hematoma. Note the low density of the liquifying clot.

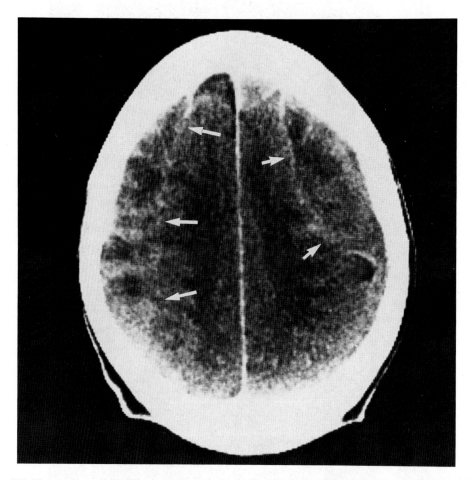

Figure 1.6.   This 87-year-old man had a CT scan to evaluate dementia. Precontrast slices showed effacement of cortical sulci and equivocal medial displacement of the white matter. Following contrast infusion, bilateral extra-axial, isodense collections are defined by the enhancing inner borders. Both were subdural hematomas. Note the inwardly bulging shape of the left-sided collection, mimicking the shape taken by acute epidural bleeds.

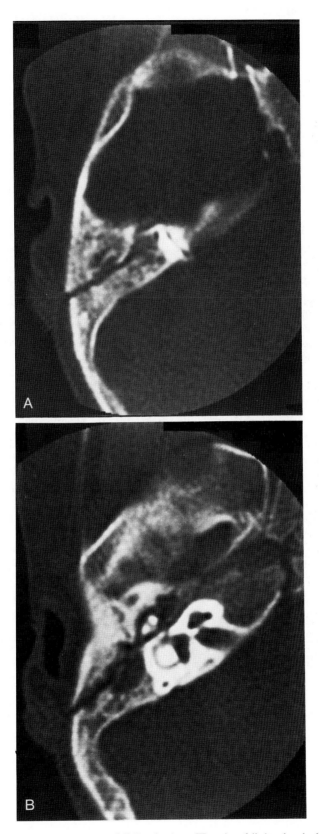

Figure 1.7. Three-year-old female suffering a two-story fall. Routine 1-cm CT sections failed to show basilar fracture, despite the presence of a right hemotympanum.
A. High-resolution CT scan done with a specific bone detail reconstruction algorithm utilizing an extended CT number scale (RE VIEW, GE CORP) showed an oblique fracture of the petrous bone.
B. At the level of the ossicles, soft tissue can be seen in the middle ear, but no evidence of ossicular disruption is noted. The fracture did not involve the inner ear structures depicted here.

Limitations

Technical limitations do occur in the scanning of head trauma victims. Some of these patients may be agitated, and motion artifact severely degrades the CT images. Sedation is occasionally contraindicated and may even produce a paradoxical response. Heavier sedation with anesthesia "standby" may be necessary to achieve diagnostic images. Yet, most patients are either cooperative or comatose, and diagnostic images are easily obtained. Bone streak artifacts may obscure optimal visualization of the temporal lobes, posterior fossa, and other anatomy; repeat slices may be necessary at affected levels.

Vascular damage, such as transection of blood vessels, formation of false aneurysm, and development of spasm, may be difficult to identify on CT scans despite contrast infusion. Thus, a limited role still exists for angiography of the head-traumatized patient.

Other limitations of computed tomography relate to the complex pathophysiology of head trauma. Thus, up to one-half of severely head-injured patients may show no abnormality on the initial CT evaluation (5, 6). Some of these patients will develop delayed intracranial hemorrhage necessitating its surgical evacuation. Thus short-interval follow-up scans in this group are mandatory (7–10), especially if the patient develops focal neurologic deficits or has persistent intracranial hypertension.

Some patients with severe head injury will remain comatose and survive in a vegetative state or die despite persistently normal CT scans. This subgroup of individuals includes those who have suffered diffuse brain damage due to the immediate impact forces, causing a shearing injury of the cerebral white matter. Such an injury may produce only minimal subcortical hematomas and punctate hemorrhages in the corpus callosum and pontine tectum, which may be difficult to visualize on CT scanning unless high-resolution, thin-section technique is employed (11–13). The mechanism of this injury will be further discussed in the next section. It should also be realized that the delayed effects of direct brain trauma—such as vascular engorgement, edema, and infarction—are quite common but are difficult to detect on CT scans obtained within the first 24 hours of injury.

Finally, CT scanning alone has been found wanting in its contribution to the early prediction of outcome in head-injured patients due to the complex interaction of multiple factors which affect the prognosis of these patients (14, 15).

Because of the above-mentioned considerations, the radiologist should not only understand the radiographic principles which apply to the interpretations of CT scans in the head trauma patient, but should have at least a broad understanding of the pathophysiologic mechanisms that lead to the radiographic expression of the abnormality on the CT image.

PATHOPHYSIOLOGY OF HEAD TRAUMA—AN OVERVIEW

Much of our understanding regarding the pathophysiology of head trauma is derived from experimental studies, the review of which is beyond the scope of this chapter. The interested reader is referred to the concise discussion of this topic offered by Jennett and Teasdale in their excellent monograph on the management of head injury (16). As these authors point out, experimental models are far from perfect. However, systematic investigation of brain trauma in animal models has yielded important information.

The structural pathology of the brain following trauma can be divided into two broad categories. The first is the "primary" impact injury, and the second is the damage produced by the "secondary" cerebral responses initiated by the original impact and/or parenchymal disruption. The general systemic response to central nervous system injury and generalized body trauma (if any) also contributes to the secondary influences encountered in the head-traumatized patient.

Primary Impact Damage

Direct impact to the cranial vault results in a skull fracture in the majority of patients who suffer fatal or severely debilitating brain injuries. Yet the presence of a skull fracture, in and of itself, is of little clinical significance, unless it traverses a meningeal vessel or produces displacement of fragments sufficient to contuse or lacerate the brain parenchyma.

Focal contusions and lacerations of the brain parenchyma occur under the point of impact, if local deformation of the bony calvarium has been severe enough. More commonly, the contusions and subsequent hematomas which develop occur due to inertial factors (Fig. 1.8). Thus, when the bony cranial vault is hit and displaced, the brain within it is transiently "left behind." This leads to contusion of those portions of the brain which are adjacent to the more angulated and roughened internal calvarial structures. The undersurface of the frontal lobe which overlies the irregular orbital roofs and the temporal lobe enclosed within the middle fossa and its protruding sphenoid wing are the regions of the cerebrum which most often show evidence of contusion and/or frank hematoma (Fig. 1.9). The relatively low incidence of such lesions in the parieto-occipital region can be explained by the smooth and gently curving nature of the parieto-occipital skull.

In addition to the focal lesions just described, diffuse brain damage can occur immediately upon impact. Extensive destruction in the white matter, especially at its junction with the gray matter, has been found at autopsy in severely traumatized brains of patients who die within a short time after impact (Fig. 1.10). The microscopic findings in these cases show axonal stretching and shearing, as well as some lac-

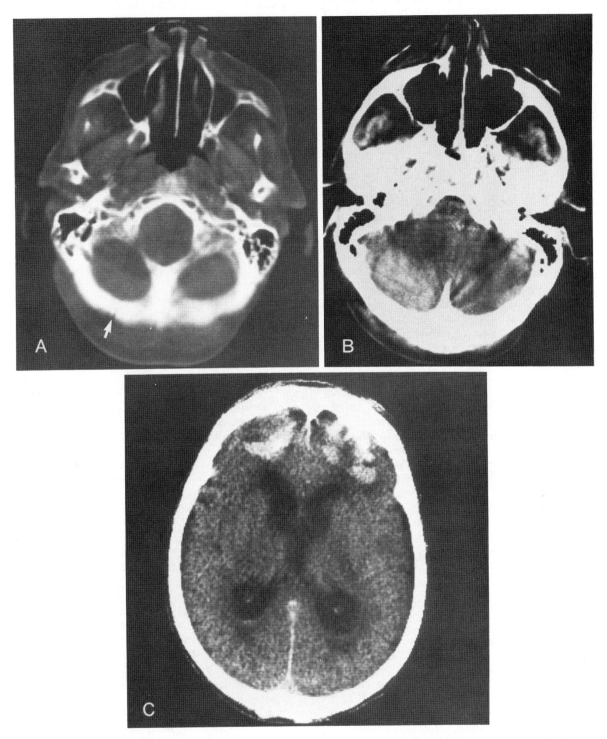

Figure 1.8. Eighty-year-old female was obtunded in the emergency room after a fall on the street. Deterioration led to this CT scan. **A, B.** A suboccipital fracture was seen on bone window settings (*arrow*), with an associated cerebellar hematoma shown on the higher cut. **C.** Supratentorial sections delineated "contre coup" hematomas in both frontal lobes. Note the hydrocephalus, with a small amount of blood in both ventricular atria. The patient recovered following surgical removal of the cerebellar hematoma.

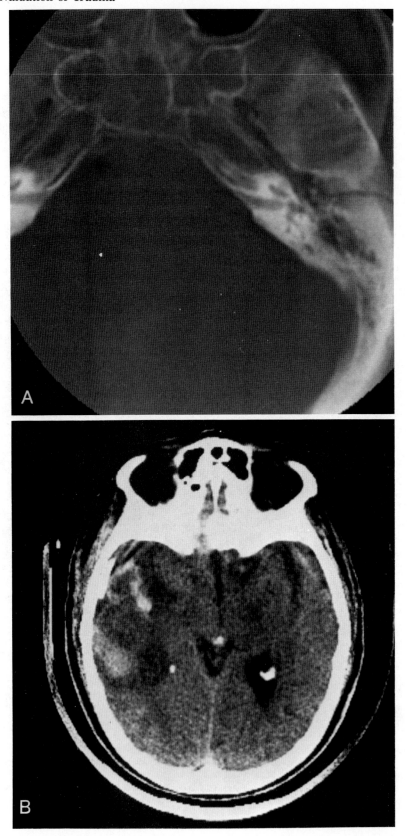

Figure 1.9.   This elderly female with an altered mental status following left-sided blow to head was noted to have blood in the left external auditory canal.
A. Bone detail CT section at the level of the left external auditory canal shows a transverse fracture traversing the collapsed canal.
B. Higher sections revealed a contralateral temporal lobe hematoma, presumably caused by contusion of the region due to sudden shift of the underlying petrous ridge.

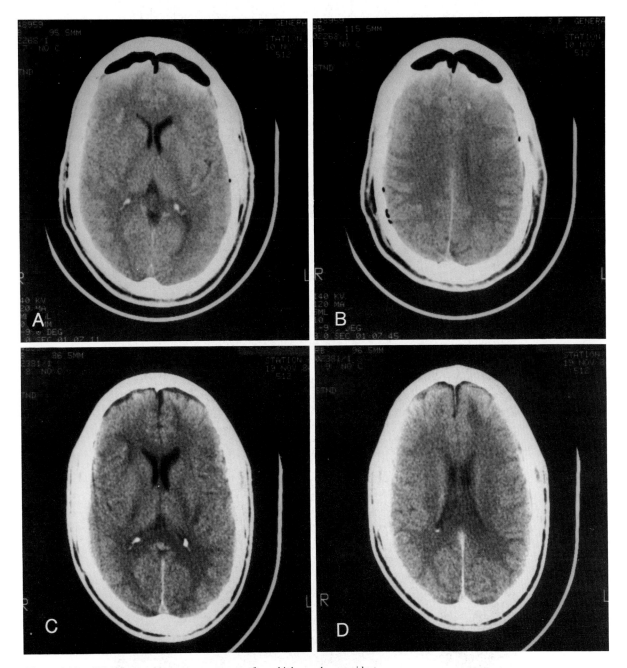

Figure 1.10.   This 25-year-old man was comatose after a high-speed car accident.
A, B. CT scan shows multiple focal hemorrhages at the junction of gray and white matter. The location and size of these hemorrhages are characteristic of shearing injury.
C, D. Nine days later the patient had not improved neurologically. Interval partial resorption of high-density hemorrhages is noted, with residual low density.

eration of brain tissue. Minor changes of this nature, i.e., axonal stretching and microvascular rupture, may be responsible for the relatively benign "concussion" seen clinically, whereas a severe generalized injury of this type heralds a uniformly bad prognosis (11). The nature of this injury relates to the structural makeup of the brain and vectors of force applied to it during impact. The brain has been compared to gelatin in consistency, since it lacks rigidity but is incompressible. This latter property allows relatively little movement or compression of different parts of the brain in linear acceleration. However, if an element of rotation is introduced during the traumatic event, there is great potential for shearing between adjacent parts of the brain which have differential densities (such as the gray and white matter) (17). The amount of brain damage sustained will relate to the amount of rotational acceleration and to the mass of the brain. The brain parenchyma is affected in a centripetal sequence, the cortex alone being damaged in milder cases, followed by the deeper structures with increas-

ing severity of injury. Not surprisingly, therefore, observations on autopsy cases of immediate impact human head injury confirm that brainstem injury is found only in conjunction with extensive subcortical and cortical damage (11). Occasionally, however, cases of primary brainstem contusion or hemorrhage can occur in isolation, if the vector of force is a linear one which shoves the pons laterally against the rigid tentorial incisura (Fig. 1.11).

Another event which occurs with impact injury is extra-axial bleeding into either the subdural or, less often, the epidural space. This is due to disruption of venous structures or arteries. Adverse effects of such bleeding arise from the secondary pressure and shift produced. The size of the bleed obviously plays a role, but is interrelated with the brain-calvarium volume relationship. Thus, older patients with "shrunken" brains may accommodate extra-axial hematomas with relatively few symptoms or neurologic signs, and the secondary damage to the brain may be slight.

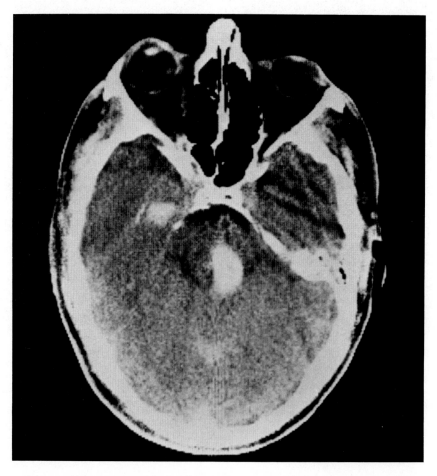

Figure 1.11.   Twenty-eight-year-old man was thrown from a car involved in a collision. Decerebrate positioning was noted on evaluation in the emergency room. The CT scan demonstrated a brainstem hematoma. The patient survived with a profound right hemiparesis. Incidentally, note the small, medial temporal hematoma.

Secondary Factors

Secondary brain damage occurs consequent to the impact and requires some time to develop; the resulting structural changes require still longer for recognition on CT scanning or at autopsy. The mediating physiologic factors of this secondary damage include loss of autoregulation of the cerebral vasculature, breakdown of the blood-brain barrier, the development of vasogenic edema, and brain shift. All of these factors may be influenced by the cardiovascular and pulmonary systems, their responses to CNS injury including initial hypertension or shock, changes in cardiac rhythm, contractility and cardiac output, and ventilatory abnormalities leading to hypoxia and hypercarbia.

The "final common pathway" of brain damage of most, if not all, of the secondary factors mentioned relates to the disruption of metabolic pathways within the brain cells. The marked metabolic demands of the brain are reflected by its enormous consumption of oxygen and glucose. This organ, which represents only 2% of the adult body weight, requires 20% of the cardiac output for its oxygen needs and 25% of the total glucose consumption of the entire body. Not surprisingly, any factor diminishing either blood flow and/or glucose delivery to the brain may severely affect its function. If such disruption persists for more than a few minutes, irreversible damage results.

Cerebral tissue perfusion depends upon the differential between systemic arterial blood pressure and the intracranial pressure. If the intracranial pressure is elevated sufficiently by mass effect, to effectively block capillary blood flow, even systemic hypertension cannot maintain cerebral perfusion. A paradoxical example of this is the diffuse cerebral swelling seen following pediatric head injury. A generalized loss of autoregulation leads to cerebral vasodilatation and increased blood volume, with little or no edema. This hyperemia may actually cause sufficient expansion of the brain's volume to cause its compression against the inner table, raising the intracranial pressure sufficiently to diminish cerebral capillary blood flow and produce tissue anoxia. Prolonged coma and even death may result (18). The CT picture in these young patients depicts loss of cerebrospinal fluid (CSF) spaces (Fig. 1.12), including the ventricles, and evidence of brainstem compression due to generalized cerebral swelling without obvious low density indicative of edema (18–20).

All elevations of intracranial pressure, whether due to the "hyperemia" just mentioned or to focal mass lesions induced by intracranial hematoma and/or contusion, may lead to diminution of regional or general cerebral blood flow (21, 22). These disturbances of circulation may lead to increasing edema, mass effect, and further infarction in a vicious cycle of events. In fact, ischemic brain damage and/or frank infarction can be found in more than 90% of severely brain-traumatized patients at autopsy (23). Infarcts in head trauma patients can be seen most often in the "watershed" areas between two arterial distributions (23) (Fig. 1.13). It is these regions of the brain, farthest removed from the major arterial feeders, that first feel the effects of diminished perfusion. Vascular occlusion due to brain shift and resulting vessel compression can produce more typical territorial infarcts. These are most often noted in a posterior cerebral artery distribution since the artery may be compressed against the tentorial edge by the shifting brain. However, they can occur in other discrete arterial territories as well (Fig. 1.14).

It is not surprising, therefore, that the high morbidity and mortality associated with intracranial hemorrhage are not necessarily due to the primary brain injury itself, but more probably due to the secondary processes, which might be modified if treatment is instituted rapidly. The relatively bleak prognosis of severely head-injured patients is related to the fact that we have only recently begun to improve treatment regimens which can effectively control the secondary processes of direct brain damage. The increasingly rapid diagnosis and evacuation of intracranial hemorrhages undoubtedly have a positive impact in some patients.

Certainly, the use of CT for rapid diagnosis of acute intracranial hemorrhage following trauma has been shown to reduce significantly the use of other imaging modalities. Also, the more rapid therapeutic intervention that CT allows has been reported to improve the morbidity and mortality statistics of patients with focal hematomas (24–26). Unfortunately, the large group of patients with severe diffuse brain damage still poses a major therapeutic problem, and the impact of CT on the management of these unfortunate patients, and on their prognosis, is minimal.

Having briefly summarized the broad concepts of pathophysiology operative in head trauma, let us now turn to more specific considerations of CT diagnosis in this context.

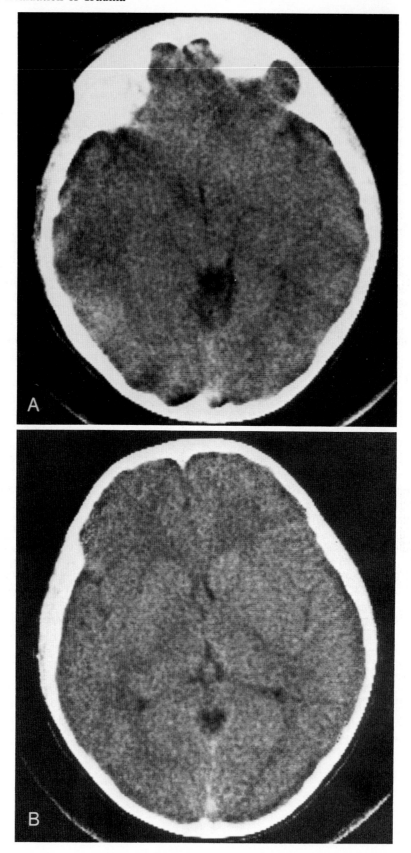

Figure 1.12.   This 6-year-old girl fell out of a third floor window. Her coma persisted for 3 weeks.
A, B. CT scan showed no focal abnormality, but the effacement of subarachnoid space, the loss of perimesencephalic cisterns, and diminutive ventricles suggested increased intracranial pressure due to diffuse loss of autoregulation.

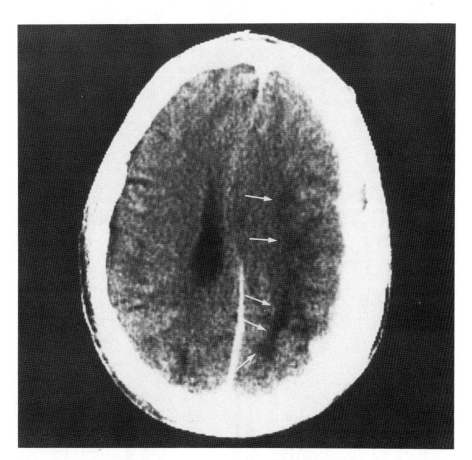

Figure 1.13.   Seventy-one-year-old male was found on the floor with a frontal scalp laceration and was thought to have suffered a cerebrovascular accident. The initial CT scan revealed a subdural hematoma overlying the left convexity, and edema in the "watershed" region posteriorly in the left hemisphere (*arrows*) indicated infarction. Note the extension of the convexity subdural into the interhemispheric subdural space along the falx. Lower sections revealed a massive temporal lobe disintegration (see Fig. 1.39).

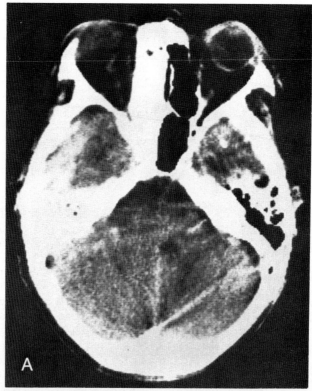

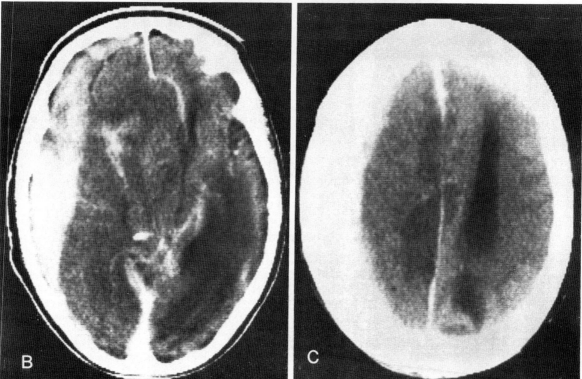

Figure 1.14.   This 69-year-old female was comatose after head trauma suffered in a motor vehicle accident. CT scan on admission depicted a massive right subdural hematoma extending from the temporal lobe up over the cerebral convexity.

A. Section at the fourth ventricle level shows its displacement to the left due to the marked midline shift supratentorially. Note the subdural collection in the middle fossa, and blood in the right mastoid air cells and in the sphenoid and ethmoid sinuses.

B. Higher section shows the massive subdural, with marked subfalcine shift of the contrast-opacified anterior cerebral artery. The tentorial incisura shows soft tissue within it, presumably herniating brain, and there is massive infarction in the distribution of the left posterior cerebral artery due to its compression at the tentorial edge.

C. Higher section shows continuation of the right subdural over the convexity and reveals infarction in the distribution of both anterior cerebral arteries, especially the right. Note that the posterior cerebral infarct extends high into the left hemisphere. The left ventricular enlargement is presumably on the basis of obstruction at the foramen of Monro due to the shift.

Skull Fracture

In the traumatized patient, an unsuspected linear fracture or suture diastasis may be demonstrated on review of the CT scan with bone window settings (Fig. 1.15 and 1.16). However, with a few noteworthy exceptions most such fractures, in and of themselves, are of no clinical importance. Rather it is the possibility of associated significant intracranial injury, seen in less than 50% of patients with skull fractures, which is of concern. Skull radiography is more accurate than computed tomography in the diagnosis of linear skull fractures. However, it is damage to the brain and not the calvarium which is of clinical concern. Therefore, computed tomography is the imaging modality of choice in any patient with suspected basilar or displaced skull fracture, transient or persistent loss of consciousness, or focal neurologic signs. In contrast to CT scanning, skull films do not effectively contribute to the evaluation, management, or outcome of acute intracranial injury. In fact, in a large series, fewer than 5% of all patients with suspected head injury studied with skull films had skull fractures, and less than half of the 5% suffered clinically important intracranial sequelae (27).

Fractures of significance include those which cross vascular channels or those which violate the dura. When a fracture injures a meningeal artery or a venous sinus, extracerebral bleeding may occur. The hematoma may be delayed in onset, especially when the initial increased intracranial pressure tamponades the bleeding site (Fig. 1.17 and 1.18). Fractures which tear the dura, particularly adjacent to the frontal and sphenoid sinuses, the cribriform plate, and the temporal bone, may cause CSF leakage (see Chapter 2) or pneumocephalus. Tension pneumocephalus results when the collection of air become large, producing mass effect on the underlying brain (Fig. 1.19). Clinically such patients develop severe neurologic compromise with symptoms of increased intracranial pressure. In almost 90% of cases, the air is subdural in location. Sequelae include focal pressure effects, rupture of bridging veins with secondary subdural bleeding, brain swelling, and venous infarction due to compromise of venous drainage (28). Computed tomography permits accurate compartmental localization of the air and an assessment of its effect on the brain.

Approximately 85% of patients with depressed skull fractures suffer additional intracranial injury (29). Therefore, a palpable calvarial depression is an absolute indication for CT. Brain contusion or laceration underlying the fracture, and contrecoup injuries are the most common findings. Diffuse cerebral hemorrhages, subarachnoid hemorrhage, or a normal examination except for the fracture is more rarely seen (Fig. 1.20 and 1.21). CT scans depict the location and number of bone fragments, as well as associated parenchymal damage.

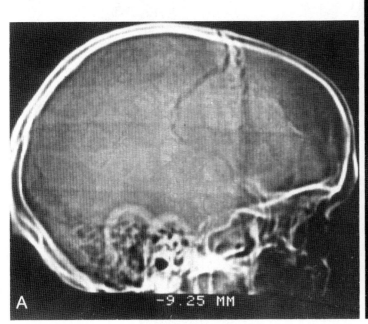
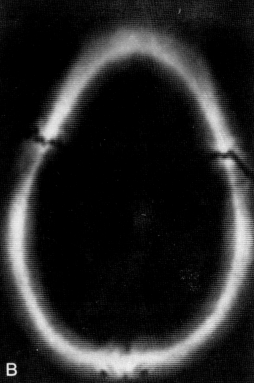

Figure 1.15.   This 27-year-old male was obtunded following a car accident.
A. The digital radiograph showed a parietal fracture extending posteriorly from the coronal sutures, which show diastasis.
B, C. Bone window settings verified the suture diastasis and left parietal fracture.

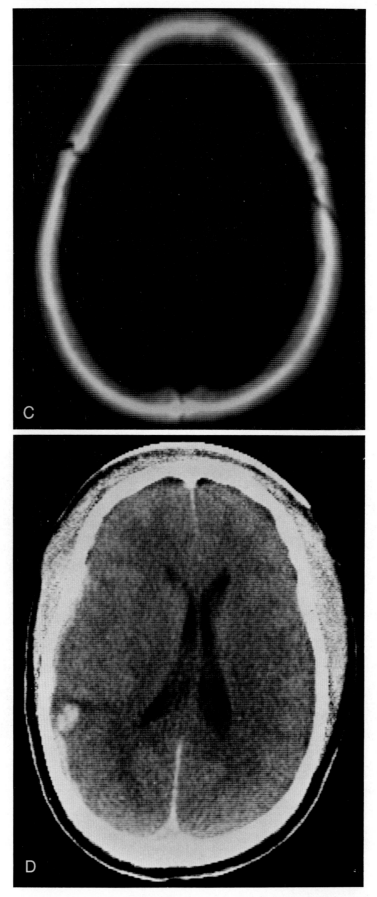

Figure 1.15.
D. The brain views showed a small right subdural collection and a focal retrosylvian hematoma. Note the midline shift.

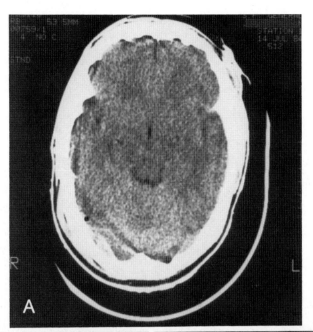

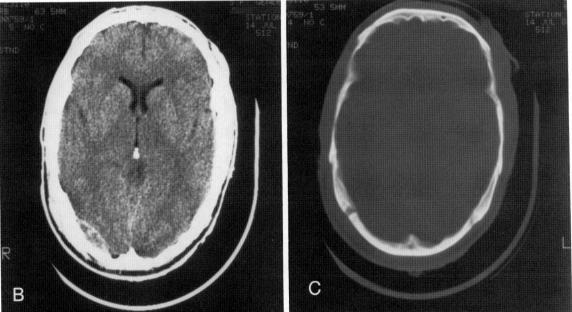

Figure 1.16.   After being thrown from his motorcycle, this 33-year-old man experienced a seizure.
A. CT scan shows focal pneumocephalus suggesting an overlying fracture.
B. At the level of the third ventricle, a small epidural hematoma is seen on the right posteriorly.
C. Bone window settings show diastasis of the right lambdoid suture.

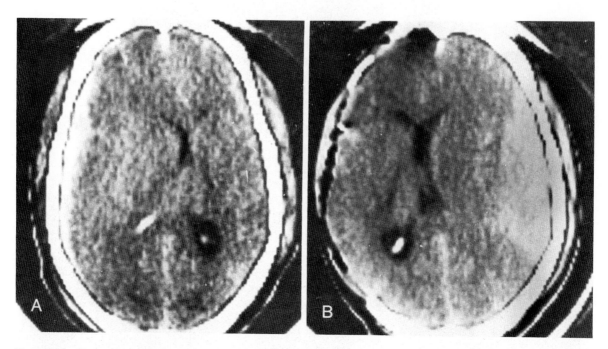

Figure 1.17.   This 12-year-old male suffered a left hemiparesis after a fall off his skate board.
A. CT scan on admission showed a right subdural hematoma with marked right-to-left shift of midline. Emergency surgery drained the collection.
B. Upon recovery, a right hemiparesis was noted. The ensuing CT scan showed a new epidural collection in the left extra-axial space. Bone window settings revealed an underlying fracture of the calvarium adjacent to this epidural. Incidentally, note the marked swelling of the brain with herniation beyond the craniectomy. Presumably, the marked initial mass effect prevented the rapid accumulation of the left epidural hematoma; subsequent decompression allowed its evolution.

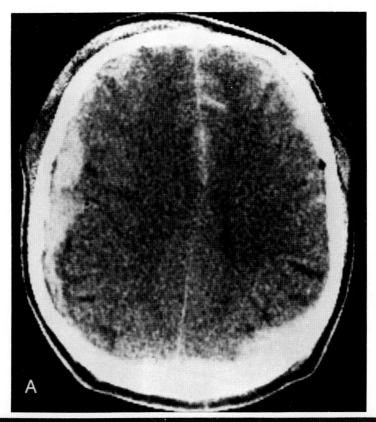

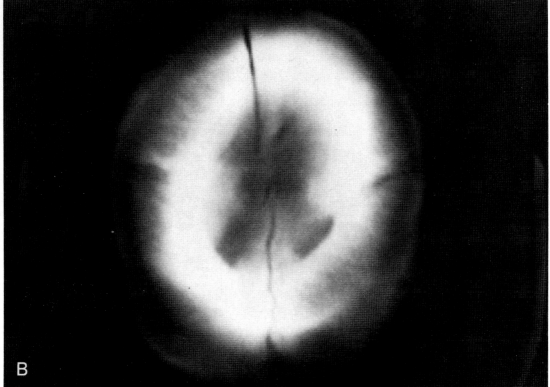

Figure 1.18.   This 57-year-old male was admitted comatose after being hit by a car.
A. A moderate right subdural hematoma was seen, with minimal interhemispheric blood and a small epidural collection along the posterior left convexity.
B. A paramedian sagittal skull fracture was seen crossing the sagittal suture on bone window settings. Although a sagittal sinus tear was suspected, none was found at surgery.

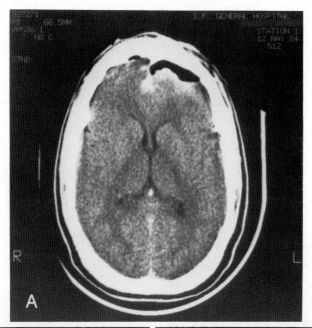

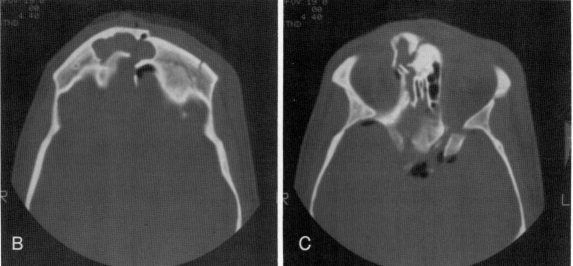

Figure 1.19.   This 25-year-old man lost control of his motorcycle at high speed. On examination, he had no light perception in his left eye.
A. CT scan shows left frontal pneumocephalus.
B. Bone window settings demonstrate a comminuted fracture of the frontal bone involving the frontal sinus. The frontal sinus is opacified with blood.
C. More inferiorly, at the level of the optic chiasm, disruption of opacified ethmoid sinuses is seen. Additionally a displaced fracture of the left anterior clinoid process is noted, with compromise of the optic canal. These findings account for the patient's post-traumatic blindness. He regained his vision after emergency decompressive surgery.

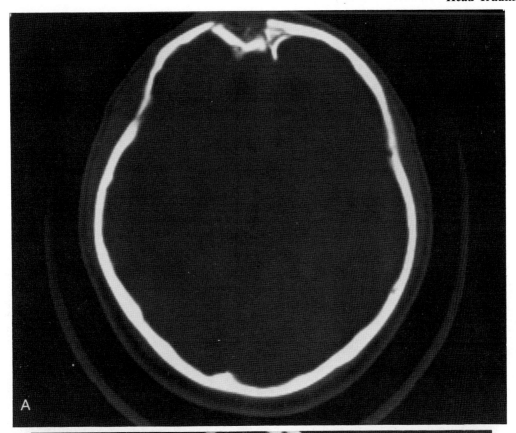

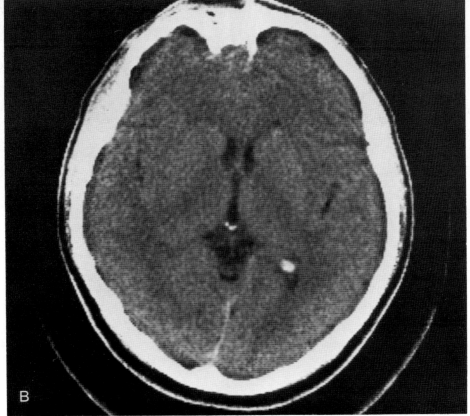

Figure 1.20. A CT scan was obtained on this 58-year-old male hit in the forehead with a ballpin hammer.
A. Bone window settings showed inward encroachment of the frontal bone at the site of trauma.
B. No significant underlying brain injury is seen.

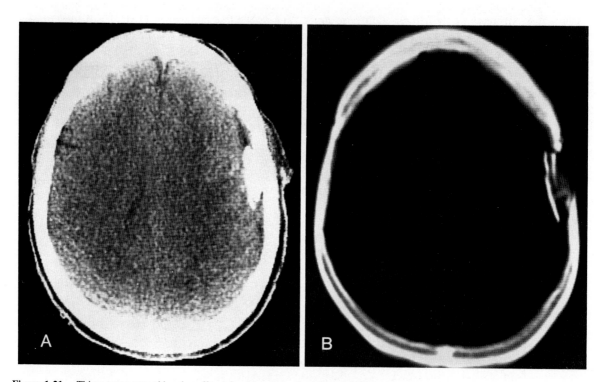

Figure 1.21. Thirty-seven-year-old male suffered focal trauma to the left parietal bone.
A. The brain is seen slightly displaced away from the inner table by a high-density collection on the CT scan.
B. Bone windows verify an inwardly displaced bone fragment. Surgery showed no significant underlying hematoma.

Basilar skull fractures may result in a variety of cranial nerve palsies, vascular injury, and leakage of CSF. Although routine head CT scans will demonstrate skull base fractures in only one-half of cases, such scans may provide clues that should arouse suspicion of such injuries and prompt more definitive study. Sinus opacification in or near the temporal bone, particularly of the mastoid or sphenoid, and other calvarial or facial fractures are frequently seen. Cerebral contusion or extra-axial hematoma, often contralateral to the basilar fracture, is commonly observed (Fig. 1.9 and 1.22). Local pneumocephalus occurs more rarely. Thin-section CT scans are required for the accurate depiction of the actual site and course of basilar fractures, and associated soft tissue findings, including blood in the middle ear or the source of CSF leakage (30, 31).

Classically, fractures of the lateral skull base are categorized with respect to the long axis of the temporal bone as longitudinal, transverse, or mixed. Longitudinal fractures, associated with direct blows to the petrous bone, comprise over two-thirds of temporal bone fractures. Such fractures begin in the temporal squamosa, course medially across the posterior aspect of the external auditory canal and middle ear, and extend along the surface of the petrous pyramid anterior to the labyrinth capsule, terminating in the middle cranial fossa (Fig. 1.7). Clinical symptomatology includes a conductive hearing loss in 65% of cases, associated with ossicular disruption in a minority; facial nerve paresis in 20% (usually transient); and CSF otorrhea, related to fracture of the tegmen tympani.

Associated with blows to the occipital or frontal area, transverse fractures constitute 20% of temporal bone fractures. Transverse fractures usually course along the internal auditory canal, extending across the pyramidal process of the temporal bone, or through the labyrinth capsule (Fig. 1.23). Sequelae include deafness, frequently sensorineural, and facial nerve paresis, each seen in about one-half of cases. Mixed temporal bone fractures follow a variable complex path, often resulting in multiple bone fragments. Clinical consequences are similarly variable, depending on the fracture course. Ossicular dislocation usually occurs in association with temporal bone fractures but may result from relatively minor head trauma. A transverse compressive force transiently deforms the tegmen inferiorly, subluxing the incus from the stapes. Rarely the entire chain may be disrupted (Fig. 1.24). Early recognition of such a complication may prompt timely intervention and prevent permanent hearing loss.

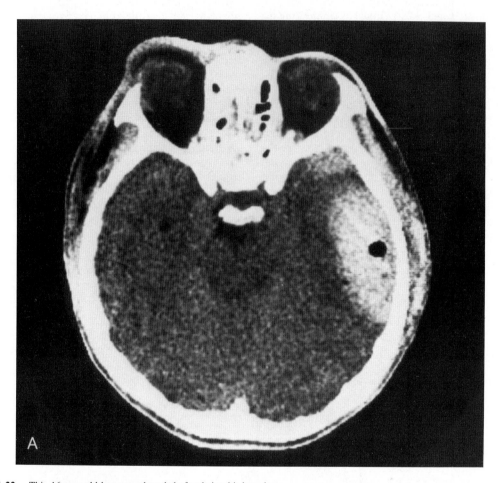

Figure 1.22.   This 16-year-old boy was obtunded after being hit by a bus.
A. CT scan on admission showed a left temporal epidural hematoma with pneumocephalus.
B. High-resolution, extended CT number temporal bone study verified a fracture through the petrous ridge seen on the highest cut. At surgery, the source of the epidural bleeding as confirmed to be at the site of the petrous fracture. Note the opacified mastoid air cells.
C. Image reformations in the coronal and sagittal plane through the ossicles (*arrows*) were done to assess conductive hearing loss. Ossicular dislocation was not found, but blood in the middle ear was seen.

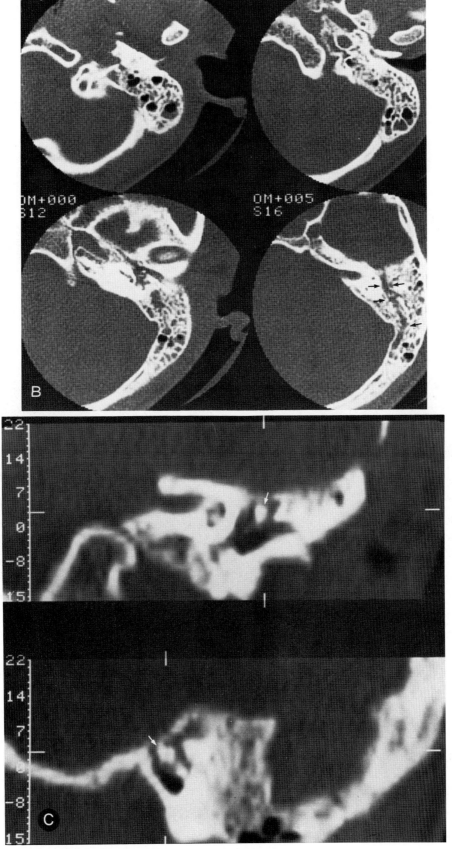

Figure 1.22.   B, C.

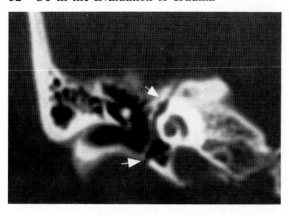

Figure 1.23. This woman suffered from post-traumatic sensorineural hearing loss. Coronal CT scan shows a transverse fracture (*arrows*), extending from medial tegmen tympani, adjacent to the cochlea, inferiorly through the floor of the middle ear.

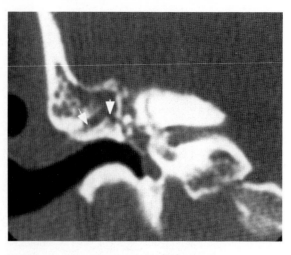

Figure 1.24. This 27-year-old man developed conductive hearing loss after a motorcycle accident. Coronal CT scan demonstrates ossicular disruption. Presumably a fracture fragment (*arrows*) compressed the ossicles acutely during impact, with secondary ossicular subluxation. Blood fills the middle ear cavity.

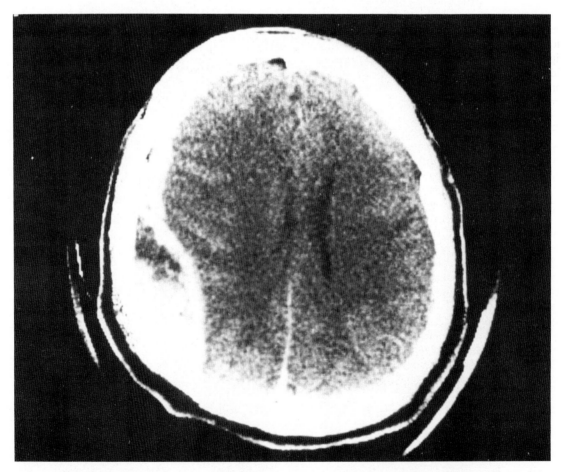

Figure 1.25. Fifty-four-year-old male admitted to the emergency room after being found on the street following an assault. Subdural hematoma, seen along the right convexity, is being invaginated by an epidural bleed in the posterior extra-axial space. Moderate midline shift is likewise noted.

Extracerebral Hemorrhage

Extra-axial hematomas are demonstrated in 8 to 25% of patients who undergo computed tomography for the evaluation of head trauma (2, 25, 32). Epidural hematomas are more often seen in the young; 40% are seen in patients under the age of 20 (16). The majority of epidural hematomas are temporal or temporoparietal and result from damage to the adjacent anterior or posterior branches of the middle meningeal vessels. Stripped from the inner table by the growing hematoma, the densely adherent outer membrane of the dura bulges inward. The most common CT appearance of such hematomas is a homogeneously dense, biconvex collection, based against the calvarium (Fig. 1.16, 1.17, 1.22, and 1.25). Active bleeding is suggested when a lucent "swirl" is demonstrated in the midst of the dense hematoma. If the epidural bleed is chronic, a mixed- or low-density collection may be seen, limited medially by a contrast-enchancing "membrane," representing the displaced, often thickened dura (33). An associated fracture is detected in up to 90% of cases (Fig. 1.16). Although most epidural hematomas are arterial in origin, a torn venous sinus accounts for a minority of such collections, most commonly in the posterior fossa (Fig. 1.26). In contrast to subdural collections which must enter the interhemispheric fissure and cross the midline under the falx to appear bilaterally, epidural hematomas can cross the midline directly by stripping the falx from its bony attachments. Most epidural hematomas occur within the first 24 hours of injury. However, delayed hemorrhage into the epidural space is occasionally seen (Fig. 1.17 and 1.27). Delayed bleeds can occur after surgical decompression of a contralateral extra-axial hematoma.

Subdural hematomas are caused by rupture of veins bridging the cortex and the sinuses. They develop more commonly in older patients, possibly because of "stretching" of these veins, crossing the large subarachnoid spaces of the aging brain (16). Subdural hematomas, interposed between the inner dural membrane and the arachnoid, appear acutely as crescentic, peripheral collections of increased density, with a concave inner margin, conforming to the shape of the inner calvarium. Their shape dictated by the underlying cerebral convexity, they may distribute themselves throughout the subdural space, including that in the interhemispheric regions and along the tentorium (Fig. 1.28). In the interhemispheric region, the extent of the subdural collection is delineated by the falx itself. Thus subdural blood cannot extend in the midline just above the corpus callosum, where the opening in the falx exists and limits the subdural space (Fig. 1.28**A**). Blood seen in this location on CT can only be in the subarachnoid space.

Secondary findings of subdural hemorrhages include mass effect, with flattening of gyri, and shift of midline toward the contralateral side. Other intracranial injuries should be sought, as they are seen in 40% of patients with extracerebral hematomas (34).

In 5% of cases, subdural hematomas may be isodense. Such hematomas may be either acute or subacute. If acute, their isodensity may be explained by bleeding in an anemic patient (with blood of inherently low hemoglobin content), or from bleeding into a pre-existing subdural hygroma, with admixture of hyperdense blood and hypodense CSF. If subacute (7 to 21 days), the isodensity of the hematoma stems from the lower X-ray attenuation of the denatured protein constituents of old blood compared with that of fresh hemorrhage. The relative isodensity of the blood to that of adjacent brain may make diagnosis by typical CT criteria difficult. However subtle clues to the presence of such a collection on noncontrast scan include obliteration of sulci, the shift of midline, or the medial shift of the white matter in the centrum semiovale (35–38) (Fig. 1.29). Contrast enhancement may demonstrate displacement of the cortical vasculature from the inner table or define a "membrane" medial to the subdural (Figs. 1.6 and 1.30).

Occasionally, a subdural hematoma may appear as a peripheral collection of two distinct densities—lucent superiorly, hyperdense inferiorly. This unusual appearance is due to the sedimentation of more solid elements into the dependent portions of the hematoma. Frequently the low-density upper position is a chronic component of the subdural collection, while the denser inferior portion is composed of acute hemorrhage (Fig. 1.31).

Extra-axial posterior fossa hematomas are rare. Most such hematomas are epidural and of venous origin, due to disruption of the torcular or transverse sinus (39) (Fig. 1.26). Subdural hematomas of the posterior fossa complicate 0.3 to 0.5% of all head injuries (Fig. 1.32). Associated findings include cerebellar or brainstem contusion, compression and shift of the fourth ventricle, and obliteration of perimesencephalic cisterns (40). Because of the relatively small volume of the posterior fossa and the importance of the structures contained therein, these hematomas are poorly tolerated. Variation of normal gray scale viewing windows and coronal reformations may aid in the recognition of these life-threatening collections (Figs. 1.1 and 1.28).

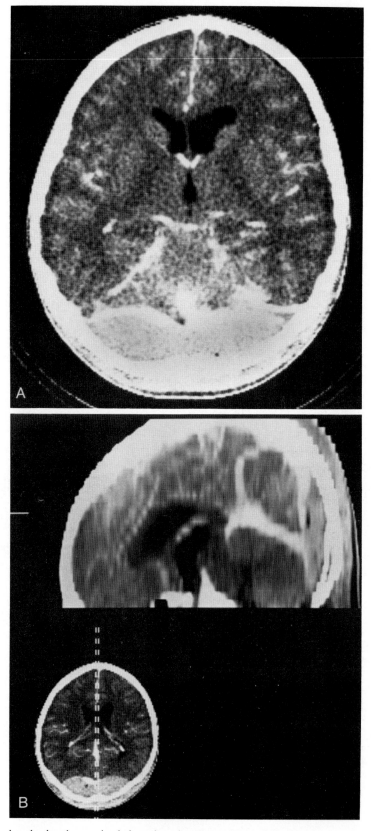

Figure 1.26.   This young boy developed severe headache and an altered mental status following a bike accident.
A. Axial views demonstrated a hematoma stripping the falx and tentorial attachment away from the internal occipital bone at the level of the torcula (contrast-enhanced scan).
B. Sagittal reformation delineates the extent of this epidural collection caused by a dural sinus tear. (Courtesy of Dr. Vince McCormack, Modesto, CA.)

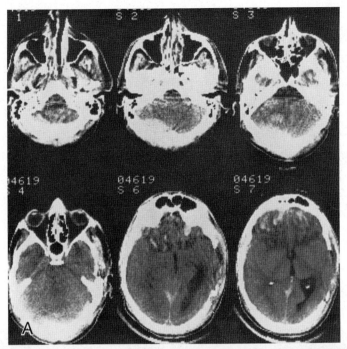

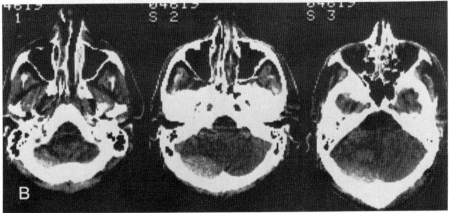

Figure 1.27.   After being found in a pile of beer cans at the bottom of a stairway in his rooming house, this 25-year-old male was admitted. An emergency craniotomy removed a large left temporal epidural hematoma shown by the admission CT. Three days later, his intracranial pressure suddenly rose.

A. CT scan 3 days after surgery shows bifrontal contusions and postoperative changes in the left temporal region, and suggests a cerebellar bleed on the lower sections. Note the absence of the fourth ventricle, effacement of the perimesencephalic cisterns, and loss of the superior cerebellar cistern in the incisura.

B. Widened gray scale settings define a new epidural collection in the right cerebellum which was not present on the admitting CT study.

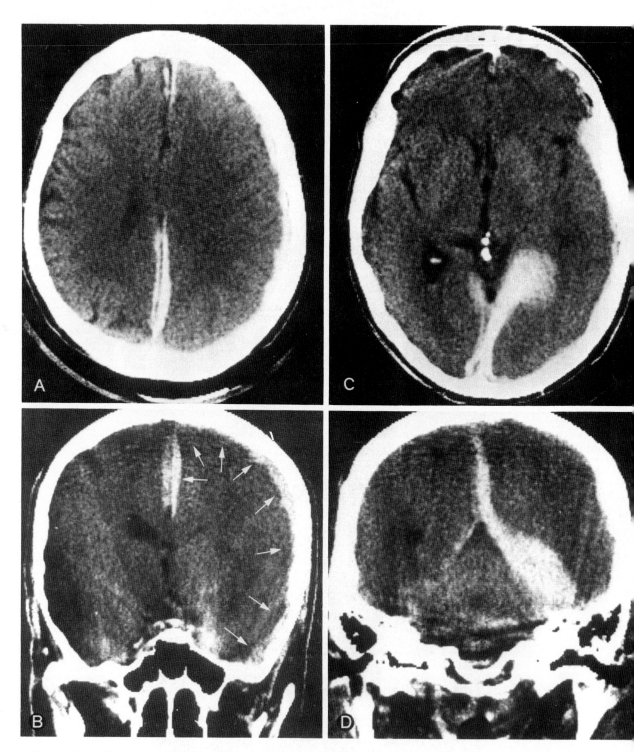

Figure 1.28.   This 54-year-old alcoholic was admitted after hitting his head on the curb.
A. Axial CT section at the level of the ventricular roofs reveals a blood collection on either side of the falx (the latter seen as a linear lucency in the anterior and posterior portions of the interhemispheric fissure). A small subdural collection continues around the left cerebral convexity adjacent to the inner table. Note the lack of extension of the interhemispheric subdural into the subarachnoid space above the corpus callosum.
B. A coronal view delineates the continuation of the interhemispheric subdural around the left convexity down to the middle fossa (*arrows*).
C. An axial view at the level of the tentorial incisura shows continuation of the interhemispheric component down to the tentorial leaf.
D. A coronal section shows the blood on top of the tentorium bulging into the left occipital lobe. Incidentally, note that the superior cerebella cistern is preserved within the incisura.

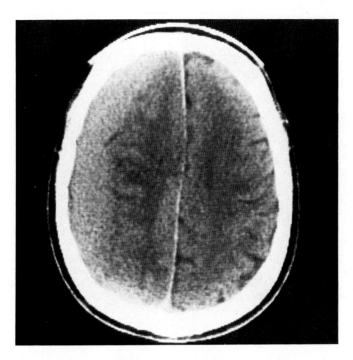

Figure 1.29. Seventy-year-old male admitted with a history of 5 days of headache and 3 days of left hemiparesis. The CT scan shows medial shift of the gray-white junction and white matter, along with mild midline shift, due to a relatively isodense extra-axial collection along the right convexity.

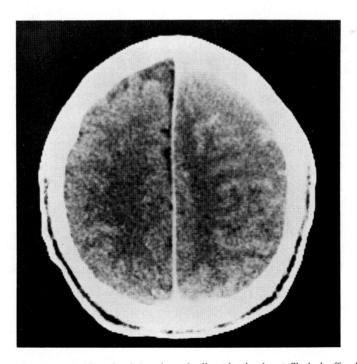

Figure 1.30. This 55-year-old female returned from South America and collapsed at the airport. She had suffered head trauma in a political demonstration 3 weeks prior to her return. Noncontrast CT scan showed equivocal medial shift of the high-convexity white matter. The contrast scan shows displacement of the enhanced gray matter away from the inner table. Note the obliteration of paramedian and frontal sulci. Contrast-enhanced meningeal vessels can be seen adjacent to the inner table, indicating that the extra-axial collection is in the subdural space. The patient recovered following drainage of the collection.

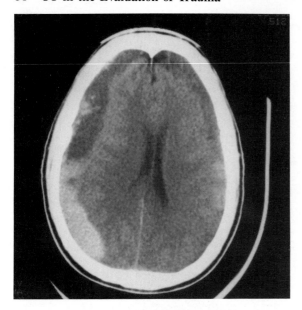

Figure 1.31. This 65-year-old man, admitted hypothermic and mumbling incoherently, demonstrated only slight left hyperreflexia on examination. CT scan shows high-density blood bilaterally at the dependent aspect of lucent extra-axial collections. Because of the bilaterality of the collections, minimal midline shift is seen. Surgery verified chronic subdural hematomas with acute clots.

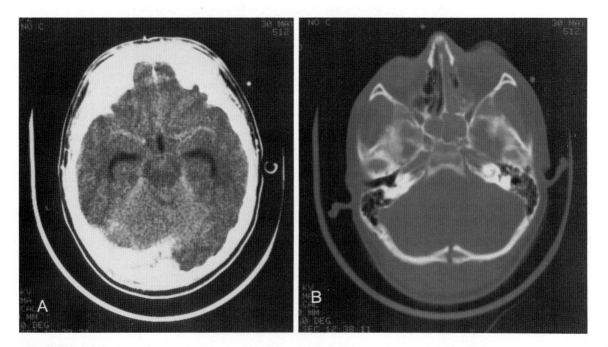

Figure 1.32. This 2-year-old boy was found unconscious after a two-story fall.
A. CT scan demonstrates a right-sided subdural hematoma of the posterior fossa. Obliteration of the perimesencephalic cisterns and dilatation of the temporal horns suggest secondary upward transtentorial herniation.
B. Bone window settings define an occipital fracture in the region of the torcular. However, no evidence of venous laceration was noted at surgery.

Extra-axial hematomas may evolve over the course of weeks through the isodense phase into hypodense collections, reflecting their high water content. Whether epi- or subdural, they may resolve spontaneously (Fig. 1.33), resorbed through a fibrovascular neomembrane lining the hematomas (41–43). In other cases, these chronic hematomas may increase in size gradually due to repeated subclinical bleeds, or acutely due to rebleeding (Figs. 1.31 and 1.34), producing focal neurologic signs mimicking stroke. These episodes of hemorrhage occur because of the persistent stretching of the bridging veins by the chronic extra-axial collection, the fragility of the proliferated capillaries lining the inner membrane of the dura enclosing the chronic collection, and an anticlotting agent found within the old hematoma (42).

Subdural hygromas may develop acutely after trauma or subacutely, 1 to 7 weeks after injury (44). The etiology of these collections of xanthochromic, proteinaceous fluid is poorly understood. Those which form acutely may be due to arachnoidal tears with secondary leakage of CSF into the subdural space or defective CSF resorption related to leptomeningeal vascular trauma. Those which are more delayed in onset may actually be effusions from damaged capillaries at the dural, arachnoidal, or pia-parenchymal level. The hygromas are frontal and bilateral in over 50% of cases. A clinically complex entity, the subdural hygroma has, in most cases, no clinical significance (Fig. 1.35) (45, 46). However, it may act as an extra-axial mass lesion, causing sufficient neurologic compromise to require surgical evacuation (Fig. 1.36). In the posterior fossa, such collections are rare and unlikely to be asymptomatic since space-occupying lesions are poorly tolerated in this tight space (Fig. 1.37). The overall mortality rate of subdural hygromas is reported to be as high as 20 to 24%, but usually reflects more serious underlying injuries.

Extracerebral fluid collections are the most common intracranial complication of child abuse. Presumably due to both direct impact injuries and rotational forces with shearing stresses, these collections are most often subdural in location, seen especially around the vascular tentorium and straight sinus (47) (Fig. 1.38). The vulnerability of the young to the development of traumatic extra-axial hematomas and hygromas is related to multiple factors permitting movement and distortion of the brain, including the increased elasticity of the infant calvarium with open sutures and the increased plasticity of the incompletely myelinated brain. The risks of rotational injury are compounded by the relatively large size of the infant head with respect to the minimal strength of the supporting neck muscles (48). Because the extracerebral collections usually result from a whiplash injury ("shaking"), skull fractures are rarely demonstrated. The long-term intracranial sequelae of child abuse include atrophy and porencephaly in addition to chronic hygromas.

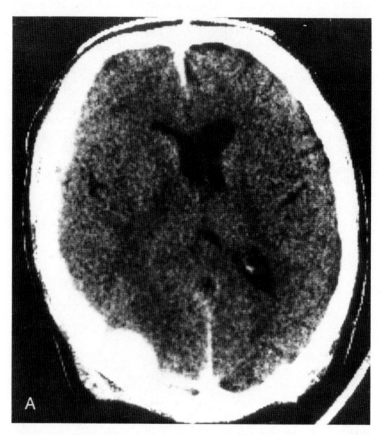

Figure 1.33. This 48-year-old male suffered head trauma during an assault. Obtundation prompted the CT scan on admission.
A. A moderate right subdural hematoma is seen producing a midline shift.
B. Study done 12 days later shows evolution of the subdural collection into a low-density fluid collection; the midline shift has not changed. The patient was discharged without surgery, and a follow-up study was performed.
C. CT scan 5 months after trauma shows normal brain and ventricles.

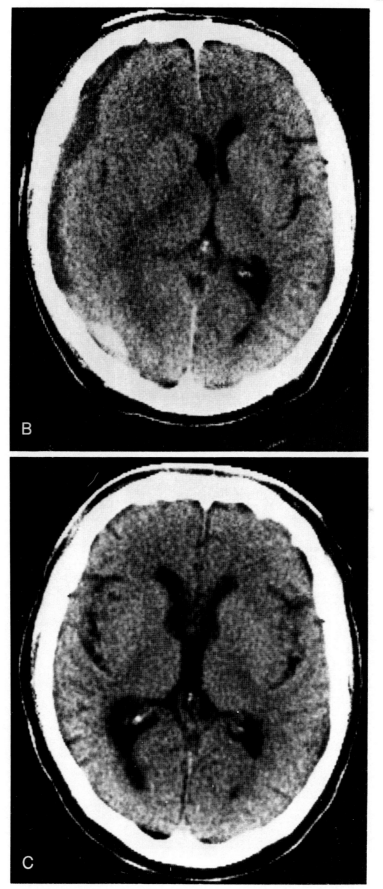

Figure 1.33.   B, C.

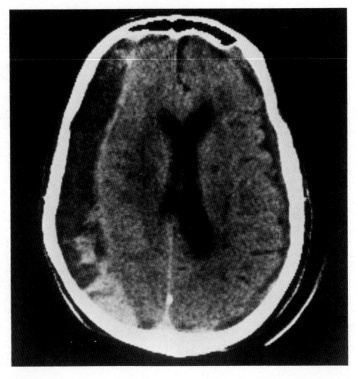

Figure 1.34.   This 81-year-old male, who was institutionalized for progressive dementia, suffered an acute left hemiparesis followed by a seizure. The subsequent CT scan showed blood density within a lucent extra-axial collection and a midline shift. Surgery verified a chronic subdural hematoma with an acute clot.

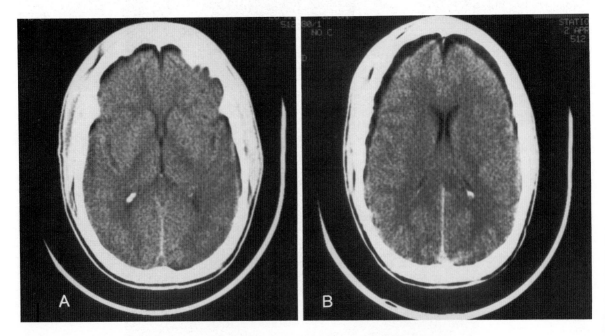

Figure 1.35.   This 23-year-old man complained only of a headache after a motor vehicle accident.
A. CT scan immediately after injury is normal.
B. Five days later, interval development of bilateral subdural hygromas is seen.

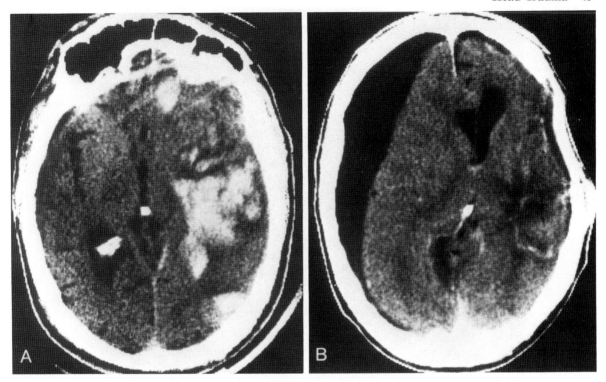

Figure 1.36.   This 51-year-old man was comatose following a car accident.
A. CT scan on admission showed a massive temporal hematoma, with a subfrontal hematoma as well. He remained comatose, despite surgical evacuation of the blood.
B. Follow-up study done 3 weeks later, when the patient developed sudden hypertension, showed a massive hygroma (autopsy proven) with marked shift of midline. Note the post-traumatic changes in the left temporal region.

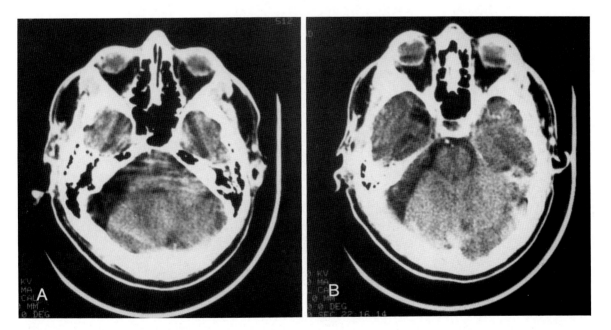

Figure 1.37.   This 28-year-old drug abuser was evaluated for fever of unknown origin. He had suffered head trauma in a motor vehicle accident 1 year prior to presentation.
A, B. CT scan 1 year after injury demonstrates a low-density extra-axial fluid collection in the posterior fossa. Since post-traumatic subdural hygromas are rarely asymptomatic, particularly of this size, this most likely represents a congenital anomaly (i.e., subarachnoid cyst, large cisterna magna).

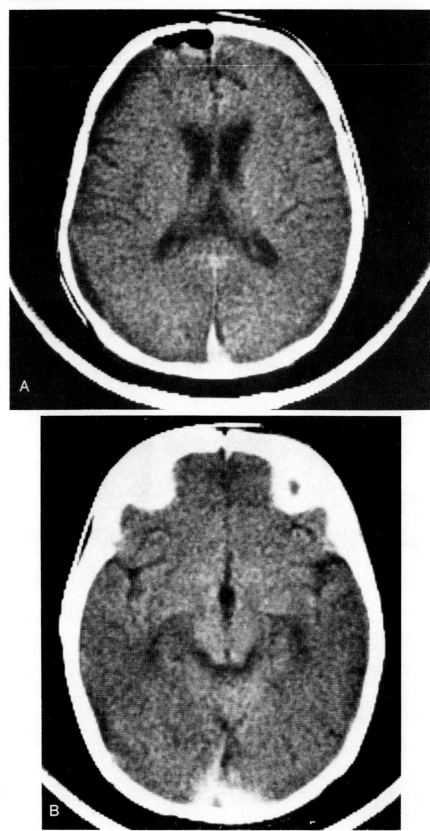

Figure 1.38.   This unfortunate 4-month-old infant suffered head trauma due to parental abuse.
A, B. CT scan obtained after an emergency subdural tap (which showed chronic hematoma) reveals some residual extra-axial fluid bilaterally and blood density along the straight sinus and tentorium on two sections.

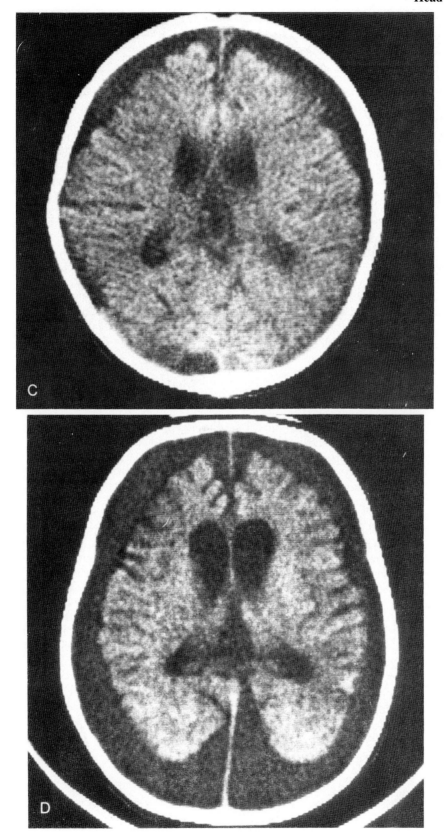

Figure 1.38.

C, D. CT scans obtained 2 weeks and 2 months after the original episode show progressive extra-axial fluid accumulation, communicating hydrocephalus, and evidence of brain atrophy.

Parenchymal Injury

Subdural bleeds are most often accompanied by intracerebral hemorrhage, especially in the temporal region where a "burst" temporal lobe may be produced (Fig. 1.39). This entity consists of a mixture of subdural and massive intracerebral clot with parenchymal disruption. Intracerebral hemorrhage may arise acutely, develop slowly from initial contusions, or appear belatedly in a region of the brain initially normal on CT (Figs. 1.40 and 1.41). Regardless of the initial benign CT findings, the CT scan should be repeated if the patient's mental status is abnormal or deteriorates, as delayed hematomas may develop in up to 20% of patients 1 to 3 days or longer after severe trauma (7–10) (Figs. 1.42 and 1.43). Incidentally, the distinction between contusion and hematoma on CT is somewhat blurred. Generally, only patchy or mixed-density lesions are termed contusion (Fig. 1.44), whereas focal homogeneous, well-circumscribed collections of blood earn the designation of hematoma (Fig. 1.45). Occasionally, in the acute phase, rather than a homogeneous dense appearance, hematomas may have a blood-fluid layer (Figs. 1.41 and 1.46).

Clinical findings are helpful in localizing the region of parenchymal bleeding. When a post-traumatic progressive deterioration in mental status is accompanied by focal motor movements or signs, one can suggest that the site of intracranial hemorrhage on CT (whether extra- or intra-axial) will most likely be contralateral to the abnormal motor findings. Pupillary dilatation and fixation more reliably localize to the side of hemorrhage, being accurate signs of laterality in more than 90% of cases (16).

As mentioned previously, the value of CT rests in its rapid delineation of focal hemorrhage amenable to surgical removal. Such therapy is especially crucial when CT scanning depicts mass shifts with compression of vessels or the brainstem by herniation. Tentorial herniation can be suggested on CT images by obliteration of the CSF spaces in and around the incisura. Thus, absence of the normal lucency in the superior cerebellar, quadrigeminal plate, and perimesencephalic cisterns should be taken as a grave radiographic sign of increased intracranial pressure and/or transtentorial herniation (Figs. 1.14 and 1.47–1.49). Complete effacement of all CSF spaces with loss of gray-white differentiation is a bad prognostic sign (Fig. 1.50). The presence of Duret's hemorrhage in the brainstem is a definitive CT sign of transtentorial herniation (Figs. 1.48 and 1.49).

Although intracranial pressure elevation can be confidently diagnosed in those patients with obvious midline shift and/or transtentorial herniation, in more subtle cases, attempts to correlate CT findings with intracranial pressure have been only partially successful (34, 49). Over half of patients with focal parenchymal or intraventricular hemorrhage by CT have intracranial hypertension. Of note, acute hematomas and mixed-density lesions appear to increase intracranial pressure more consistently than post-traumatic low-density lesions such as edema, infarct, or resolving contusion. Ventricular compression or ventricular shift with dilatation of the contralateral temporal horn seem to correlate best with intracranial hypertension (Figs. 1.46 and 1.47). More importantly, elevated intracranial pressure may exist even in the presence of an entirely normal CT scan. Consequently, intracranial pressure catheters are still routinely used in severely traumatized patients. In the vast majority of cases, such monitoring greatly aids in the clinical management of these patients, especially when combined with serial CT scans (34, 50, 51). Rarely, these catheters may produce iatrogenic damage, evident on CT (Fig. 1.51).

The temporal evolution of focal untreated intracerebral hemorrhage is similar to that of an abscess. The production of granulation tissue along the periphery of the hematoma accounts in part for the peripheral enhancement seen on follow-up studies (Figs. 1.5 and 1.52). The nonspecific ring-enhancing pattern may simulate abscess or neoplasm if the history of recent trauma is not elicited. However, the relative lack of mass effect or vasogenic edema associated with typical abscesses may be a distinguishing feature of resolving hematoma. The density of the hematoma gradually decreases with time as described above for extra-cerebral collections. The size of the bleed and its accessibility to the circulation dictate the duration of the process of resolution.

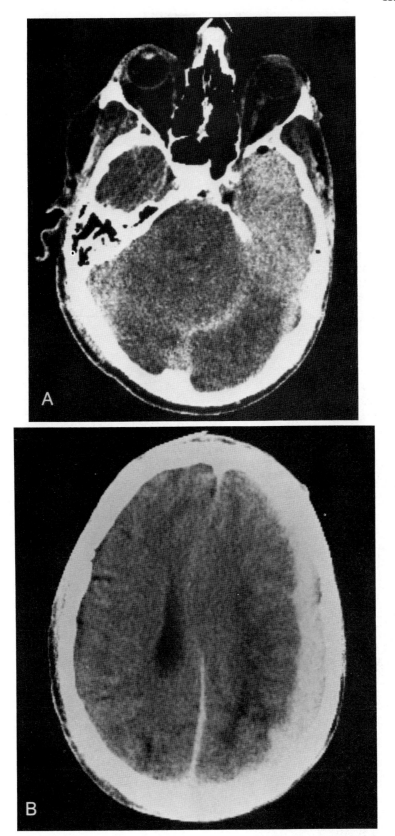

Figure 1.39. Seventy-one-year-old male found on the floor with a frontal scalp laceration was admitted in a coma.
A. CT scan showed diffuse, homogeneous opacification of the temporal pole, with a small pocket of air in the anterior middle fossa.
B. Higher section depicts the associated subdural hematoma and "watershed" infarction in the left parietal region. Incidentally, note the effacement of the perimesencephalic cisterns on the lower section suggesting increased intracranial pressure. At surgery, a disintegration of the temporal lobe was found, in addition to the subdural hematoma (same patient as Fig. 1.13)

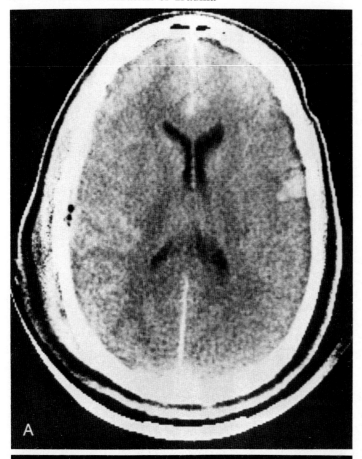

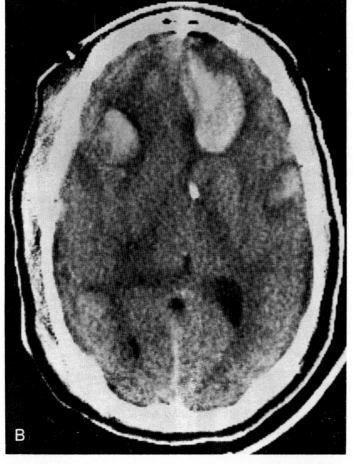

Figure 1.40. Thirty-five-year-old male suffered coma during a motor vehicle accident.

A. Admitting CT scan showed a small contusion in the left sylvian region and suggested a basilar fracture by virtue of small air collections in the right extra-axial space. A minimal right subdural hematoma was likewide present.

B. Progressive elevation of intracranial pressure led to a repeat study on the next day. Striking new bifrontal hematomas are seen, as is blood in the right ventricle's atrium. The paramedian punctate density is the tip of an intraventricular pressure monitor.

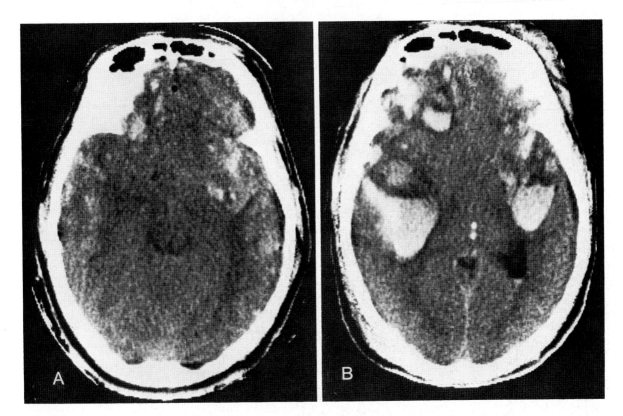

Figure 1.41.   Fifty-five-year-old man admitted following an assault. The patient became progressively unresponsive.
A. Initial CT scan shows scattered areas of high density throughout both subfrontal and temporal regions. A punctate air collection just behind the crista galli suggested basilar skull fracture.
B. Continued deterioration led to the follow-up study the next day. The previous contusions have evolved into large hematomas, with a "hematocrit effect" being seen in the large right temporal collection. Note the subtle blood-CSF level in the atrium of the left ventricle.

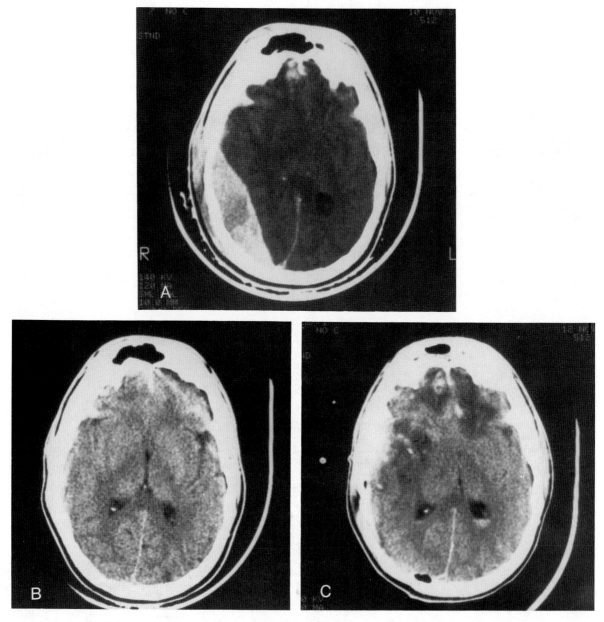

Figure 1.42.   This 34-year-old man was comatose after a motorcycle accident.
A. A large right epidural hematoma is shown with associated mass effect.
B. CT scan immediately after surgical evacuation of hematoma is normal.
C. Two days later, multiple contusions are seen. Note blood in atria of lateral ventricles.

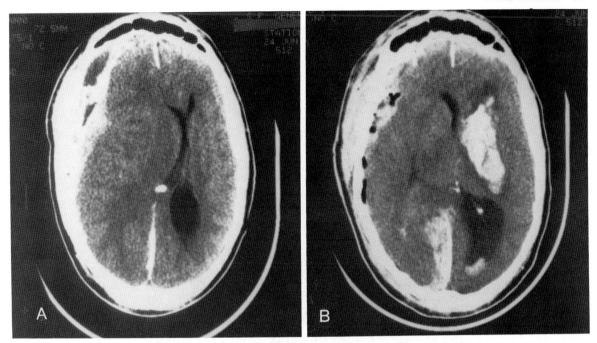

Figure 1.43.   This 58-year-old man was found unresponsive after falling and striking his head.
A. CT scan shortly after injury shows a large mixed-density subdural hematoma. Massive subfalcine herniation is seen.
B. The patient's clinical condition continued to deteriorate after surgical evacuation of the extraaxial hematoma. Although the right subdural collection is smaller, the patient has developed a massive left basal ganglia hemorrhage. In addition, note intraventricular hemorrhage and subdural blood along the falx posteriorly. The patient died shortly after this examination.

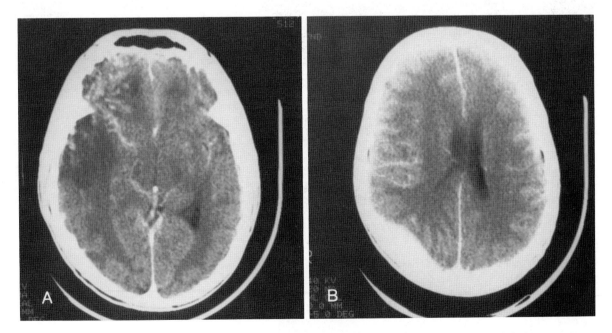

Figure 1.44.   This 42-year-old drug abuser was initially admitted to the psychiatry service because of his bizarre behavior.
A. CT scan shows right frontotemporal contusion of heterogeneous density. Note effacement of perimesencephalic cisterns.
B. An axial section at level of lateral ventricles demonstrates an unsuspected small right occipital epidural hematoma with mass effect and slight midline shift.

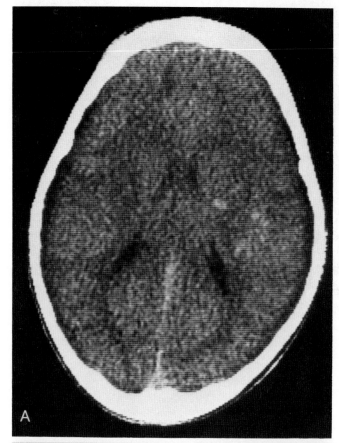

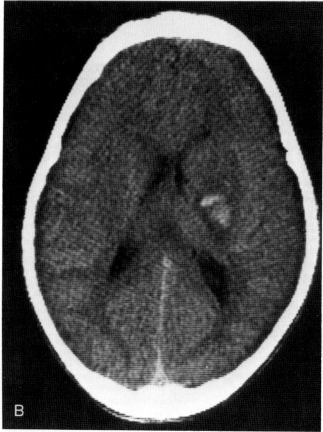

Figure 1.45.   This 6-year-old girl was hit be a car and suffered right hemiparesis.
A. CT scan on admission showed only subtle, punctate densities in the deep left hemisphere.
B. The next day's study depicted a hematoma which had evolved from the initial contusion, centered near the posterior limb of the internal capsule on the left.

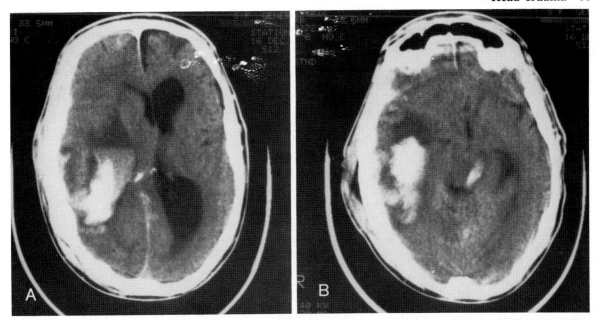

Figure 1.46. This 67-year-old man was admitted lethargic but arousable.
A. A large, right, parieto-occipital hematoma is shown. Blood-fluid level confirms that acute nature of the hemorrhage. Note the midline shift with "trapping" of the left lateral ventricle.
B. The brain stem is compressed with focal hemorrhage laterally. Obliteration of the perimesencephalic cisterns and dilatation of the left temporal horn suggest impending transtentorial herniation.

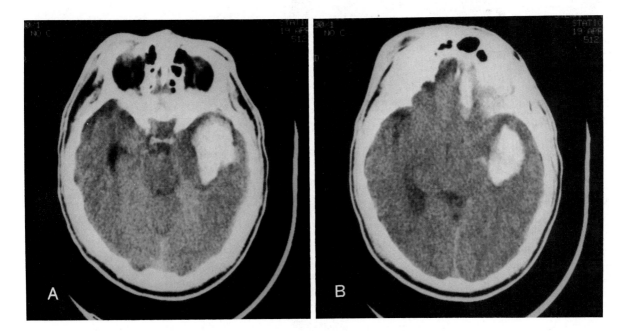

Figure 1.47. Confused and slightly lethargic, this 42-year-old alcoholic presented with minimal ataxia.
A. CT scan shows left temporal hematoma. Compression of the brain stem with dilatation of the right temporal horn suggests impending transtentorial herniation.
B. More superiorly, an additional hematoma is seen in the left frontal lobe. Notice obliteration of the perimesencelphalic cisterns and the third ventricle.

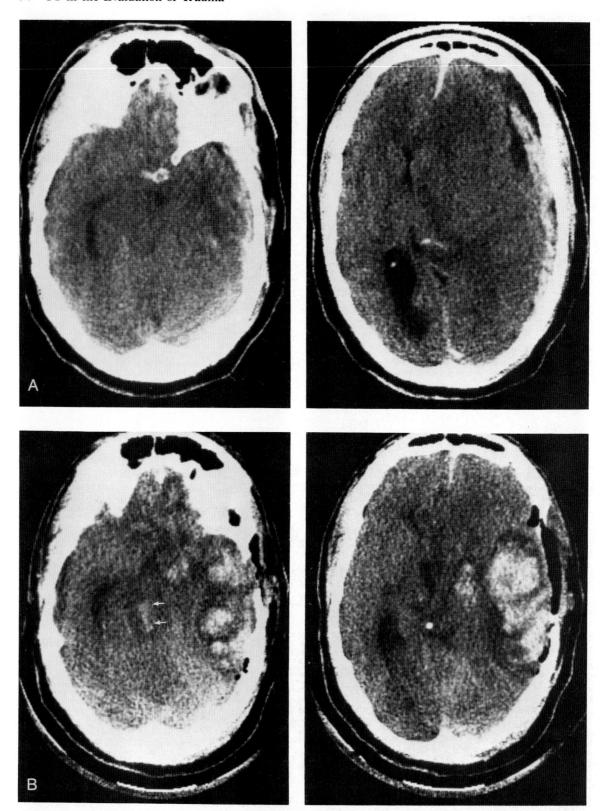

Figure 1.48.   This 49-year-old male was found comatose on the street.

A. Admission CT scan showed a subdural collection with a marked midline shift. Note obliteration of the perimesencephalic cisterns and suggestion of dilatation of the right ventricle's atrium.

B. Following surgery, the patient became decerebrate, and a repeat CT study showed a new, massive hematoma in the temporal lobe. Also noted was further compression of the brain stem with blood density at the level of the cerebral peduncles (*arrows*). Duret's hemorrhages were found at autopsy, where evidence of downward tentorial herniation was also seen.

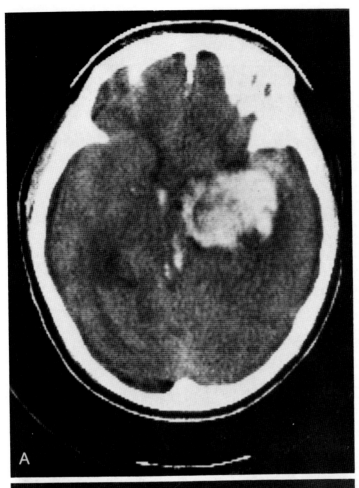

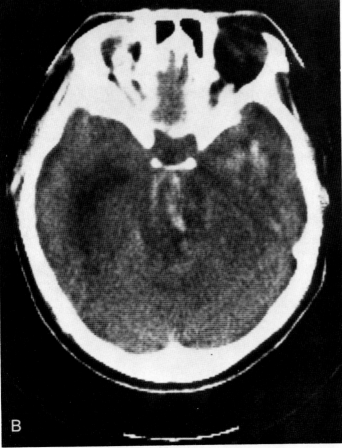

Figure 1.49.   Fifty-seven-year-old female, found on the floor, died shortly after admission and CT scanning.

A. A deep temporal hematoma is seen on the left. Note the absence of any perimesencephalic cisterns and nonvisualization of the superior cerebellar cistern, which would be expected in the midline in the incisura at this level.

B. Hemorrhage is seen in the brain stem just behind the dorsum sella. Note the effacement of the perimesencephalic cisterns. Autopsy verified the transtentorial herniation with Duret's hemorrhages.

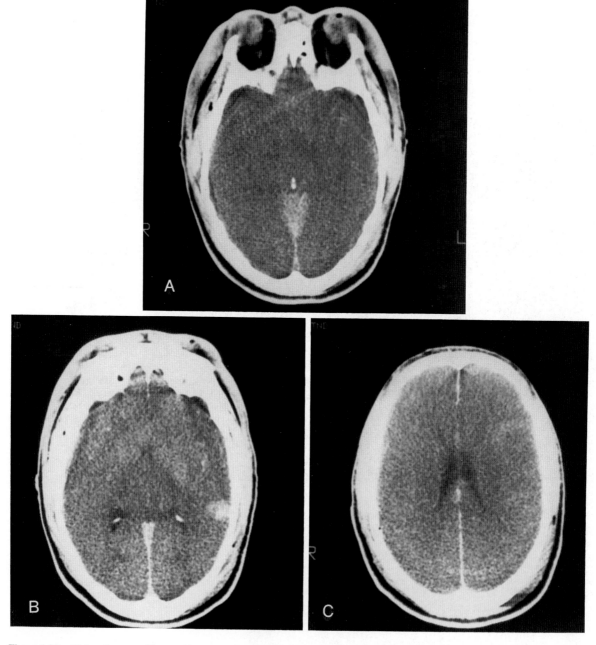

Figure 1.50. This unfortunate 29-year-old man was found unresponsive at the site of a "hit and run" accident.
A. Complete obliteration of perimesencephalic cisterns with loss of gray-white differentiation is seen, suggesting diffuse cerebral edema with raised intracranial pressure. Note blood along the tentorium.
B. Small left parietotemporal hematoma is demonstrated.
C. Lateral ventricles are compressed by edematous, featureless brain. Minimal subarachnoid blood extends along the interhemispheric fissure. The patient was pronounced dead 24 hours later.

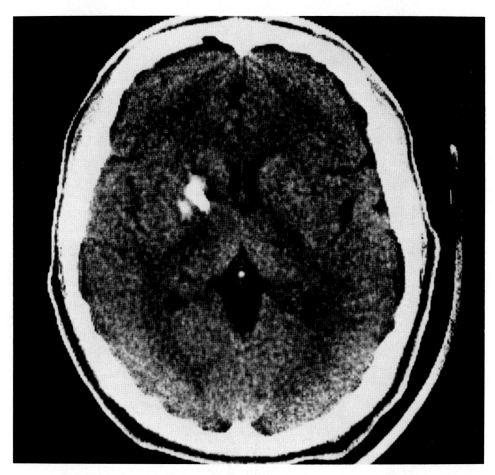

Figure 1.51. This young male was comatose following a motorcycle accident, and a catheter to monitor intracranial pressure was introduced through a right-sided burr hole. As the patient recovered, a left hemiparesis was noted. A CT scan showed the tip of the catheter in the region of the right internal capsule, with surrounding punctate hemorrhage. The catheter was removed, and the patient's hemiparesis resolved.

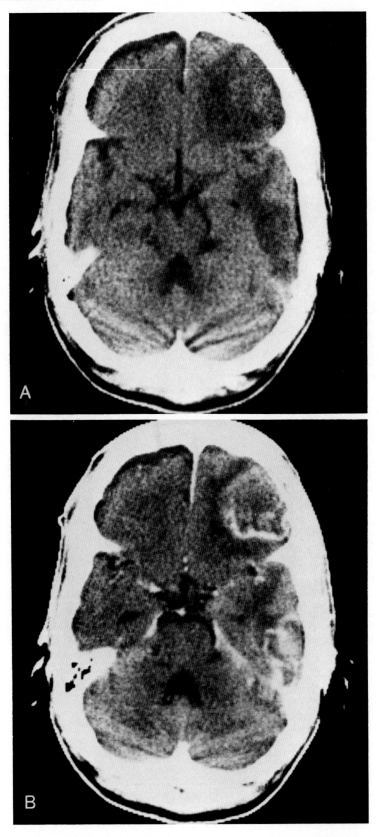

Figure 1.52.   This 45-year-old male was aphasic on admission and had a history of 6 weeks of progressive mental deterioration.
A, B.   CT scan on admission showed low-density regions in the temporal and low frontal lobes with surrounding peripheral enhancement after contrast administration. Given the size of the lesions, relatively little surrounding edema or mass effect are noted. Angiography showed only mass effect. The patient developed a fever while in the hospital, and an open biopsy of the left frontal lesion was performed. This revealed evolving hematoma.

Shearing injury, due to nonuniform rotational stresses at the juncture of gray and white matter discussed above, results in severe neurologic deficits. CT findings include diffuse brain swelling with ventricular and cisternal compression, eccentric hemorrhage in the corpus callosum, and subarachnoid hemorrhage (Fig. 1.10). Additionally, small focal hemorrhages may occur within the white matter or adjacent to the third ventricle. Thin CT sections are occasionally required to identify these small hemorrhages (19).

Intraventricular hemorrhage is detected in only 3% of head-injured patients studied with CT (Fig. 1.43). The majority of such patients are comatose on admission, with an overall mortality rate approaching 75%. In most cases, the intraventricular hemorrhage is due to disruption of the ventricular wall by adjacent intracerebral hematoma. However, rupture of subependymal veins due to pressure changes at the time of impact may play a role in a minority of cases. Significantly, more than half of patients with post-traumatic intraventricular hemorrhage have diffuse brain damage (52).

Delayed follow-up scans of head-injured patients may show secondary focal encephalomalacia (Fig. 1.53), porencephaly (Fig. 1.54), or generalized atrophy. Diffuse atrophy will appear as an overall increase in cerebral CSF spaces, including the ventricles. In fact, up to 30% of patients with severe injuries will develop ventricular dilatation as early as 90 days postinjury (53). In a small percentage of cases, post-traumatic hydrocephalus is due to extraventricular obstruction rather than atrophy. The presumed mechanism of communicating hydrocephalus is partial blockage of CSF absorption pathways due to the chemical meningitis induced by subarachnoid blood (Fig. 1.38).

Lastly, the use of CT in the evaluation of patients with missile or other penetrating injury of the brain is self-evident. CT can delineate the tract of the object through the parenchyma and show damage to vital structures (Fig. 1.55). Fragments of missile and bone can be accurately localized, aiding in debridgement. Of note, wooden objects may appear as low-density foci due to their attenuation properties on CT (54).

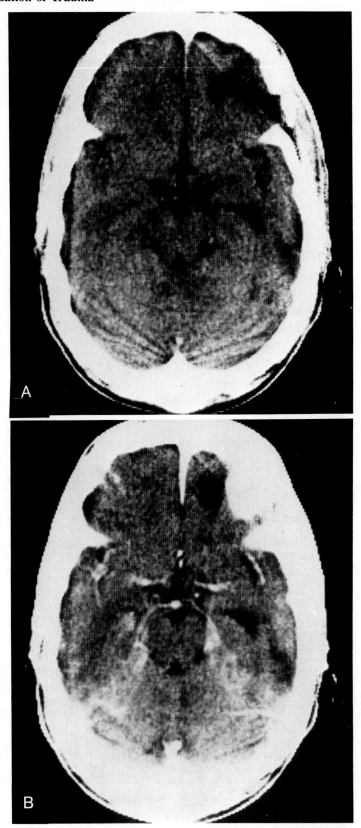

Figure 1.53.
A, B.   Follow-up CT scan (before and after contrast enhancement) 4 months after discharge showed only residual encephalomalacia in the left temporal region. Surgical changes in the left frontal lobe were also seen.

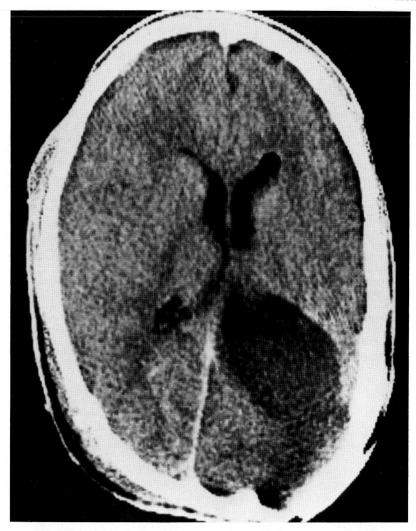

Figure 1.54. Six-year-old male with a history of birth trauma was admitted following a car accident. The CT scan at the level of the ventricles shows a porencephalic cyst in the left posterior parietal region. An overlying calvarial defect is likewise present. This coincided with the site of trauma at the time of delivery. The relative increased density of the CSF within the porencephalic cyst was caused by a small intraventricular hemorrhage due to the recent motor vehicle accident.

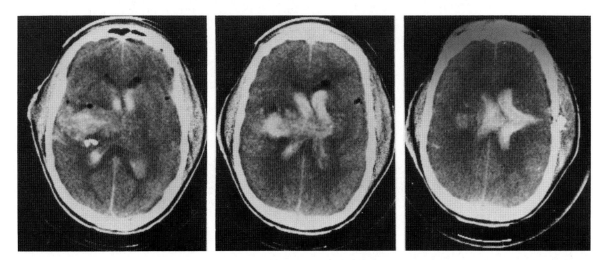

Figure 1.55. This middle-aged female died shortly after a self-inflicted gunshot wound. A CT scan was done on admission and showed a transcranial bullet wound with fragments and blood traversing both hemispheres and ventricles.

SUMMARY

As evidenced by the above discussion and illustrations, CT is of great value in the initial evaluation of the head trauma victim. Its chief virtue is the ability rapidly to detect intracranial hemorrhage, thus permitting its emergency evacuation. Unfortunately, the development of secondary pathophysiologic alterations consequent to intracranial hemorrhage and other diffuse brain trauma renders the prognosis of these victims bleak in many instances. Recent improvements in CT resolution, densitometric ability, and data manipulation may allow more insight into the pathophysiology of head injury, and improved methods of monitoring and treating the traumatized patient.

REFERENCES

1. Kalsbeek WD, McLaurin RL, Harris BSH, Miller JD: The national head and spinal cord injury survey: Major findings. *J Neurosurg* 53:519, 1980.
2. Dublin AB, French BN, Rennick JM: Computed Tomography in head trauma. *Radiology* 122:365, 1977.
3. Rose J. Valtonen S, Jeunett B: Available factors contributing to death after head injury. *Br Med J* 2:615, 1977.
4. Hoff JT, Spetzler R, Winestock D: Head injury and early signs of tentorial herniation. *West J Med* 128:112, 1978.
5. Snoek J, Jennett B, Adams JH, Graham DI, Doyle D: Computerised tomography after recent severe head injury in patients without acute intracranial haematoma. *J Neurol Neurosurg Psychiatry* 42:215, 1979.
6. French BN, Dublin AB: The value of computersized tomography in 1000 consecutive head injuries. *Surg Neurol* 7:171, 1977.
7. Lipper MH, Kishore PRS, Girevendulis AK, Miller JD, Becker DP: Delayed intracranial hematoma in patients with severe head injury. *Radiology* 133:645, 1979.
8. Diaz FG, Yock DH Jr, Larson D, Rockswold GL: Early diagnosis of delayed posttraumatic intracerebral hematomas. *J Neurosurg* 50:217, 1979.
9. Brunetti J, Zingesser L, Dunn J, Rovit RL: Delayed intracerebral hemorrhage as demonstrated by CT scanning. *Neuroradiology* 18:43, 1979.
10. Kishore PRS, Lipper MH, Domingues da Silva AA, Gudeman K, Abbas SA: Delayed sequelae of head injury. *CT* 4:287, 1980.
11. Adams JH, Mitchell DE, Graham DI, Doyle D: Diffuse brain damage of immediate impact type. *Brain* 100:489, 1977.
12. Zimmerman RA, Bilaniuk KT, Gennerelli T: Computed tomography of shearing injuries of the cerebral white matter. *Radiology* 127:393, 1978.
13. Catiff JH, Williams AL, Krigman MR, Whaley RA: CT recognition of subcortical hematomas. *Am J Neuroradiol* 2:49, 1981.
14. Young B, Rapp RP, Norton JA, Haack D, Tibbs PA, Bean JR: Early prediction of outcome in head-injured patients. *J Neurosurg* 54:300, 1981.
15. Narayan RK, Greenberg RP, Miller JD, Enas GG, Choi SC, Kishore PRS, Selhorst JB, Lutz HA, Becker DP: Improved confidence of outcome prediction in severe head injury. *J Neurosurg* 54:751, 1981.
16. Jennett B, Teasdale G. Dynamic pathology. In *Management of Head Injuries*. Philadelphia, FA Davis, 1981, pp 45–75.
17. Holburn AHS: Mechanics of head injuries. *Lancet* 2:438, 1943.
18. Bruce DA, Alavi A, Bilaniuk L, Dolinskas C, Obrist W, Uzzel B: Diffuse cerebral swelling following head injuries in children: The syndrome of "malignant brain edema." *J Neurosurg* 65:170, 1981.
19. Zimmerman RA, Bilaniuk LT, Bruce D, Dolinskas C, Obrist W, Kuhl D: Computed tomography of pediatric head trauma. Acute general cerebral swelling. *Radiology* 126:403, 1978.
20. Veiga-Pires JA, v Nieuwenhuizen O, Kaiser MC: Brainstem compression in a child with acute progressive brain edema following trauma. *J Comput Assist Tomogr* 4:121, 1980.
21. Overgaard J, Tweed WA: Cerebral circulation after head injury. *J Neurosurg* 41:531, 1974.
22. Overgaard J, Mosdal C, Tween WA: Cerebral circulation after head injury. *J Neurosurg* 55:63, 1981.
23. Graham DI, Adams JH, Doyle D: Ischaemic brain damage in fatal non-missile head injuries. *J Neurol Sci* 39:213, 1978.
24. Cordobes F, Lobato RD, Rivas JJ, Munoz MJ, Chillon D, Portillo JM, Lamas E: Observations on 82 patients with extradural hematoma: Comparison of results before and after the advent of computerized tomography. *J Neurosurg* 54:179, 1981.
25. Zimmerman RA, Bilaniuk LT, Gennarelli T, Bruce D, Dolinskas C, Uzzell B: Cranial computed tomography in diagnosis and management of acute head trauma. *AJR* 131:27, 1978.
26. Seelig JM, Becker DP, Miller JD, Greenberg RP, Ward JD, Choi SC: Traumatic acute subdural hematoma. *N Engl J Med* 304:1511, 1981.
27. Masters SJ: Evaluation of head trauma: Efficacy of skull films. *AJNR* 1:329, 1980.
28. Pop PM, Thompson JR, Zinke DE, Hasso AN, Hinshaw DB: Tension pneumocephalus. *J Comput Assist Tomogr* 6:894, 1982.
29. Healy JR, Crudale AS: Computed tomographic evaluation of depressed skull fractures and associated intracranial injury. *Computerized Radiol* 6:323, 1982.
30. Holland BA, Brant-Zawadzki M: High-resolution CT of temporal bone trauma. *AJNR* 5:291, 1984.
31. Johnson DW, Hasso AN, Steward CE, Thompson JR, Hinshaw DB: Temporal bone trauma: High resolution computed tomographic evaluation. *Radiology* 151:411, 1984.
32. Koo AH, LaRoque RL: Evaluation of head trauma by computed tomography. *Radiology* 123:345, 1977.
33. Zimmerman RA, Bilaniuk LT: Computed tomographic staging of traumatic epidural bleeding. *Radiology* 144:809, 1982.
34. Kishore PRS, Lipper MH, Becker DT, Domingues da Silva AA, Narayan RK: Significance of CT in head injury: Correlation with intracranial pressure. *AJNR* 2:307, 1981.
35. Moller A, Erickson K: Computed tomography of iso-attenuating subdural hematomas. *Radiology* 130:149, 1979.
36. Hayman LA, Evans RA, Hinck VC: Rapid-high-dose contrast computed tomography of isodense subdural hematoma and cerebral swelling. *Radiology* 131:381, 1979.
37. Kim KS, Hemmati M, Weinberg PE: Computed tomography in isodense subdural hematoma. *Radiology* 128:71, 1978.
38. Amendola MA, Ostrum BJ: Diagnosis of isodense subdural hematomas by computed tomography. *AJR* 129:693, 1977.
39. Garza-Mercado R: Extradural hematoma of the posterior cranial fossa. *J Neurosurg* 59:664, 1983.
40. Tsai FY, Teal JS, Habashi HH, Huprich JE, Hieshima GB, Segall HD: Computed tomography of posterior fossa trauma. *J Comput Assist Tomogr* 4:291, 1980.
41. Weaver D, Pobereskin L, Jane JA: Spontaneous resolution of epidural hematomas. *J Neurosurg* 54:248, 1981.
42. Markwalder T-M: Chronic subdural hematomas: A review. *J Neurosurg* 54:637, 1981.
43. Pang D, Horton JA, Herron JM, Wilberger JE, Vries JK: Nonsurgical management of extradural hematomas in children. *J Neurosurg* 59:958, 1983.
44. French BN, Cobb CA, Corkill G, Youmans JR: Delayed evolution of posttraumatic subdural hygroma. *Surg Neurol* 9:145, 1978.
45. Stone JL, Lang RGR, Sugar O, Moody RA: Traumatic subdural hygroma. *Neurosurgery* 8:542, 1981.
46. St Jone JN, Dila C: Traumatic subdural hygroma in adults. *Neurosurgery* 9:621, 1981.
47. Zimmerman RA, Bilaniuk LT, Bruce D, Schut L, Uzzell B, Goldberg HI: Computed tomography of craniocerebral injury in the abused child. *Radiology* 130:687, 1979.
48. Merten DB, Osborne DRS: Craniocerebral trauma in the child abuse syndrome. *Pediatr Ann* 12:882, 1983.

49. Tabaddor K, Danziger A, Wissof HS: Estimation of intracranial pressure by CT scan in closed head trauma. *Surg Neurol* 18:212, 1982.

50. Clifton GL, Gross RG, Makela ME, Miner ME, Handel S, Sadhu V: Neurological course and correlated computerized tomography findings after servere closed head injury. *J Neurosurg* 52:611, 1980.

51. Galbraith S, Teasdale G: Predicting the need for operation in the patient with an occult traumatic intracranial hematoma. *J Neurosurg* 55:75, 1981.

52. Cordobes F, de la Fuente M, Lobato RD, Roger R, Perez C, Millan JM, Barcena A, Lamas E: Intraventricular hemorrhage in severe head injury. *J Neurosurg* 58:217, 1983.

53. Gudeman SK, Kishore PRS, Becker DP, Lipper MH, Girevendulis AK, Jeffries BF, Butterworth JF: Computer tomography in the evaluation of incidence and significance of post-traumatic hydrocephalus. *Radiology* 141:397, 1981.

54. Mori K, Handa H, Itoh M, Okuno T: Benign subdural effusion in infants. *J Comput Assist Tomogr* 4:466, 1980.

Chapter 2

CT of Maxillofacial Injury

ROBERT DeLaPAZ, M.D.
MICHAEL BRANT-ZAWADZKI, M.D.
LEE D. ROWE, M.D.

The face is one of the most functional and, at the same time, one of the most visible structures of the human body. Maxillofacial injuries may disturb such basic functions as vision, self-nourishment, and self-expression. The cosmetic disfigurement that often accompanies facial injury can be psychologically crippling. Therefore, the primary goals in treating injuries to the face are to restore function to facial structures and to restore appearance. The role of diagnostic imaging in the evaluation of facial trauma is to provide the clinician with sufficient information to attain these goals.

Perhaps no anatomic region in the body challenges the diagnostic capabilities of an imaging modality more than the facial skeleton and its contents. This is especially true in the assessment of trauma. The complexity of the facial architecture is due not only to the multiplicity of its components, but also to the intricacy of their geometric relationships. The fragile nature of such structures as the orbital floor and the lamina papyracea permits their disruption in relatively mild trauma and taxes the spatial resolution capability of any imaging modality used to evaluate their integrity. The importance of soft tissue structures, such as the eye, its yoke muscles, and the optic nerve, emphasizes the need for an imaging modality which can also provide optimal contrast resolution, thus enabling visualization of soft tissue disruption. Initial plain film screening may be sufficient for the detection of gross facial trauma. However, the associated contusions, lacerations, and edematous areas within the soft tissue structures of the face, as well as hemorrhage into the sinuses, may make a tomographic modality necessary for definitive evaluation of the facial skeleton's disruption. Conventional tomography has continued to be the traditional method for evaluating facial trauma, mainly due to its superior spatial resolution capability.

The recent introduction of computed tomography allowed the application of this modality to the evaluation of maxillofacial trauma (1–7). Further refinements of beam collimation and detector technology have greatly improved the spatial resolution of CT and, combined with its superior contrast resolution which allows direct visualization of soft tissue, have established CT as the primary diagnostic tool in the evaluation of complex maxillofacial pathology in our institution (6, 7).

Optimal reconstruction of complex facial trauma depends not simply on stabilizing the areas of bony disruption and correcting any dental malocclusion, but also on restoring the three-dimensional relationships so important in the most visible of all human structures. It is precisely this ability of CT to graphically display the facial superstructure and its derangements in a format easy to appreciate for radiologists and clinicians alike that is enabling it to supplant a technique as time proven as conventional tomography in the evaluation of maxillofacial trauma. Thin-section CT images, along with sophisticated computer software, allow great flexibility of image manipulation. Axial cuts can be "stacked" and dissected in any desired plane, and can now even be rotated on any desired axis. Such image manipulation easily discloses major structural derangements, such as malar eminence depressions associated with tripod fractures or midfacial implosions in the Le Fort category, as well as minor fractures in the orbital wall or floor. Finally, CT has the ability to obtain such important diagnostic information at relatively little radiation exposure to the patient when compared with conventional tomography. Considering the relative sensitivity of such structures as the lens and the thyroid to radiation, and the relative frequency of trauma in the younger population, minimizing radiation exposure while maintaining a high quality of diagnostic imaging is an added advantage of computed tomography when compared to pluridirectional tomographic technique (7).

TECHNIQUE

Although early work with CT in the diagnosis of facial trauma utilized positioning of the patient's head in a coronal orientation, such positioning is often difficult to achieve (especially if cervical trauma accompanies the facial injury), and may be impossible to maintain for the period of time the study requires. In our experience, thin axial sections are sufficient, especially if one has a CT unit capable of multiplanar reformation. Very thin sections are essential for adequate spatial resolution, both on the original and the reformatted images. Current generation equipment allowing sections of 1.5 mm permits optimal image reformation. We generally begin the scan at the level of the alveolar ridge and proceed superiorly with 1.5-mm contiguous sections. Our previous equipment limited the vertical extent of such a study to 6.7 cm. This was usually sufficient for the evaluation of midfacial injury. Occasionally, when high front-oethmoidal injuries accompanied the midface trauma, we utilized thicker sections, 5 mm in width, but overlapped them by 2 mm using contiguous table incrementation of only 3 mm. This doubled our vertical range, at the expense of slight loss of spatial resolution. Our current CT imager (G.E. 9800) permits acquisition of 3 mm thick, contiguous slices when the vertical range cannot be covered by 1.5-mm slices.

CT reconstruction algorithms have been developed which allow scan data to be assigned to a smaller pixel matrix with an expanded CT number range (8). The resolution of images so produced rivals any conventional tomographic modality and surpasses previously available CT resolution of osseous structures and their disruption (Fig. 2.1). These algorithms are finding a major application in facial trauma work, as will be seen below.

Since image reformation depends upon maintenance of alignment between each successive axial section, any patient motion during the study detracts from the resolution on reformatted images. Therefore, rapid-sequence scanning is desirable. This can be achieved by automatic table incrementation, available in certain models of CT equipment. Additionally, one can diminish the time between the separate axial scans by minimizing heat load on the X-ray tube. This is done by utilizing very low exposure settings. In our experience, 160 mAs technique is sufficient for the visualization of osseous and even soft tissue in the facial skeleton; the disparate density of soft tissue structures in the face (orbital fat versus muscle versus air) permits the detection of contrast alteration at the junction of these tissues even at low exposure settings. Such low milliampere-second settings would be insufficient for the detection of subtle contrast alterations

in the brain, however. In the face, the combination of low milliampere-second technique with automatic table incrementation allows very rapid studies. Up to 45 slices can be taken in less than 12 minutes of patient time. Motion between slices is minimized, thus optimizing the quality of image reformations while allowing faster patient through-put.

Image reformation is of great benefit, especially in particular aspects of trauma. For example, images in the plane of the inferior rectus muscle (the true sagittal plane of the orbit) evaluate the extent of orbital floor displacement optimally; such displacement is difficult to assess on axial cuts as these are close to the plane of the floor itself. Coronal reformations help to delineate the exact degree of inferior rectus herniation through any defect in the floor that may exist. True coronal reformations of the face are best obtained by relating the plane of section to retrofacial bony landmarks, such as the sphenoid wings or the petrous pyramids. This insures detection of posterior displacement of facial structures, such as the zygoma, without overly worrying about exact patient positioning in the head holder. Such coronal reformations can also easily depict vertical alveolar fractures, disruption of the frontozygomatic suture, pterygoid plates, etc. Direct coronal projection can be utilized in patients with less extensive injuries, if they are able to maintain that position.

Reformation of axial sections can be carried a step further than the planar sagittal and coronal images. True three-dimensional information is present in a set of contiguous axial sections and can be displayed by using pixel intensity to display spatial information. In Figure 2.2 pixel intensity is used to encode depth in a frontal view. High intensities indicate proximity to the viewer, and low intensities are points distant from the viewer. The result is a visual impression of depth and a "3D display" of facial bony anatomy. The data can be further manipulated by the computer to create multiple perspective angles and give the viewer the impression of "rotating the facial anatomy in space." This technique is currently under development, and some problems are yet to be resolved. As with planar reformations, spatial resolution is degraded relative to the in-plane resolution of the antecedent axial sections and thin fracture lines may not be visualized. Due to the partial volume averaging of thin bones with adjacent soft tissues (e.g., orbital floor), artifactual defects may be displayed in the 3D reformations.

Finally, one should not neglect evaluation of the brain itself in routine fashion. Up to 33% of significant facial trauma may have an associated intracranial injury (3), such as extracerebral or parenchymal hematomas, encephaloceles, and cavernous-carotid fistula (Fig. 2.3). Evaluation of the brain is imperative in the presence of a sphenoid sinus effusion with acute head trauma. Over 90% of cases with effusion have associated intracranial abnormalities, including intracerebral and extracerebral hematomas, cerebral edema, and pneumocephalus (4).

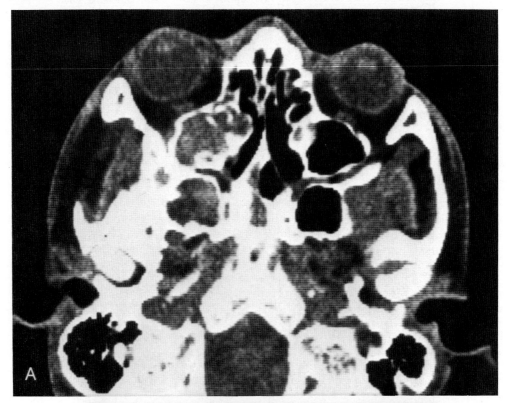

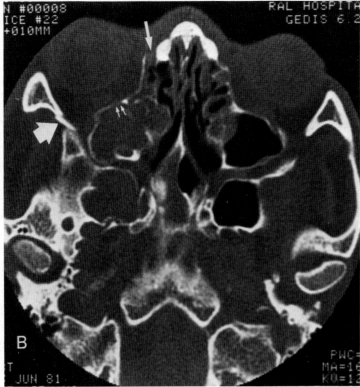

Figure 2.1. Conventional reconstruction versus reconstruction utilizing decreased pixel size and extended CT number range (ReView, G.E. Corporation).

A. Conventional reconstruction depicts soft tissue within the maxillary antral roof; bony detail is insufficient to make a specific diagnosis.

B. ReView reconstruction shows discontinuity of bone at the maxillary roof-orbital floor level (*small arrows*); note also the fracture of the frontozygomatic suture (*white arrowhead*) and disrupted lacrimal bone (*white arrow*). Incidentally, note the sharp detail of the foramina at the base of the skull and the temporomandibular joints (same patient as Fig. 2.15).

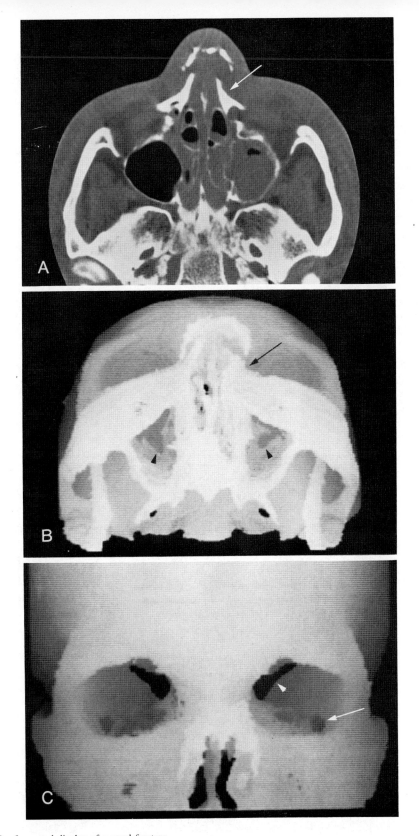

Figure 2.2. "3D" reformatted display of a nasal fracture.

A. Axial section shows a comminuted fracture of the nasal bones bilaterally with medial displacement of the frontal process of the left maxilla (*arrow*).

B. Reformatted display of an axial CT set using pixel intensity to indicate depth (higher intensities are closer to the viewer) gives the visual impression of three spatial dimensions. This view is approximately equivalent to a Water's projection. The elevation of the nasal bones and depression of the left maxillary frontal process (*arrow*) are seen. The small fracture lines in the nasal bones seen in the axial section are not clearly seen here. The apparent defects in the orbital floors (*arrowheads*), seen through the maxillary sinuses, are artifacts due to the thin bone in these regions.

C. 3D reformatted display in an approximate Caldwell projection shows the elevation of the nasal bones bilaterally. The superior orbital fissures are also clearly seen at the orbital apices (*arrowhead*). The apparent defects in the orbital floors (*arrow*) are artifacts due to the thin bone in these regions.

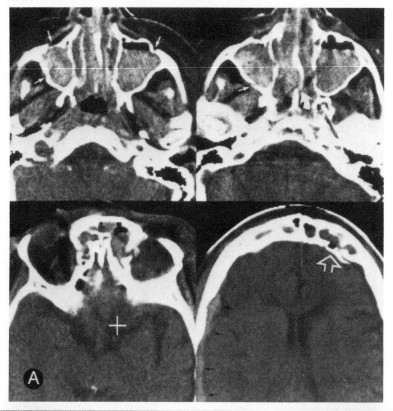

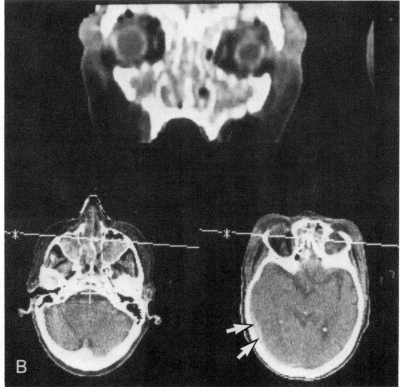

Figure 2.3. Le Fort II fracture with frontoethmoidal sinus component and subdural hematoma.
A. Selected axial cuts demonstrate disruption of maxillary antra and inferior orbital rim (*small white arrows*), vomer (*curved arrowhead, top right*), ethmoid sinuses (*lower left*), and posterior wall-frontal sinus fracture on the left (*open arrow*).
B. Right subdural hematoma (*large white arrows*) was unsuspected clinically.

NASAL FRACTURES

Simple nasal fractures can easily be diagnosed clinically, although routine plain films do play a supporting role. These fractures are usually reduced via mechanical manipulation under general or local anesthesia. Open reduction and direct wiring are only rarely indicated, except in instances where a deviated cartilagenous portion of the septum cannot be stablized in the maxillary groove. Since such fractures are often seen as a component of complex facial trauma, they will be discussed briefly here. The radiologist should be able to ascertain the level of the nasal fracture, whether there is any displacement, and whether the fracture is comminuted.

Fractures of the nasal bones rarely involve the strongly reinforced upper portion and primarily involve the nasal tip. Most nasal fractures are due to blows which strike the nose from the side. In such cases, both nasal bones are fractured at a horizontal level and dislocated to one side. This permits their detection on axial cuts or reformatted coronal images (Figs. 2.2 and 2.4). Only the more severe impact will produce a fracture of the nasofrontal angle region and nasal-ethmoid complex.

Severe fractures of the nasal bone are almost always associated with fractures of the frontal process of the maxilla (Figs. 2.2 and 2.4), which are usually not detectable on plain films but can be easily identified and characterized with CT (5). When evaluating nasal fractures, one must rule out associated fracture of the lacrimal bones, the lamina papyracea, the cribriform plate, and/or the orbital plate of the frontal bone. Occasionally, even the optic foramen can be disrupted, with partial or complete blindness resulting from compression of the optic nerve (Fig. 2.5). Progressive decrease in vision immediately after facial trauma necessitates careful evaluation of the optic foramen.

Nasoethmoidal fractures, if neglected, can result in severe deformities. Flattening of the bridge of the nose, widening of the intercanthal distance, and disruption of the lacrimal sac with subsequent dacrocystitis may occur.

Nondisplaced hairline nasal fractures may be difficult to see with CT; however, these do not require reduction, and, if uncomplicated, their X-ray diagnosis is not vital.

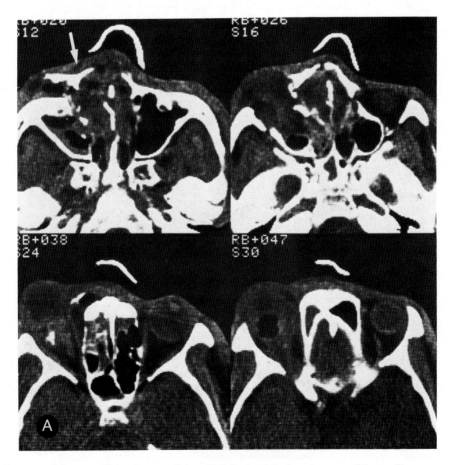

Figure 2.4. Severe nasal fracture with involvement of the orbital floor and the frontal process of the maxilla.
A. Sequential axial cuts demonstrate fracture and rotation of the right nasal bone and the frontal process of the maxilla including a portion of the medial orbital rim (*arrow*). Note bone fragments in the maxillary antrum roof, as well as in the retrobulbar region of the orbit (*lower left*). Retrobulbar hematoma and emphysema accompany the findings. Metal over nose is from patient's oxygen mask.

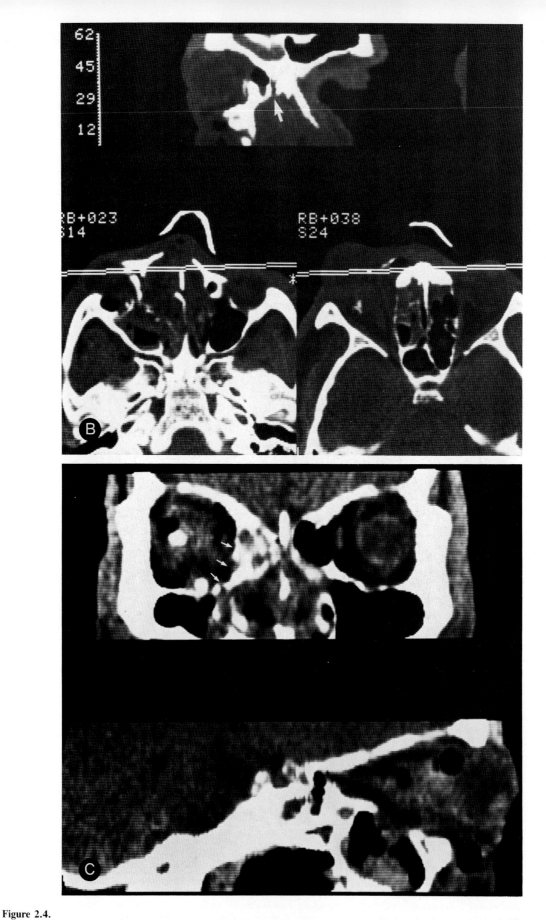

Figure 2.4.

B. Coronal section demonstrates the disrupted right nasal bone (*arrow*).

C. Coronal (*top*) and para-axial reformations along the plane of the inferior rectus (*bottom*) define the orbital floor injury to better advantage and show the bony fragment and retrobulbar hematoma and emphysema. Note that the coronal reformation defines extension of the fracture from the frontomaxillary process into the right lacrimal bone and lamina papyracea (*arrows*).

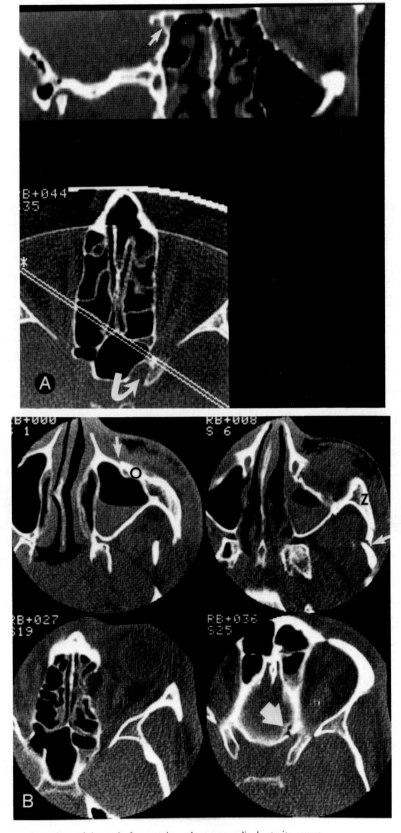

Figure 2.5.   ReView reconstructions of the optic foramen in a plane perpendicular to its course.
A. Normal optic foramen (*arrow*) seen on an image reformation perpendicular to the axis of the foramen (*curved arrow*).
B. Selected sequential CT sections show a partial left tripod fracture (*bold arrows*) and a medial orbital blowout in a patient rendered blind with the trauma (*z*, zygoma; *o*, orbital rim). Note suggestion of sphenoid fracture adjacent to the optic canal (*arrowhead, lower right*).

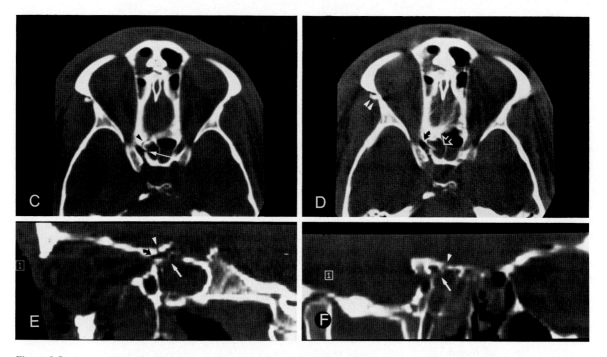

Figure 2.5.
C, D. Axial sections (1.5 mm thick) in another patient with traumatic blindness show fractures of the medial right optic foramen (**C,** *arrow*) and the adjacent planum sphenoidale (**C,** *arrowhead*). A low-attenuation area (**D,** *curved arrow*) indicates air in the optic foramen arising from the sphenoid sinus (now filled with hemorrhage; **D,** *open arrow*). A fracture fragment (**D,** *double arrowhead*) at the right frontozygomatic suture and hemorrhage in the ethmoid sinuses are also present.
E. Oblique sagittal reformation in the axis of the right optic foramen shows the fractures in the inferior foramen (sphenoid sinus wall, *arrow*) and superior foramen (planum sphenoidale, *arrowhead*). The air within the foramen is also seen (*curved arrow*).
F. Oblique sagittal reformation perpendicular to the axis of the right optic foramen shows the fractures of the inferior foramen (sphenoid sinus wall, *arrow*), and planum sphenoidale (*arrowhead*).

ORBITAL TRAUMA

In this section isolated fractures of the orbit and trauma to the intraorbital contents will be discussed. As will be seen subsequently, fracture of the orbital floor may commonly occur as a component of massive zygomaticomaxillary complex injury, as well as trauma to the frontoethmoidal region. However, the typical blowout fracture is caused by a very rapid increase in intraorbital pressure, usually due to a blunt object directed at the globe and lids (e.g., a fist or ball) that is slightly larger than the orbital inlet. The sudden increase in pressure fractures the bony orbit at areas of weakness, usually at the paper-thin orbital floor or the medial wall. The medial half of the orbital floor is not only thin but is further weakened by the canal or groove for the passage of the infraorbital nerve. When the orbital floor disrupts, herniation of orbital fat and incarceration of the connective tissue investments of the inferior rectus and/or oblique muscles may occur, causing subsequent limitation of eye movement. Direct entrapment of extraocular muscles, however, is a rare finding. Occasionally, a direct blow to the inferior orbital rim may cause elevation and buckling of the orbital floor with compression of the muscle. Because the late sequelae of orbital fracture—such as enophthalmos, diplopia, and ptosis—are difficult to treat surgically, it is important for the radiologist to identify not only the disruption of the orbital floor but its relationship to the important soft tissue structures within that disruption. CT is of great help in the thorough evaluation of such injuries.

Many variations of the orbital floor fracture have been described (Figs. 2.6–2.12). There may be an eggshell fracture with a hammock-like sagging of the floor into the maxillary sinus, with a trapped piece of bone hanging on a periosteal hinge in the maxillary sinus (Fig. 2.6). A comminution of the floor with buckling may cause pinching of the undersurface of the orbital contents (Fig. 2.7). A typical radiologic finding, delineated nicely with CT imaging, is the "hanging drop" opacity produced by herniation of the orbital tissues into the maxillary sinus. Although this finding is obscured by a clouded sinus in conventional radiography, CT can clearly delineate this type of fracture (Figs. 2.10 and 2.11). Direct coronal views may be obtained, but reformation of axial images in a plane defined by the inferior rectus muscle shows the degree of orbital floor depression best, while the plane perpendicular to this defines the degree of herniation further. Such reformations will generally show disturbance of the normal anatomic orientation of the orbital floor, with the lower anterior portion showing a defect in the gentle downward convexity. The posterior portion is normally bulged upward by the roof of the maxillary antrum, and any fragmentation here is also easily seen. Orbital hematoma or emphysema is easily appreciated on CT, when present (Figs. 2.4 and 2.12). Subperiosteal hematomas of the orbital roof following trauma can produce ocular displacement and pressure on the optic nerve, and need rapid evaluation.

Medial wall blowout can only be suggested on plain films by opacification of the adjacent ethmoid air cells; however, actual bony fragmentation of the lamina papyracea can be appreciated with conventional axial CT images (Figs. 2.7, 2.8, and 2.10). Since plain films may miss isolated orbital floor fracture, CT should be obtained in the appropriate clinical setting when unexplained restriction of orbital extraocular muscle function is present following trauma.

Direct intraorbital injury can occur with either a foreign body or bullet (Fig. 2.13) or with direct puncture caused by a stick or an antenna (Fig. 2.14). CT can delineate the relationship of the foreign body to the globe and optic nerve or the status of such structures after a transient puncture with a sharp object.

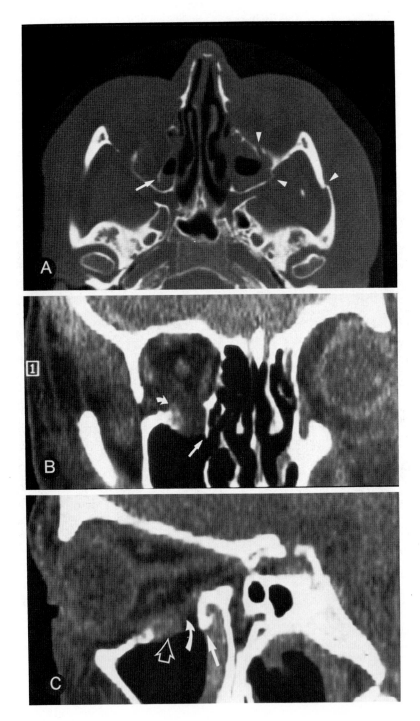

Figure 2.6.   Orbital floor blowout fracture.
A. Axial section shows medial and posterior displacement of a right orbital floor fracture fragment (*arrow*). Note the reduced size of the right maxillary antrum. Two components of a tripod fracture (anterior and posterior antral wall with a zygomatic arch fracture) are present on the left (*arrowheads*).
B. Oblique coronal reformation shows the medial periosteal "hinging" of the right orbital blowout fracture fragment (*arrow*). The inferior rectus muscle appears to be partially displaced into the lateral portion of the orbital floor defect (*curved arrow*).
C. Oblique sagittal reformation shows the left orbital floor defect with inferior displacement of the inferior rectus muscle (*curved arrow*). Posterior displacement of the orbital floor fracture fragment is also seen (*arrow*). The associated tissue in the floor defect probably represents hematoma (*open arrow*).

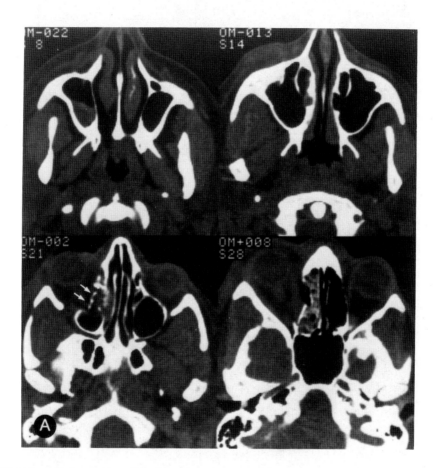

Figure 2.7. Orbital blowout fracture with medial component.
A. Selected axial sections reveal an air-fluid level in the maxillary antrum on the lowest cut, disruption of the orbital floor-maxillary antrum interface (*lower left, small arrows*), and medial blowout of the lamina papyracea (*lower right*).

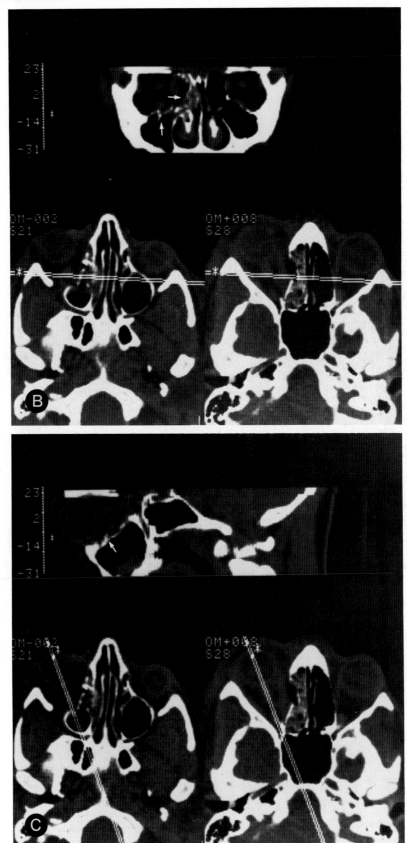

Figure 2.7.
B. Coronal reformation shows the irregularity of the orbital floor and the medial blowout of the right orbit to better advantage (*arrows*).
C. Reformation along the plane of the inferior rectus muscle shows the irregularity of the orbital floor, with a jagged protrusion upward impinging on the inferior rectus muscle (*arrow*). The patient had limitation of gaze clinically.

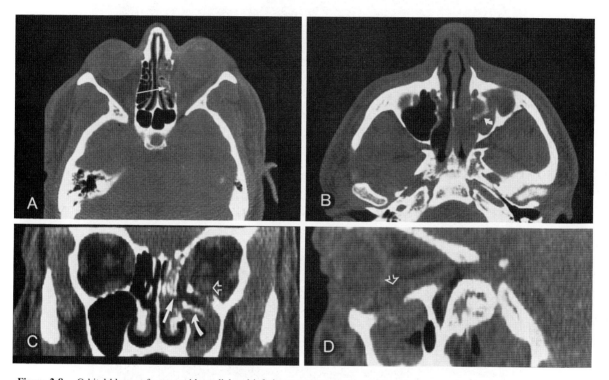

Figure 2.8.   Orbital blowout fracture with medial and inferior components.
A, B. Axial sections show the blowout fracture with medial deviation of the lamina papyracea (*arrow*). The soft tissue density in the ethmoid air cells represents hemorrhage. An inferior component to the fracture can be questioned due to the apparent posterior displacement of an orbital floor fragment (*curved arrow*). However, this finding is not diagnostic in the axial plane.
C. Coronal reformation clearly shows the medial components of the left blowout fracture (*arrow*). The break in the orbital floor and the inferiorly displaced bone fragment (*curved arrow*) are apparent. The inferior rectus muscle is seen in normal position (*open arrow*). Hematoma is present in the maxillary sinus and medial left ethmoid sinuses.
D. Sagittal reformation along the axis of the inferior rectus muscle (*open arrow*) and fracture line shows the defect in the orbital floor and adjacent maxillary sinus hematoma. The inferior rectus muscle is not displaced into the floor defect.

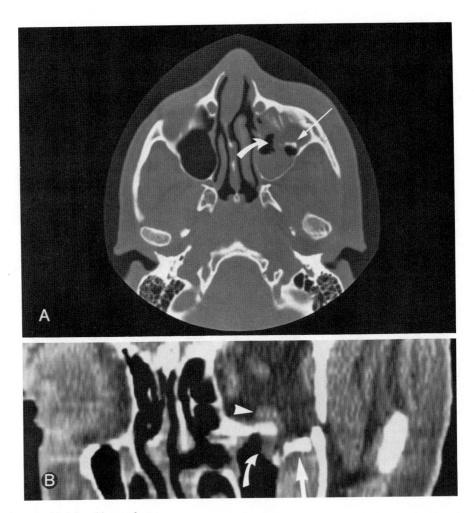

Figure 2.9.   Lateral orbital floor blowout fracture.
A.   Axial section shows a bone fragment in the lateral orbital floor (*arrow*). The linear soft tissue density adjacent to it may represent either inferior displacement of the inferior rectus muscle or hematoma (*curved arrow*).
B. Coronal reformation shows inferior displacement of the lateral orbital floor fracture fragment (*arrow*). The inferior rectus muscle lies in normal position medial and superior to the fracture (*arrowhead*). The linear density seen on the axial sections represents hematoma medial to the fracture fragment and below the intact orbital floor (*curved arrow*).

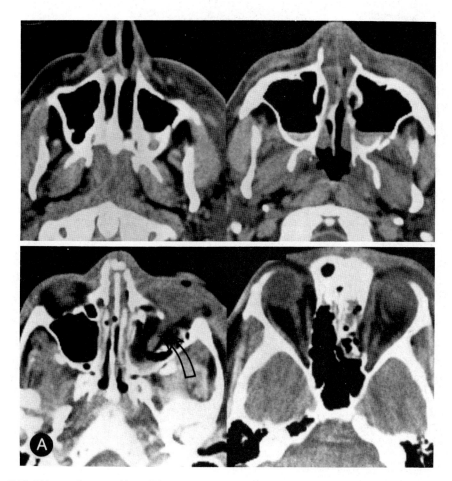

Figure 2.10.   Orbital blowout fracture with medial component, with associated nasal and maxillary antral fractures.
A. Selected sequential axial cuts show bimaxillary air-fluid levels and fractures of the left maxillary antral walls (*upper row*). The higher cuts demonstrate inferior displacement of the left inferior rectus into the maxillary antrum roof (*curved arrow, lower left*), indicating a floor disruption. Medial blowout is also shown (*lower right*). Note the incidential nasal fracture (*lower left*) and medial blowout (*lower right*).

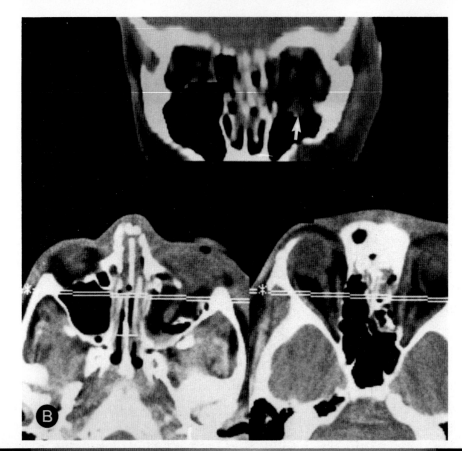

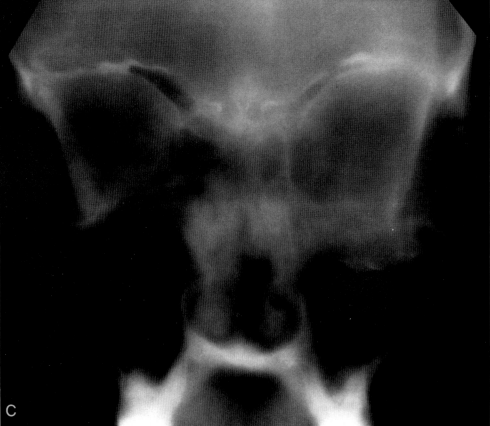

Figure 2.10.

B. Coronal reformation verifies the hammock-like displacement of the inferior rectus into the orbital floor defect (*arrow*).

C. Conventional anteroposterior tomographic section shows soft tissue opacification of the upper maxillary antrum with bone fragment. Note that the CT directly identifies inferior rectus muscle within the defect, whereas the conventional study cannot differentiate various types of soft tissue.

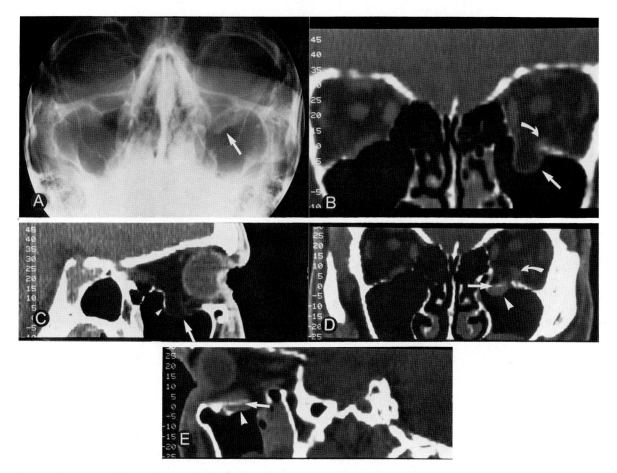

Figure 2.11.   Orbital blowout fracture with repair.

A. Water's view plain film shows an abnormal soft tissue density in the superior left maxillary sinus (*arrow*).

B, C. Coronal and sagittal reformations show herniations of fat ("hanging drop") through the orbital floor defect (*arrows*). The inferior rectus muscle appears to lie at the lateral edge of the defect on the coronal reformation (**B,** *curved arrow*). The sagittal reformation shows a posteriorly hinged orbital floor fragment (**C,** *arrowhead*). This was not appreciated on the plain film due to the orientation of the plane of the fragment perpendicular to the central beam on the Water's view.

D, E. Coronal and sagittal reformations following repair of the orbital floor by placement of a Teflon plate (*arrows*) under the inferior rectus muscle. The inferior rectus muscle is seen in a normal position on the coronal reformation (**D,** *curved arrow*). The soft tissue density inferior to the plate represents postoperative hematoma (*arrowheads*).

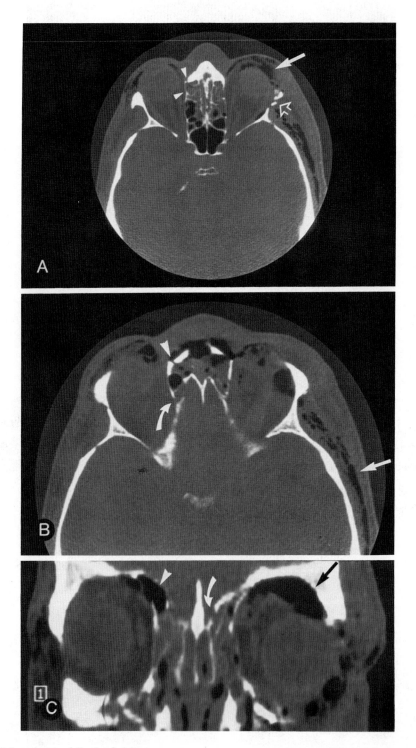

Figure 2.12.   Orbital emphysema following facial trauma.
A, B. Axial sections show extensive orbital and subcutaneous emphysema (*arrows*). Comminuted nasal and ethmoid fractures (*arrowheads*) with a right cribriform plate fracture (**B,** *curved arrow*) are present. The comminuted fracture of the left zygoma (**A,** *open arrow*) was associated with a tripod fracture.
C. Coronal reformation shows inferior displacement of the left globe with lateral orbital rim disruption and a preseptal, extraconal orbital air collection which may be under tension (*arrow*). A left cribriform plate fracture (*curved arrow*) is present. Extensive hemorrhage is seen in the ethmoid sinuses with air in the right supraorbital ethmoid air cell (*arrowhead*).

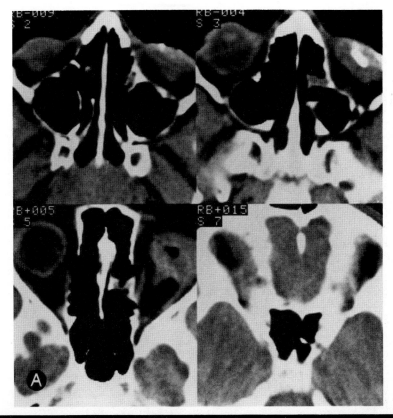

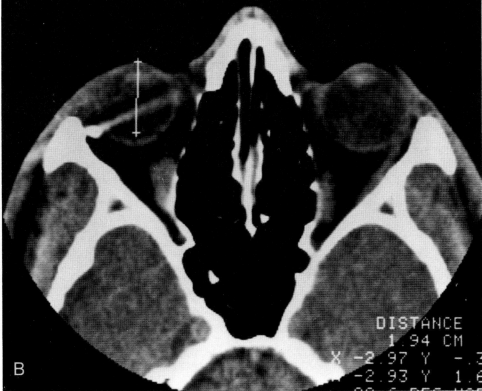

Figure 2.13.   Gunshot orbital trauma.
A. This unfortunate teenager was blinded by a bullet fragment. Sequential axial CT sections show the fragment inside the left globe, with shrinkage of the eyeball.
B. A BB can be seen in the outer aspect of the right orbit (outside the globe) in another patient. Its localization and retrieval were facilitated by the measurement capabilities of the CT scanner.

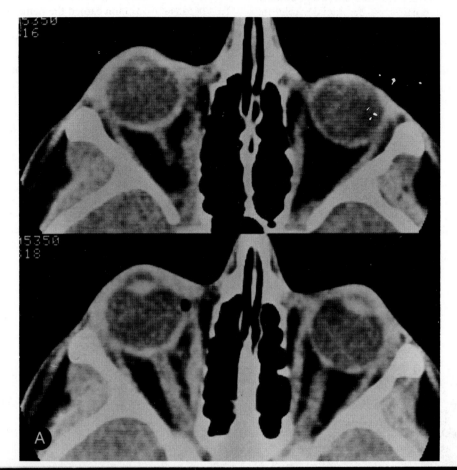

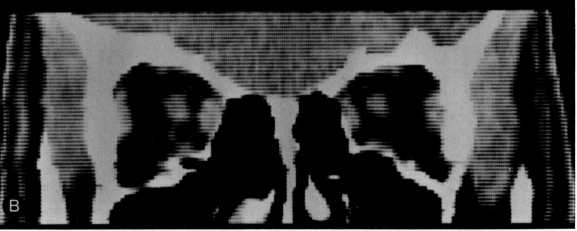

Figure 2.14.   Puncture injury of the orbit. A car antenna penetrated the orbit in this young patient, with resulting blindness.
A. Adjacent axial sections revealed only thickening of the right medial rectus, with increased density of the surrounding retrobulbar fat and a small amount of air. The findings are indistinguishable from an inflammatory process except for the air.
B. Coronal section verifies the asymmetry of the findings in the right orbit.

FRACTURES OF THE ZYGOMA

The zygoma or cheek bone is an important cosmetic structure in the face and forms a strong buttress for the midlateral portion of the facial skeleton. Zygomatic complex fractures usually occur as the result of a force striking the prominence of the zygomatic bone (malar eminence). The zygomatic complex is comprised of the bone itself and its articulations, including those with the frontal, maxillary, and temporal bones superficially and with the greater wing of the sphenoid bone dorsally. The zygomatic bone forms the lateral wall and most of the inferior rim of the orbit. It also helps to form the superolateral border of the maxillary sinus and guards the temporal and infratemporal fossa.

Fractures in this region are usually due to direct impact and commonly manifect themselves clinically as flatness of the cheek with downward drooping of the eye. The malar eminence usually fractures as a unit, the disruptions generally occurring at the sites of its articulations. Medially, the fracture occurs through the maxillary antrum at the infraorbital foramen, also involving the floor of the orbit. Superiorly, the frontozygomatic suture is disrupted, while posterolaterally the fracture generally involves the zygomatic arch. This tripartite disruption earned the name tripod fracture. Multiple fractures of the lateral maxillary wall almost always accompany these disruptions (Fig. 2.15). The degree of displacement and rotation of the malar eminence produced by its separation from normal articulations is easy to appreciate and conceptualize in a three-dimensional sense with the use of computed tomography. This is of great help in planning the vector of forces to be exerted in the surgical reduction of all the fragments. The degree of orbital floor disruption and herniation of its contents can likewise be assessed. When the tripod fracture is incomplete, for instance, when the zygomatic arch is not disrupted, the malar eminence displacement may be limited (Figs. 2.16 and 2.17). The tripod fracture may appear as an isolated injury; however, it is also often a component of the more complex Le Fort midface fracture.

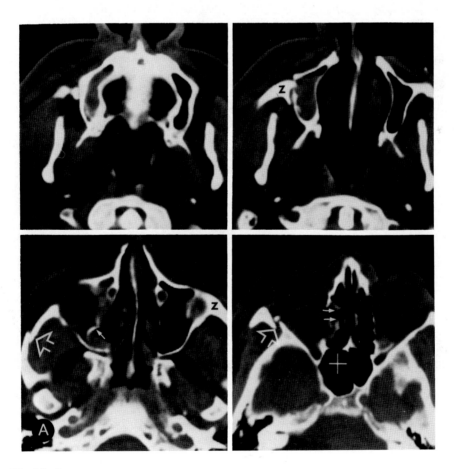

Figure 2.15.   Tripod fracture.
A. Selected sequential axial CT sections show disruption of the zygoma (*z*) from its maxillary articulation, and the resulting inferomedial rotation (*upper row*). The zygomatic arch fracture and frontozygomatic suture disruption are likewise seen (*open arrows*). Note the associated orbital floor and medial wall fractures (*lower row, small arrows*).

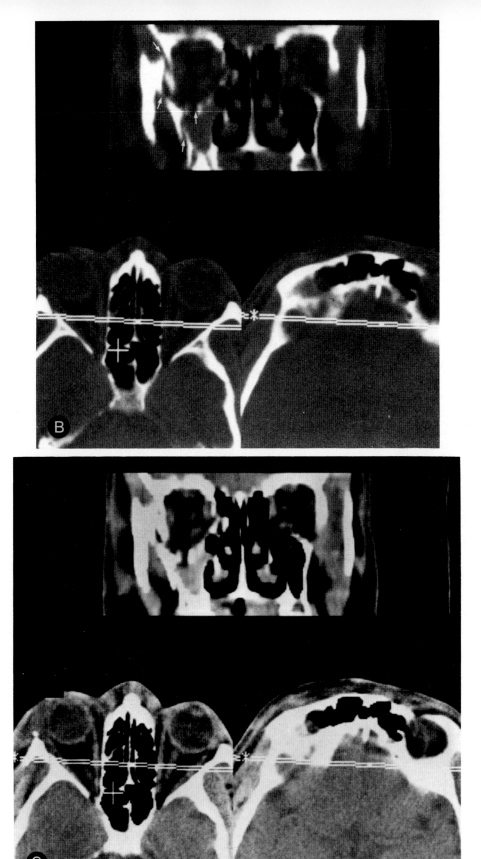

Figure 2.15.

B. Coronal reconstruction nicely delineates the frontozygomatic and maxillary, including inferior orbital rim, components of the tripod fracture (*arrows*). Note that the malar eminence is seen on the right in the same plane as the zygomatic arch on the left, indicating the former's posterior displacement.

C. Soft tissue windows of the reformation shown in **B** verify the orbital floor fracture with slight downward displacement of the inferior rectus muscle.

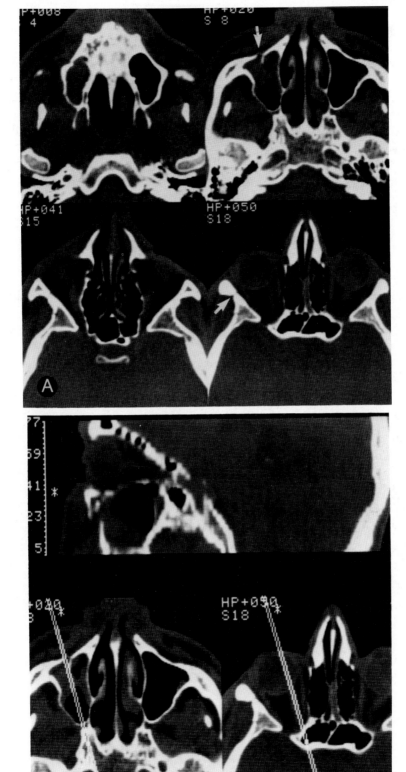

Figure 2.16.   Partial tripod fracture.
A. Selected sequential axial sections depict fracture of the inferior orbital rim and frontozygomatic suture on the right (*arrows*) with minimal displacement. Note absence of zygomatic arch fracture.
B. Image reformation in a plane defined by the optic nerve shows the associated disruption of the anterior maxillary wall and orbital floor. Note the hyperaerated orbital roof.

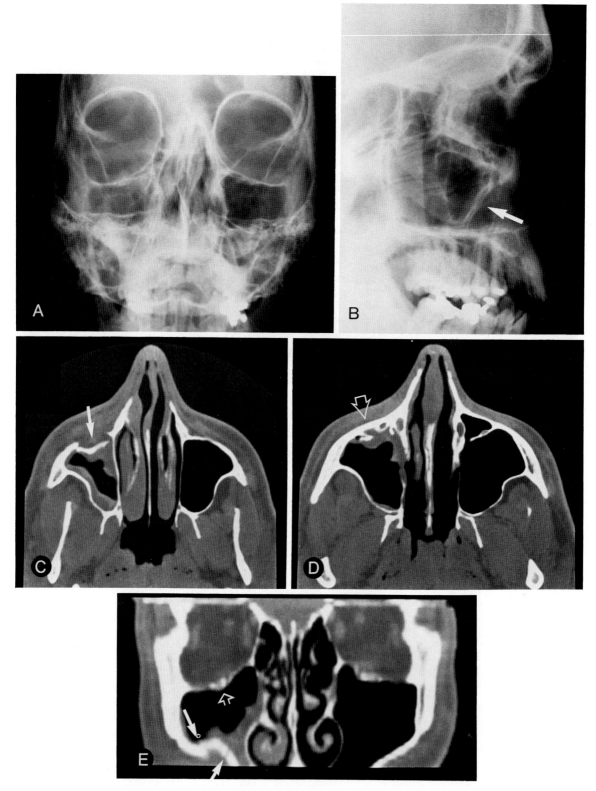

Figure 2.17. Anterior maxillary fracture.
A, B. Anteroposterior and lateral radiographs show clouding of the right maxillary sinus and suggest posterior displacement of the anterior wall of a maxillary sinus (**B,** *arrow*) but are not definitive.
C, D. Axial sections show an intact inferior orbital rim (**D,** *open arrow*) with a clear, posteriorly displaced fragment of the anterior right maxillary sinus wall (**C,** *arrow*).
E. Coronal reformation shows additional fractures in the inferior aspect of the right maxillary sinus (*arrows*). The right orbital floor is intact (*open arrow*).

Acute fractures of the zygomatic bone are usually easily reduced. The fractured osseous complex is elevated into position through various approaches, and the zygomatic bone snaps into place and remains stable. If the zygomatic bone does not snap into place or remain reduced, there is probably either soft tissue interposed along the fracture line or osseous comminution at the fracture site. Open reduction and stabilization with wire sutures in at least two fracture areas, such as the frontozygomatic suture and the fracture line along the infraorbital rim, are then required. Proper reduction generally accomplishes restoration of the ophthalmic disfigurement. Such disfigurement is due either to orbital blowout (Fig. 2.15) or to the inferior displacement of the lateral canthal ligament which attaches to the zygomatic bone on the frontal process, approximately 1 cm below the zygomaticofrontal suture line. This ligament, when displaced inferiorly with the tripod fracture, pulls the outer canthal line downward. Of course, direct orbital floor injuries must be reduced if they are present; otherwise enophthalmos may persist.

MIDFACE FRACTURES

The appropriate therapeutic approach to the reconstruction of midfacial fractures requires an accurate understanding of the vector of the applied traumatic force and the precise delineation of resulting osseous dislocation, particularly in cases of maxillary alveolar involvement. The classical work in this field was accomplished by Rene Le Fort at the turn of the century, in a masterful series of papers based upon cadaver studies of midfacial bone fracture (9). His precise analysis of the lines of weakness in the facial skeleton provided the method of classification of midfacial fractures into transverse (Le Fort I), pyramidal (Le Fort II), or complete craniofacial separation (Le Fort III). Unfortunately, subsequent medical and surgical textbooks have generally applied Le Fort's observations too rigorously, implying that the midface fracture occurs completely along only one of these lines, despite the fact that Le Fort described complex combinations of these fractures which could be complete or incomplete, depending on the nature and vector of the trauma.

In our increasingly violent society, complex combinations of Le Fort fracture lines frequently occur, often with additional fractures of the supporting buttresses of the maxilla. Appropriate stabilization of these injuries aimed at preserving midfacial height, permitting functional occlusion, and avoiding facial asymmetry depends upon a three-dimensional understanding of the fragmentation pattern. Reference to Figure 2.18 will help the reader's understanding of the following discussion.

Midfacial osseous injuries may involve any or all of the bones forming the midfacial skeleton: the two maxillae, the two palatine bones, the two nasal bones, the two lacrimal bones, the vomer, the ethmoid bone and its perpendicular plate and turbinates, the two

inferior turbinates, the pterygoid processes of the sphenoid bone, the two zygomatic processes of the temporal bone, and the two zygomatic bones and their temporal processes. The paired maxillae constitute the major portion of the midface, and their support is found in three main buttresses which transmit the load of any force delivered to the maxilla to the cranial vault: the frontonasomaxillary buttress, the zygomaticomaxillary buttress, and the pterygomaxillary buttress. Further support is obtained from the vomer, perpendicular plate of the ethmoid, lamina papyracea, and ethmoid sinuses (maxilloethmoidal buttress), and the pyramidal process of the palatine bone.

By definition, Le Fort fractures of the midface involve the dentoalveolar component of the upper jaw. They may involve the pterygoids at variable levels or incompletely transverse the maxilla. They may be unilateral. All three major fracture lines may have associated sagittal or parasagittal fracture of the hard palate. Often, a coexisting fracture of the bony nasal septum is encountered. This complexity of involvement necessitates use of a standard nomenclature. A complete Le Fort fracture indicates disruption along an entire single line of great weakness (I, II, III) and may have associated or additional fractures in other parts of the maxillary supporting buttresses. Incomplete Le Fort fractures include bilateral fractures along a single line of great weakness which do not fully involve the entire line. Pure Le Fort injury of the midface is defined as a complete fracture involving only one of the lines of great weakness without additional involvement of the facial skeleton. Unilateral or hemi-Le Fort fractures involve the pterygoid laminae and traverse the maxilla only to the anterior midline, in one of the three configurations. Alveolar fractures are vertical fractures of the dental arch of the maxilla where two or more teeth are included in osseous block of bone, and they may be isolated or part of a Le Fort injury (Fig. 2.19).

Le Fort I Fracture

The fracture line about to be described results in detachment of the entire lower portion of the maxilla and pterygoid processes from the rest of the midface in a transverse plane. The line of disruption begins just under the anterior nasal aperture, passes above the canine fossa, drops beneath the zygoma, transverses the anterolateral wall of the maxilla, and ascends posteriorly across the pterygomaxillary fossa to fracture the pterygoid laminae at the junction of the lower third of these processes. In addition, it courses along the medial wall of the maxillary antrum, joining the lateral fracture line behind the maxillary tuberosities. Such a complete fracture would result in a Le Fort I occlusal fragment (Fig. 2.20). Axial CT images depict fractures in the lower portion of the maxillary antrum and the degree of the occlusal fragment's posterior displacement. Multiplanar reformations show vertical alveolar fractures to better advantage (Fig. 2.19).

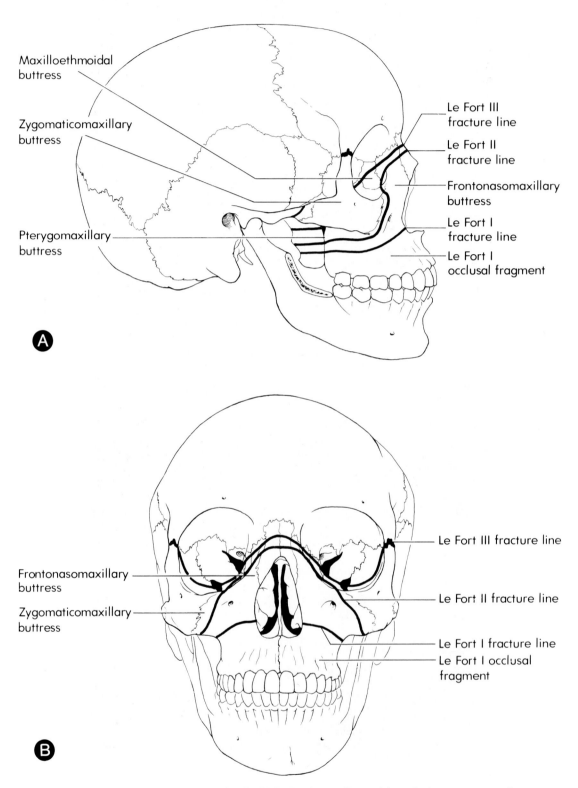

Figure 2.18. Anteroposterior and lateral depiction of skull with Le Fort fracture lines and the major buttresses annotated.

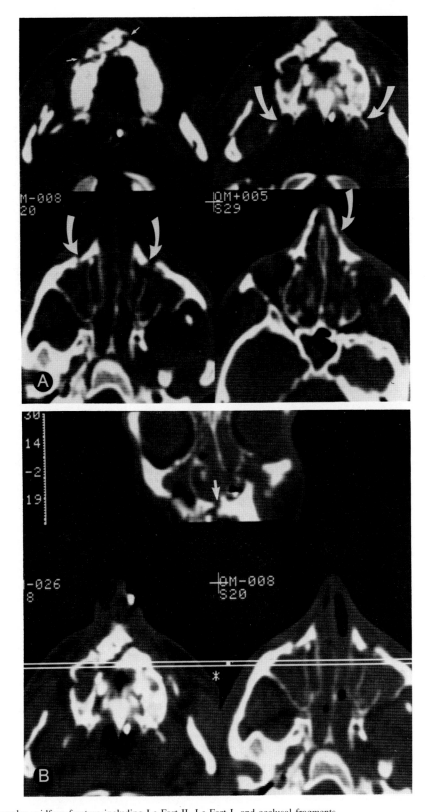

Figure 2.19. Complex midface fracture including Le Fort II, Le Fort I, and occlusal fragments.
A. Selected sequential axial CT scans depict the alveolar ridge fractures including a block containing the right incisors and canines (*arrows, upper left*); in addition, the cuts show fractures through the pterygoid plates, inferior orbital foramina, and nose (*curved arrows*). Incidentally noted is a right mandibular neck fracture (*upper row*).
B. Coronal reformation shows the vertical component of the alveolar fracture (*arrow*), multiple maxillary fractures, and a displaced left malar eminence, suggesting a superimposed tripod injury.

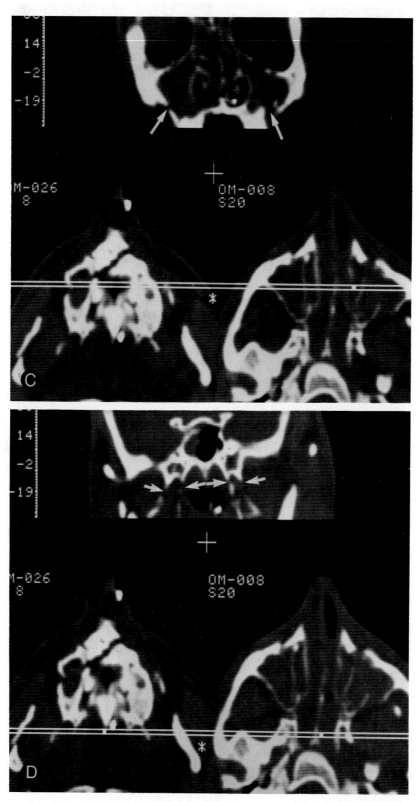

Figure 2.19.
C, D. Coronal reformations posteriorly show maxillary and pterygoid plate fractures (*arrows*).

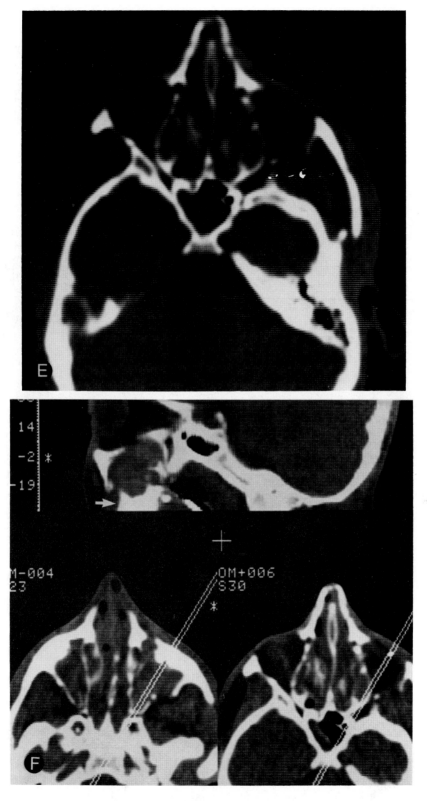

Figure 2.19.
E. Axial cut at the level of the left zygomatic arch showing its disruption. This verifies the tripod injury superimposed on the complex Le Fort fracture.
F. Reformation in the plane of the inferior rectus muscle shows posterior displacement of the left alveolar ridge (*arrow*) due to the Le Fort I injury.

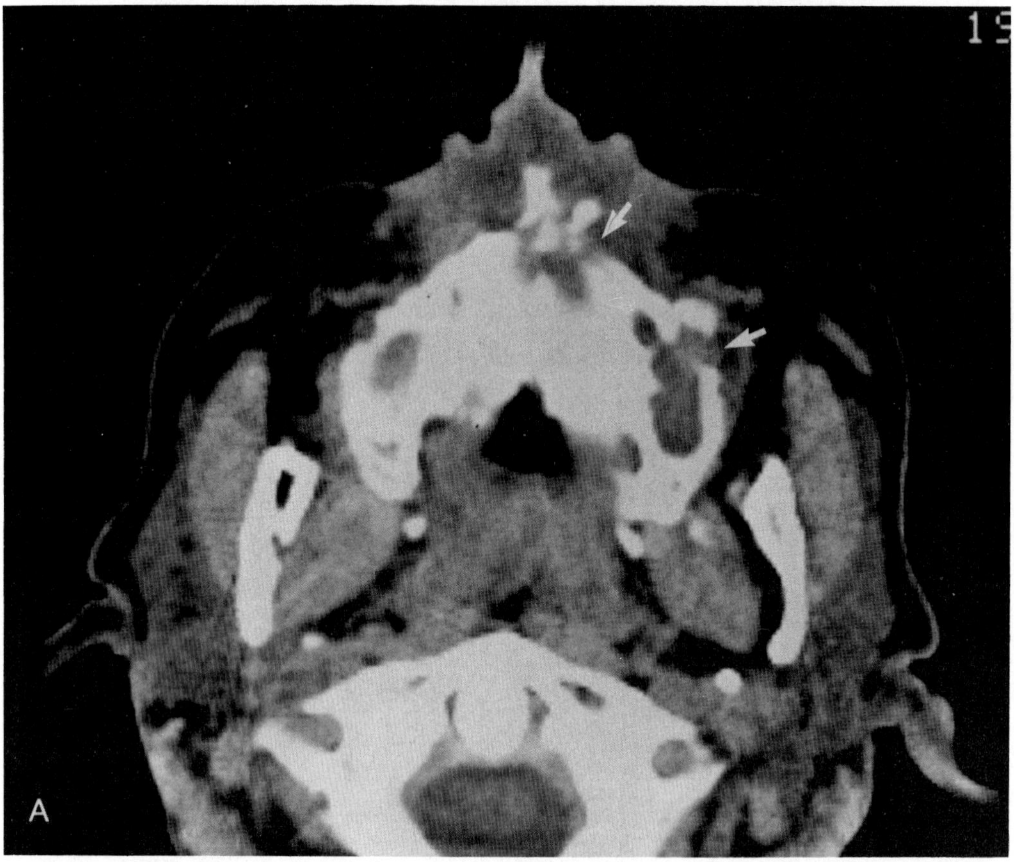

Figure 2.20.   Le Fort I fracture.
A. Axial section at the level of the hard palate shows a fracture through the nasal process of the maxilla in the midline, extending laterally to involve the left maxillary antrum floor (*arrows*).
B. Higher section depicts multiple maxillary fractures bilaterally, with fracture of the left lateral pterygoid plate (*p*).
C. Section at the level of the inferior orbital rim shows no evidence of disruption of these structures, although both pterygoid plates are involved. No other fractures superior to this level were identified. Note the blood density in both maxillary antra, right greater than left.

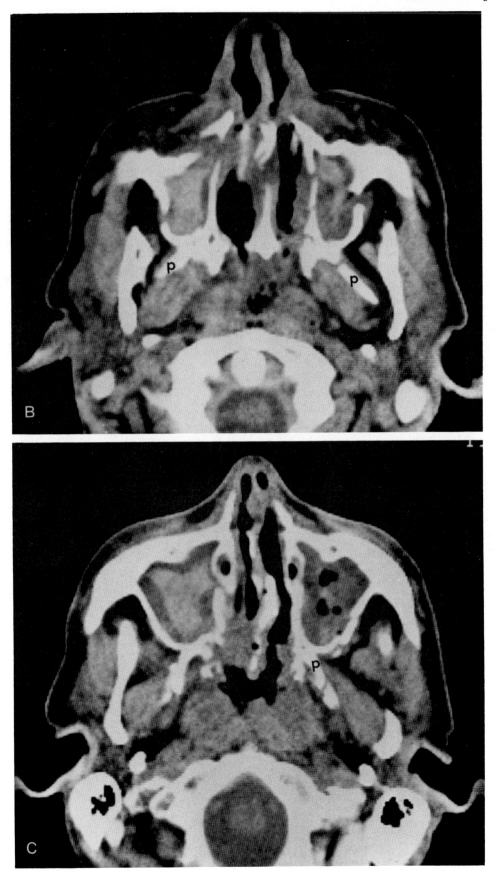

Figure 2.20. B, C.

Le Fort II Fracture

Le Fort described this second great line of weakness as descending from the lower portion of the nasal bones in the midline, across both frontal processes of the maxilla in a horizontal plane to include the lacrimal bones. The fracture line then descends to involve the inferior orbital margin at the zygomaticomaxillary suture, in the vicinity of the infraorbital foramen. It then drops to the anterolateral wall of the antrum curving posterolaterally beneath the zygomatic buttress. Posteriorly, it proceeds above the plane of the lower line of weakness (Le Fort I), crossing the pterygomaxillary fossa at a higher level. This fracture is often referred to as a pyramidal fracture, since the bilateral disrupted midfacial segment is grossly shaped like a pyramid. Backward displacement of the pyramid is common in these fractures, causing midfacial implosion and associated naso-orbital fractures as well. Computed tomography can show multiple sites of skeletal disruption both in the axial and reformatted para-axial planes (Fig. 2.19). Associated orbital floor and frontoethmoidal injury, and even brain damage, is easily and rapidly depicted

(Fig. 2.3). The ultimate category of fracture may depend on subtle nondisplaced disruptions. Since appropriate therapy is important, high-resolution reconstruction algorithms should be used in equivocal cases (Fig. 2.21).

Le Fort III Fracture

In the Le Fort III fracture, there is a complete separation of the middle portion of the face from the cranium. The fracture line originates at the frontonasal suture and extends backward through the frontal processes of the maxilla, lacrimal bone, and lamina papyracea of the ethmoids. At this point, in the posterior depths of the inferior orbital fissure, the fracture line forks into two major branches. One branch of the fracture crosses laterally to involve the lateral orbital wall adjacent to the sphenozygomatic junction and separates the zygoma from the frontal bone. The inferior branch of the fracture descends from the inferior orbital fissure (which is also the superolateral edge of the maxillary sinus) across the back wall of the maxilla near the pterygomaxillary fossa and fractures the pterygoid laminae near the

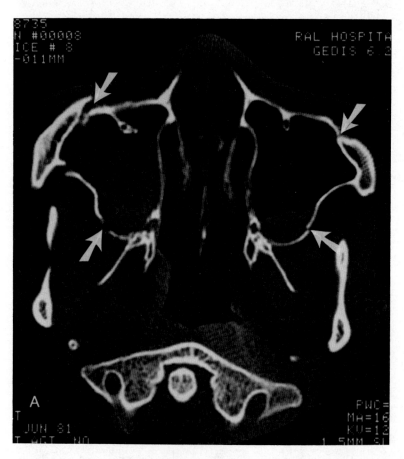

Figure 2.21. Le Fort II fracture—ReView reconstruction study. Conventional reconstruction algorithm showed an apparent right tripod fracture with left maxillary antrum posterior wall fracture only.

A, B. Lower sections show fractures through both inferior orbital rims, maxillary walls, and both pterygoid plates (*arrows*).

C. Slightly higher cut shows similar findings, with additional fracture of the vomer in its anterior portion (*arrow*).

D, E. Higher cuts reveal fracture of the lacrimal bone (**D**, *open arrow*) and the nasoethmoidal disruption characteristic of a Le Fort II injury. Incidentally, note the slight disturbance of the right frontozygomatic suture (**D**) and zygomatic arch (**C**) thought to represent a healed tripod fracture (history verified this impression).

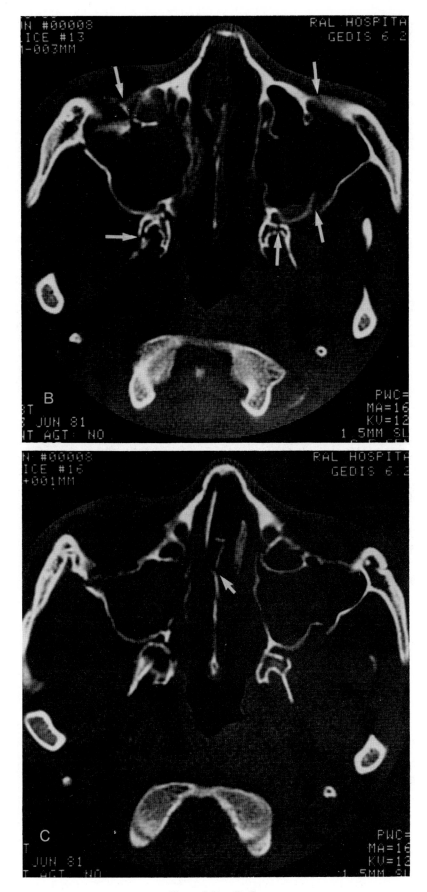

Figure 2.21. B, C.

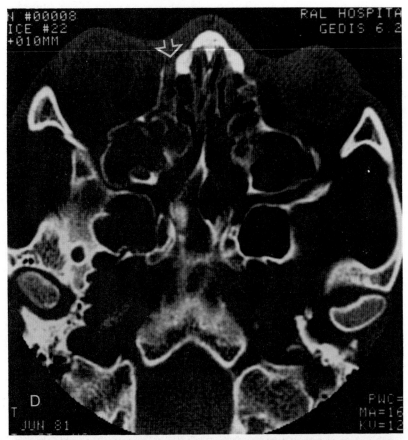

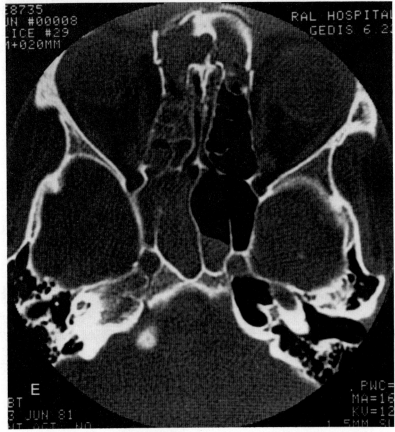

Figure 2.21.   D, E.

base of the sphenoid. Separation of the face from the cranial vault is completed by bilateral fractures of the zygomatic arches and fracture of the perpendicular plate of the ethmoid below the cribriform plate. This last type of fracture generally results from the more forceful traumatic injuries of the maxillofacial region and is often associated with involvement of the cribriform plate and the frontal sinuses, as well as the brain parenchyma itself (Fig. 2.22).

In our experience, isolated pure Le Fort I or Le Fort III fractures are distinctly unusual. Even the Le Fort II fracture was seen as a pure injury in only one-fifth of the patients we studied over a 3½-year period (6). In our series, Le Fort II and III fractures were commonly associated with additional tripod, frontal sinus, and/or nasoethmoidal disruption (Figs. 2.3, 2.19, 2.21, and 2.22). Complete Le Fort II fractures represented by far the largest group of injuries encountered. This finding is echoed by numerous other investigators (9, 10). Overall, tripod fractures were the most common addi-tional fractures in midfacial injuries, presumably be-cause both the Le Fort II and III fracture lines contain components of the tripod fracture (6, 10–13).

In our study, additional fragmentation of the max-illa into complete or unilateral Le Fort I fracture lines was seen in more than one-third of the patients with a complete Le Fort II fracture. This interrelationship of the Le Fort I and II fracture lines may be understood by remembering that they circumscribe the frontal processes of the maxilla (II). Le Fort showed that anterolateral blows directed against the malar bone frequently resulted in three fragments including not only the frontal process of the maxilla and alveolar arch, but also the malar eminence disruption in the tripod pattern.

Because the maxillary and ethmoid sinuses weaken the supporting buttresses of the maxilla to the skull, concomitant fractures of the nasoethmoidal and max-illoethmoidal buttresses should be anticipated (Fig. 2.3).

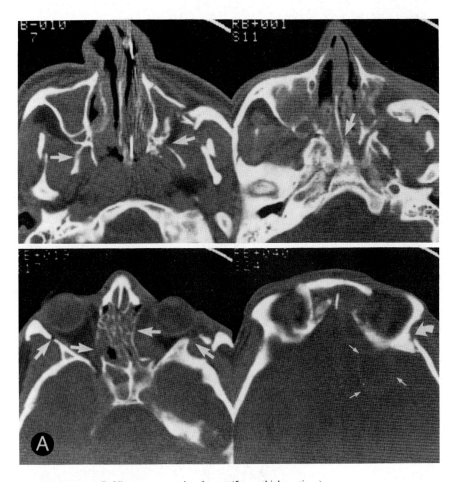

Figure 2.22. Le Fort III fracture—ReView reconstruction format (5 mm thick sections).
A. Selected sequential CT sections obtained 2 weeks after facial trauma show disruption of the pterygoid plates, both frontozygomatic sutures, vomer, and the medial orbital walls (*bold arrows*), indicating a Le Fort III fracture. Note associated fractures of both mandibles (*upper left*), frontal sinus (*lower right*), and sphenoid wing (*curved arrow*). Also seen is a posteriorly displaced left tripod fracture.

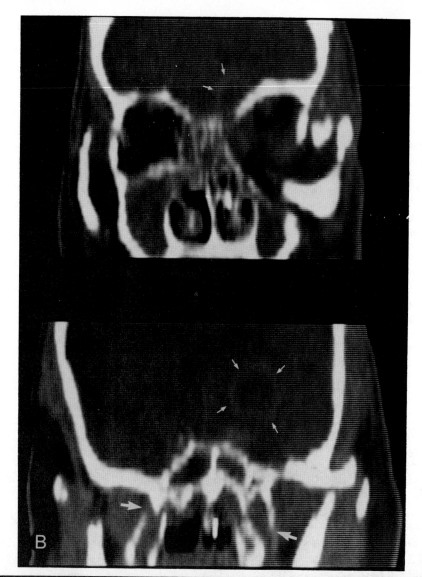

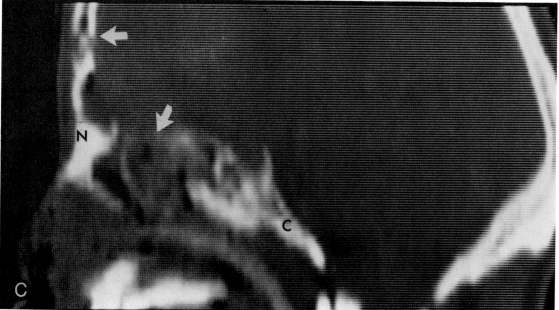

Figure 2.22.

B. Coronal reformations show the tripod fracture and pterygoid disruption (*bold arrows*) to better advantage. A left frontal lobe resolving hematoma (*small arrows,* **A** and **B**) was better seen on brain windows.

C. Sagittal reformation depicts the comminution of the frontal and ethmoid sinuses (*arrows*) (*N*, nasion; *C*, clivus).

FRONTOETHMOIDAL FRACTURES

Fractures in this region are again usually the result of blunt trauma and are more apt to occur in patients with exuberant aeration of the sinuses within the bones in the superomedial aspect of the orbit. Major disruptions here can cause communication with the intracranial space via either the cribriform plate or the posterior frontal sinus wall. Encephaloceles can sometimes result (Fig. 2.23). Also, fragmentation may be sufficient to impinge upon the superior rectus muscle or even the globe itself. Computed tomography delineates these complications beautifully (Fig. 2.24). If the orbital roof is sufficiently comminuted, an intracranial hematoma may result in either the intra-axial or extra-axial space.

Posterior wall frontal fractures of the frontal sinus are important to diagnose accurately (Figs. 2.3 and 2.25), since an intracranial surgical approach is necessary to treat these injuries. Otherwise, cerebrospinal fluid (CSF) leakage with meningitis and/or epidural abscess formation can result. CSF leak can be demonstrated if metrizamide, introduced into the subarachnoid space, is detected in the paranasal sinuses (Fig. 2.26). Only 5 ml of iso-osmolar metrizamide introduced into the lumbar space are needed to demonstrate such a leak, with the patient positioned head down for 2 minutes prior to obtaining coronal CT sections, with the patient in the prone position.

GUNSHOT INJURY OF THE MAXILLOFACIAL REGION

The proliferation of handguns in recent years has resulted in a significant increase in gunshot injury to the maxillofacial region. Such injuries can be quickly and completely evaluated with computed tomography. Relationship of bony fragmentation of metallic fragments to the globe and optic nerve can be quickly assessed. Associated intracranial penetration and injury are likewise easily evaluated (Fig. 2.27). One disadvantage of computed tomography is the streak artifact produced by metallic fragments. The information lost in such cases is generally insignificant when compared to the amount obtained in a very short period of time in patients who usually are in critical need of emergency assistance.

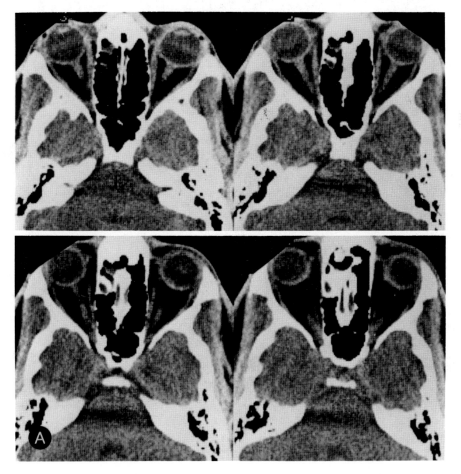

Figure 2.23. Encephalocele with CSF leak. Meningitis 6 months after facial trauma led to this study. **A.** Selected contiguous axial sections show minimal opacification of right ethmoid air cells.

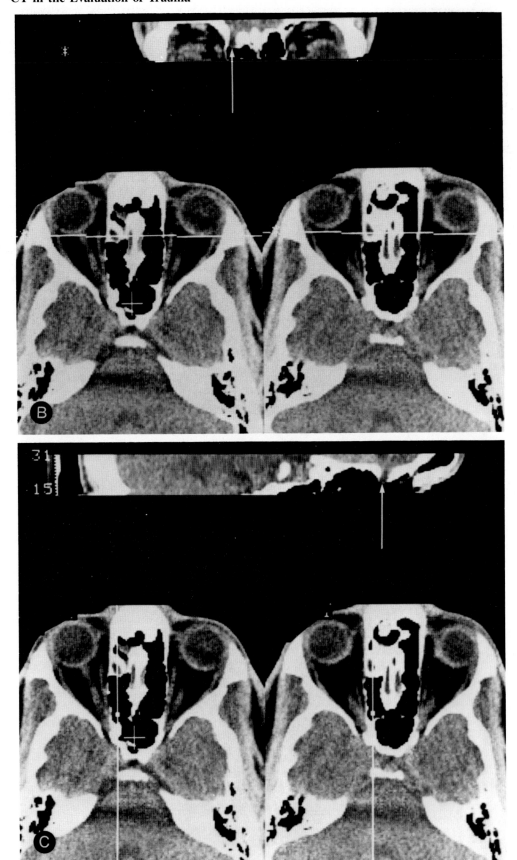

Figure 2.23.
B, C. Coronal and sagittal reconstructions through the involved ethmoid sinuses depict a dehiscence in the fovea ethmoidalis, with intracranial soft tissue protruding down through the defect (*arrows*). Surgery verified a 5 mm encephalocele.

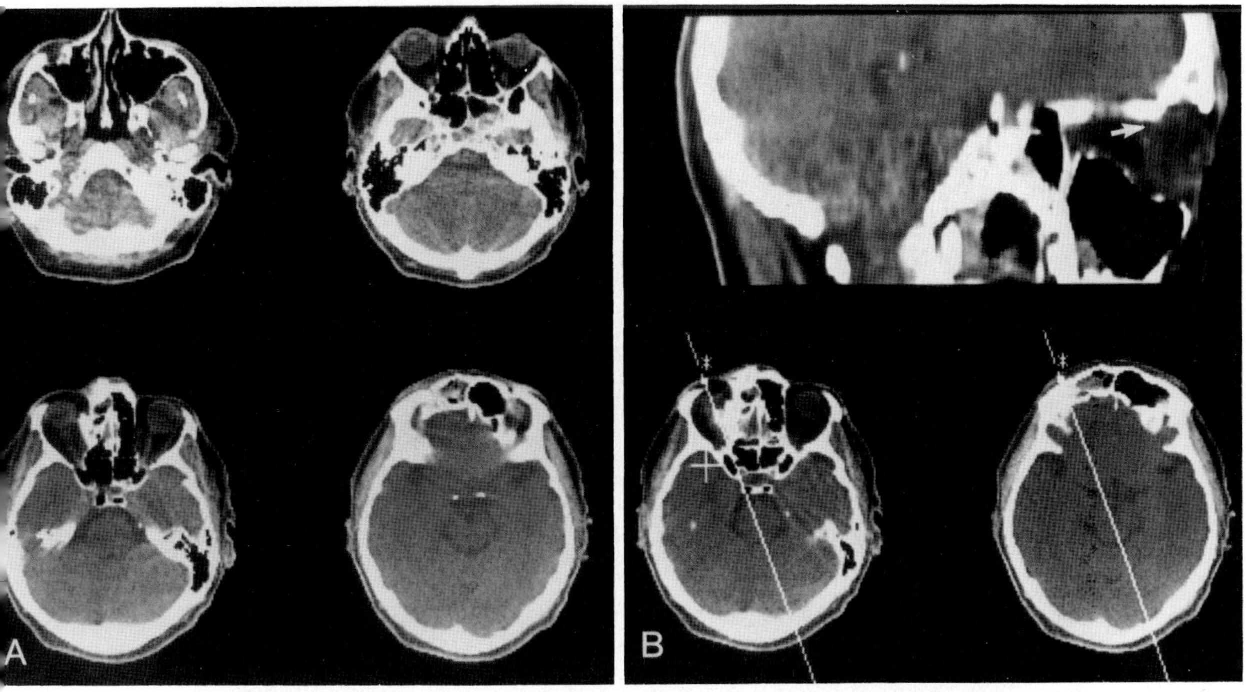

Figure 2.24.   Frontoethmoidal injury.
A. Selected axial sections show no abnormality below the orbits but do reveal lateral rotation of the lamina papyracea on the right, with suggestion of impingement on the right globe. The frontal sinus is also opacified (higher cuts showed the posterior wall fracture).
B. Reformation in the plane defined by the inferior rectus muscle verifies bony fragment impinging on the posterior-superior aspect of the globe (*arrow*). The patient's limitation of eye motion was initially attributed to an orbital blowout; the CT study defined the true nature of the injury.

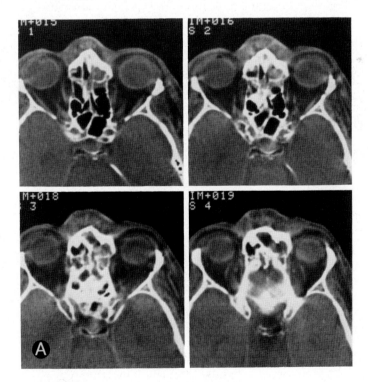

Figure 2.25.   Frontoethmoidal sinus injury.
A, B. Successive axial sections demonstrate the disrupted ethmoid and frontal sinuses.
C. Sagittal reformation through the frontal sinus fracture verifies the posterior wall disruption (**C**, *open arrow*). Note the artifact produced by patient motion between scans. This is easily seen to be artifactual since the back of the skull is artificially displaced as well as the frontal bone region (**C**, *arrows*).

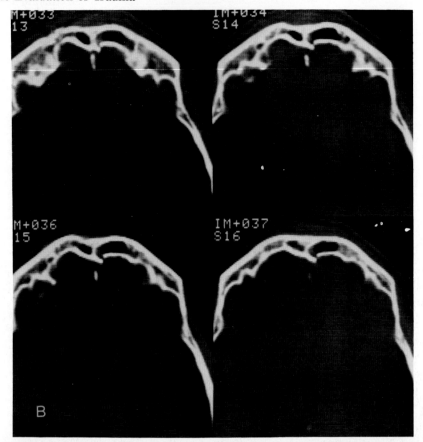

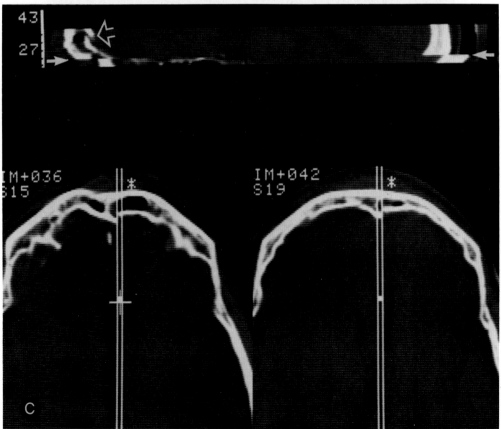

Figure 2.25.   B, C.

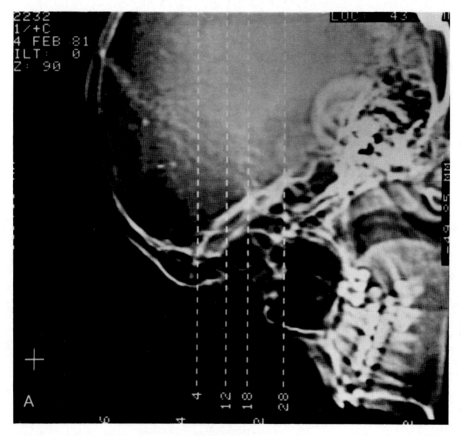

Figure 2.26.   CSF leak—demonstration with intrathecal metrizamide.
A. Preliminary digital radiograph with annotation of the sections scanned. Patient prone, chin down on scanning couch. No gantry angulation.

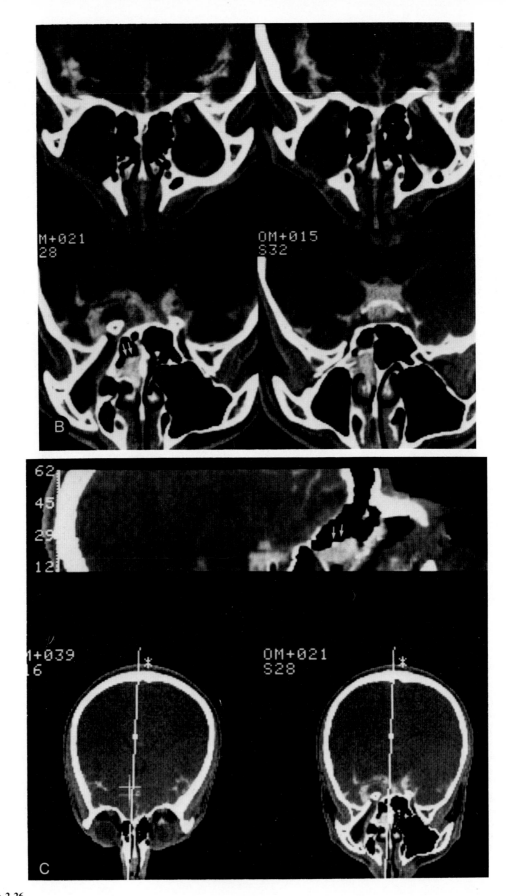

Figure 2.26.
B. Resulting sections show intracranial metrizamide, with leakage into the posterior ethmoid region seen on the more anteroinferior sections (*lower row, arrows*).
C. Sagittal reformation shows pool of metrizamide in the posterior ethmoid sinus region (*arrows*). Surgery corrected the planum sphenoidale defect.

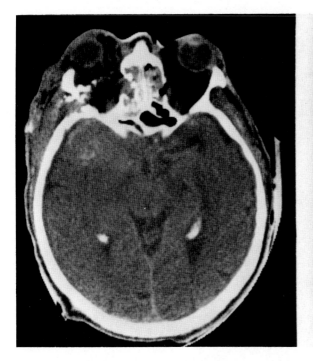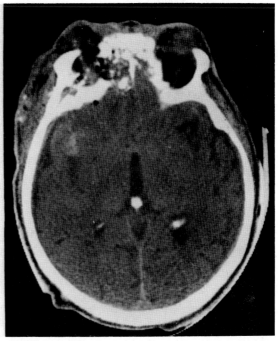

Figure 2.27. Self-inflicted gunshot wound. Bullet and bone fragments are seen extending from the right temporal region into the orbit, ethmoids, and anterior cranial fossa. The patient survived, with blindness. Brain windows verified intracranial hematoma on the affected side.

SUMMARY

Computed tomography has the ability to evaluate maxillofacial trauma quickly. The well-known contrast resolution capabilities of CT play a role in the usefulness of this modality. However, it is the image manipulation capability which is of singular advantage in these cases. The spatial resolution of computed tomography has matched that of conventional pluridirectional tomography in current generation equipment. Since a set of axial CT sections can be obtained with automatic table incrementation within 12 minutes, the information content per time of study ratio is improved over that of conventional tomography, despite the fact that image reformation requires extra time on the part of the radiologist. Radiation savings are significantly in favor of computed tomography as well. In our experience, computed tomography is the primary diagnostic imaging modality used in the evaluation of complex facial trauma, after routine screening films are obtained.

REFERENCES

1. Grove AE, et al: Orbital fracture evaluation by coronal computed tomography. *Am J Ophthalmol* 85:679, 1978.
2. Claussen C, Singer R: Progress in the diagnosis of craniofacial injuries and tumors by computer tomography. *J Maxillofac Surg* 7:210, 1979.
3. Rowe LD, Miller E, Brant-Zawadzki M: Computed tomography in maxillofacial trauma. *Laryngoscope* 91:745, 1981.
4. Quinn SF, Smathers RL: The diagnostic significance of posttraumatic sphenoid sinus effusions: Correlation with head computed tomography. *J Comput Assist Tomog* 8:61, 1984.
5. Johnson DH Jr, Colman M, Larsson S, Garner OP, Hanafee W: Computed tomography in maxillo-orbital fractures. *J Comput Assist Tomog* 8:416, 1984.
6. Rowe LD, Brant-Zawadzki M: Spatial analysis of midfacial fractures with multidirectional and computed tomography: Clinicopathological correlates in 44 cases. *Otolaryngol Head Neck Surg* 90:651, 1982.
7. Brant-Zawadzki M, Minagi H, Federle MP, Rowe LD: High resolution CT with image reformation in maxillofacial pathology. *AJNR* 3:31, 1982.
8. Littleton JT, Shaffer KA, Callahan WP, Durizch ML: Temporal bone: Comparison of pluridirectional tomography and high resolution computed tomography. *AJR* 137:835, 1981.
9. Le Fort R: Etude experimentale sur les fractures de la machoire superieure. *Rev Chir Paris* 23:208, 360, 479, 1901.
10. Gwyn PP, Carraway JH, Horton CE, et al: Facial fractures—associated injuries and complications. *Plast Reconstr Surg* 47:225, 1977.
11. Morgan BDG, Madan DK, Bergerot JPC: Fractures of the middle third of the face—a review of 300 cases. *Br J Plast Surg* 25:247, 1972.
12. Landin K, Ridell A, Sandberg N, et al: One thousand maxillofacial and related fractures at the ENT Clinic in Gothenburg. *Acta Otolaryngol* 75:359, 1973.
13. Tessier P: Commentary on Le Fort's papers. *Plast Reconstr Surg* 50:605, 1972.

Chapter 3

CT of Laryngeal Trauma

R. BROOKE JEFFREY, M.D.

INTRODUCTION

Computed tomography has made a significant contribution to the radiologic assessment of the injured larynx (1, 2). CT is an accurate, noninvasive modality that can rapidly diagnose both soft tissue and cartilaginous injuries. CT of the larynx involves a minimal degree of patient manipulation and discomfort and can be performed in conjunction with CT evaluation of intracranial or facial injuries.

CT and laryngoscopy are complementary procedures for evaluating laryngeal injuries (3). Direct laryngoscopy affords optimal visualization of the mucosal surface and can readily detect functional impairment of the vocal cords (4, 5). However, cartilaginous and deep soft tissue injuries cannot be diagnosed. At times, marked supraglottic soft tissue swelling may preclude adequate examination by direct laryngoscopy. CT may be utilized as the initial noninvasive screening procedure to direct the laryngoscopist. The transverse plane of CT is ideal for assessing the true extent of airway encroachment by edema or hematoma and may aid in the therapeutic decision to perform intubation or tracheostomy.

Conventional radiologic studies (anteroposterior and lateral soft tissue films of the neck, tomograms, or xerograms) are capable of demonstrating some cartilaginous fractures but are of limited value in defining the extent of soft tissue injury (6). In the acute trauma setting, laryngography is often technically difficult to perform because of patient discomfort and inability to cooperate. Although the overall experience is somewhat limited, CT appears to overcome many of the limitations of these conventional radiologic methods. The following is a discussion of the role of CT scanning in evaluating injuries to the larynx and cervical soft tissues.

CT ANATOMY

Anatomically, the larynx may be subdivided into supraglottic, glottic, and subglottic regions (Figs. 3.1–3.7). The paired thyroid cartilages provide the major structural support to the supraglottic portion of the larynx including the pyriform sinuses and

laryngeal vestibule. In addition, they provide important anatomic landmarks for localizing the level of various laryngeal structures. The superior cornua of the thyroid cartilage attaches to the hyoid bone via the lateral thyrohyoid ligament. Sections at the level of the superior cornua demonstrate the laryngeal vestibule, valleculae, pre-epiglottic space, and pyriform sinuses. The inferior cornua are seen at the subglottic level and articulate with the cricoid cartilage to form the cricothyroid joint. There is considerable variation in the degree of mineralization of the thyroid cartilage. This variability must be taken into account before diagnosing either cartilaginous fractures or destructive changes. In addition, a well-developed anterior thyroid notch in the midline may mimic a pathologic process since axial sections at this level will show discontinuity of the thyroid cartilage (Fig. 3.4).

In the supraglottic larynx the laryngeal vestibule is formed by the epiglottis anteriorly and the aryepiglottic folds laterally. The aryepiglottic folds separate the laryngeal vestibule from the pyriform sinuses. Anterior to the epiglottis are the paired valleculae. Below the level of the valleculae the fat density pre-epiglottic space is identified anterior to the epiglottis (Fig. 3.4). Normally, there is no soft tissue density in the pre-epiglottic space, and hematomas involving this area are well evaluated by CT.

On scans obtained at the glottic level both the true and false vocal cords can be identified by CT. The true cords are located just inferior to the false cords and may be identified by their attachment to the vocal process of the arytenoids (Fig. 3.5). The triangular-shaped arytenoid cartilages articulate with the superior aspect of the cricoid cartilage to form the cricoarytenoid joints. Dislocation of either the cricoarytenoid or cricothyroid joint is a well-recognized sequela of blunt trauma to the glottic region and may result in significant vocal impairment (6, 7). Lateral to the arytenoid and cricoid cartilages is the paralaryngeal space. Superiorly, the paralaryngeal spaces are contiguous anteriorly with the pre-epiglottic space. This is an important area of deep soft tissue infiltration that can be diagnosed by CT.

The signet-shaped cricoid cartilage forms the major structural support of the subglottic region (Figs. 3.6

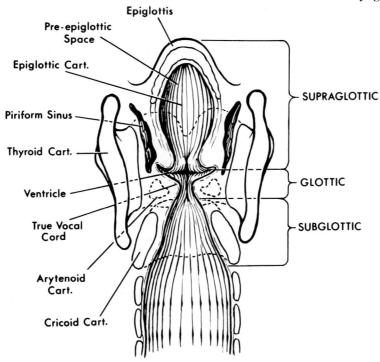

Figures 3.1 to 3.8.   Normal laryngeal anatomy.

Figure 3.1.   Coronal view of normal larynx depicting supraglottic, glottic, and subglottic areas.

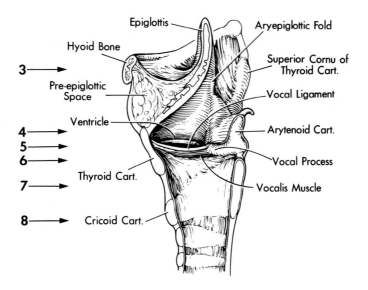

Figure 3.2.   Sagittal view of normal larynx. Numbers *3* through *8* indicate approximate level of plane of section for Figures 3.3 to 3.8.

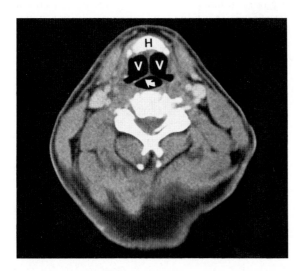

Figure 3.3.   Normal supraglottic larynx at level of hyoid (*H*) and valleculae (*V*). Note epiglottis designated by *curved arrow*.

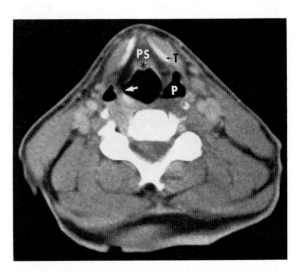

Figure 3.4.   Normal supraglottic larynx at level of pyriform sinuses (*P*). (*T*, thyroid cartilage.) *Asterisk* denotes epiglottis. *White arrow* indicates aryepiglottic fold. Note the normal fat in the pre-epiglottic space and normal thyroid notch anteriorly.

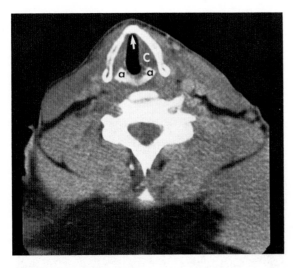

Figure 3.5.   Scan at level of true vocal cords (*C*), (*a*, arytenoid cartilage.) Note symmetry of cords and lack of tissue anteriorly at the anterior commissure (*arrow*).

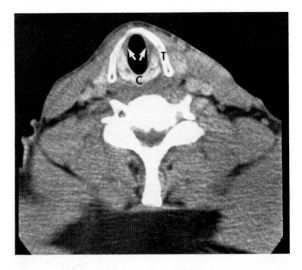

Figure 3.6.   Scan at level of undersurface of true cords (*arrows*). (*T*, thyroid cartilage; *C*, cricoid cartilage.)

and 3.8). Because of its ring-like configuration, it invariably breaks in two parts when fractured. Soft tissue injuries to the subglottic portion of the larynx are confined to the conus elasticus, which is located immediately below the mucosal surface and permits circumferential extension of edema and hemorrhage.

INDICATIONS AND TECHNIQUE FOR LARYNGEAL CT

Following the initial clinical and radiologic assessment, CT of the larynx may be performed as a separate examination or at the same time as CT evaluation of intracranial or facial injuries. While the patient is in the CT scanning area, there must be close clinical observation by the radiologist, technician, and clinical team to ensure both a patent airway and optimal management of other life support systems. As noted by Schaefer and Brown (8), the main indications for CT following blunt laryngeal trauma are to assess possible fractures or dislocations of the laryngeal cartilage and to determine the full extent of soft tissue hemorrhage and edema. In general CT is reserved for patients with significant trauma but not requiring immediate surgery for massive injuries.

Optimal CT technique is essential for accurate diagnosis. CT sections in patients with laryngeal trauma are generally obtained during quiet breathing at 5 mm intervals. If possible, slight neck extension will aid in visualizing supraglottic soft tissues by eliminating overlying bony structures such as the mandible. Scan localization is facilitated by initially obtaining an anteroposterior scout digital radiograph ("Scoutview"). Scans generally are performed from the subglottic region to the level of the hyoid bone. Rapid sequential scanning allows the study to be done in a minimal amount of time with excellent registration of the scans. Intravenous contrast is generally not administered for evaluation of the larynx per se. In penetrating injuries of the neck, it may be used to determine the patency of the great vessels and their relationship to bony injuries or foreign objects. Scan quality can be improved by removal of overlying ECG or intravenous lines and, if possible, performing the study without an endotracheal or nasogastric tube in place.

In general, axial scans are sufficient for adequate diagnosis of cartilaginous and soft tissue injuries. In selected cases, coronal or sagittal reformations may be of benefit in demonstrating the extent of soft tissue injury or airway encroachment.

PATHOLOGY

Because of the complexity of laryngeal injuries, it is useful to classify both the anatomic site and extent of laryngeal injuries. Mancuso and Hanafee (1) outlined the CT features of acute laryngotracheal injuries according to the classification by Ogura et al, (9). Injuries to the trachea and larynx may be subdivided into five main categories.

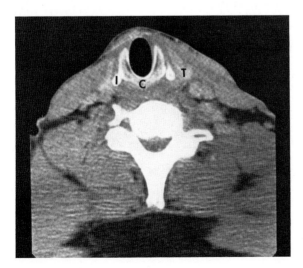

Figure 3.7. Scan at superior level of subglottic larynx. Note normal U-shaped cricoid cartilage (*C*). (*I*, inferior cornua of thyroid cartilage; *T*, superior pole of thyroid gland. Note lack of visible tissue at interface between airway and cricoid cartilage.

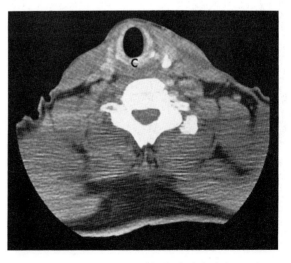

Figure 3.8. Scan at more caudal level of subglottic larynx demonstrating cricoid (*C*) as a complete cartilaginous ring.

1. *Soft tissue injuries:* These include lacerations, hematomas, and edema involving the mucosal surface (Figs. 3.8–3.10). Direct laryngoscopy is still essential to identify mucosal lacerations. However, identification of deep soft tissue extension of hematoma and edema from laryngeal injuries is an important contribution of CT. Subglottic extension is limited by the conus elasticus and tends to spread circumferentially. Above the glottis, extension tends to occur in a cephalocaudal direction lateral to the vocal cords and aryepiglottic folds. The lateral paralaryngeal space is continuous anteriorly with the pre-epiglottic space, providing a free means of communication anteriorly across the midline (1). Spreading hematomas and edema in these deep spaces may narrow the airway.

Soft tissue trauma alone may cause vocal cord dysfunction due to a variety of mechanisms. These include laceration of the cord itself, injury to the recurrent laryngeal nerve, fixation by hematoma, or disruption of the cricoarytenoid or cricothyroid joints.

2. *Supraglottic injuries:* Supraglottic injury to the laryngeal skeleton includes cartilaginous fractures of the thyroid cartilage and soft tissue injuries with either laceration or avulsion of the epiglottis. CT can accurately detect the presence of fractures of the thyroid cartilage (Figs. 3.11 and 3.12) and demonstrate extension of hematoma and edema into the pre-epiglottic space or along the aryepiglottic folds. Both transverse and vertical fractures of the thyroid cartilage may occur. These are generally surgically repaired by direct suture approximation. However, in cases of severely comminuted fractures, an endolaryngeal stent may be used for support prior to definitive repair of the cartilaginous fragments.

3. *Glottic injuries:* These include mucosal lacerations or hematomas of the true and false çords (Fig. 3.13) as well as dislocation of the arytenoid cartilages. Glottic injuries are frequently associated with thyroid cartilage fractures. Dislocation of the cricoarytenoid joint generally causes anterior displacement of the arytenoid with apparent foreshortening and widening of the cord simulating a paralyzed vocal cord. Posterior arytenoid dislocations may also be diagnosed. With glottic injuries there is frequent extention of hematomas and swelling into the paralaryngeal space.

4. *Subglottic injuries:* Subglottic trauma usually results from fractures of the cricoid cartilage when compressed against the cervical spine. As noted previously, the cricoid cartilage is a ring-like structure which fractures in two places (Fig. 3.13**B**). In addition, dislocation of the cricothyroid joint may occur. Because of the close proximity of the recurrent laryngeal nerve to the cricothyroid joint, dislocation may cause paralysis of the vocal cord. Soft tissue trauma to the subglottic region may significantly encroach upon the airway as the hematoma extends circumferentially within the conus elasticus. The axial plane of CT optimally demonstrates the extent of airway obstruction.

5. *Tracheal injuries:* These include partial or complete disruption of the tracheal rings or bronchi.

In summary, CT is an extremely useful method to evaluate the injured larynx. It is complementary to laryngoscopy and provides unique diagnostic information unavailable by any other single modality.

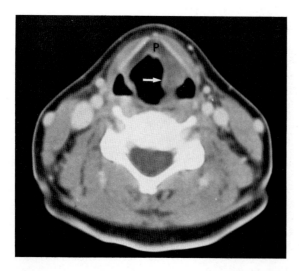

Figure 3.9. Supraglottic soft tissue injury. Hematoma and/or edema involves left aryepiglottic fold (*arrow*) extending into left pre-epiglottic space (*P*). This resolved spontaneously.

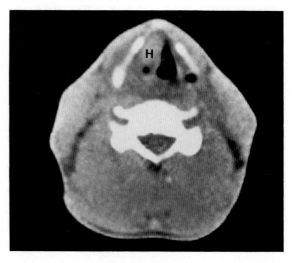

Figure 3.10. Supraglottic soft tissue injury with right side hematoma (*H*) at level of right pyriform sinus and pre-epiglottic space.

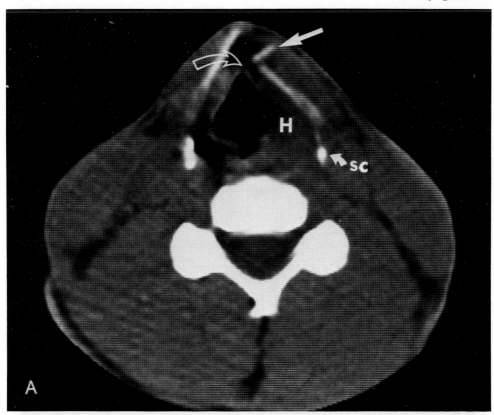

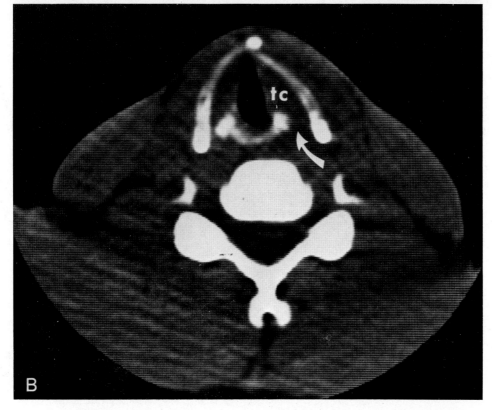

Figure 3.11.
A.   Strangulation injury to larynx. Comminuted fracture of left thyroid cartilage (*white arrow*). Hematoma (*H*) involves left paralaryngeal space and the pre-epiglottic space (*open arrow*), (*sc*, superior cornua.)
B.   Subtle thickening of left true cord (*tc*) and left paralaryngeal space (*arrow*). Separation of the left cricothyroid joint was noted on the subadjacent section.

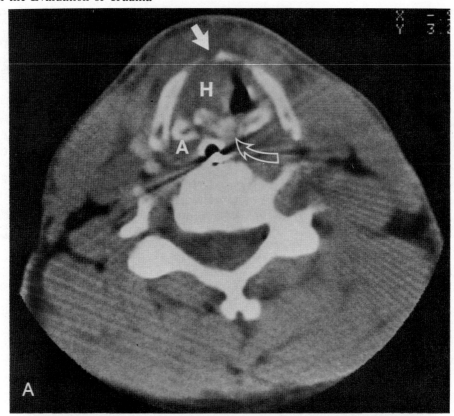

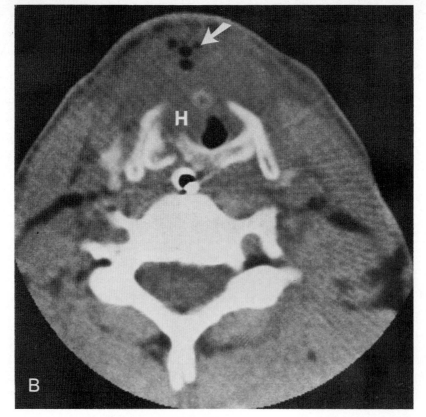

Figure 3.12.
A. Steering wheel injury to larynx. Fracture of thyroid cartilage anteriorly (*white arrow*) and cricoid cartilage posteriorly (*open arrow*). Hematoma (*H*) of right true cord. Posterior dislocation of right arytenoid (*A*).
B. Subcutaneous emphysema anteriorly (*arrow*). The cricoid cartilage is sprung apart due to the fracture. Hemorrhage (*H*) within the conus elasticus causes encroachment on the subglottic airway.

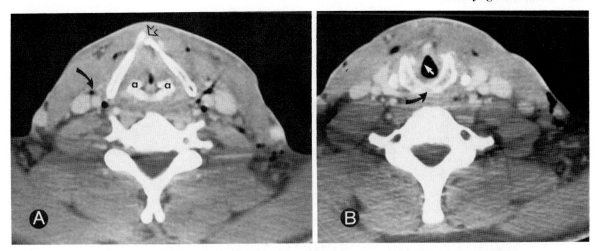

Figure 3.13.
A. Thyroid and cricoid cartilage fractures associated with extensive soft tissue injury. **A** demonstrates circumferential narrowing of the airway at level of true vocal cords from glottic hematoma. (*a*, arytenoids.) *Open arrow* shows fracture of thyroid fracture anteriorly. *Black arrow* demonstrates subcutaneous emphysema.
B. Scan at subglottic level in same patient as **A.** Note subglottic extension of edema and hemorrhage within the conus elasticus (*white arrow*). Fracture of posterior cricoid ring (*black arrow*) with splaying of ring anteriorly.

REFERENCES

1. Mancuso AA, Hanafee WH: Computed tomography of the injured larynx, *Radiology* 133:139, 1979.
2. Mancuso AA, Calcaterra TC, Hanafee WN: Computed tomography of the larynx. *Radiol Clin North Am* 16:195, 1978.
3. Mancuso AA, Hanafee WN: A comparative evaluation of computed tomography and laryngography. *Radiology* 133:131, 1979.
4. Harris HH, Lobin HA: Acute injuries of the larynx and trachea in 49 patients. *Laryngoscope* 80:1376, 1970.
5. Cohn AM, Larson DL: Laryngeal injury: A critical review, *Arch Otolaryngol* 102:166, 1976.
6. Greene R, Stark P: Trauma of the larynx and trachea. *Radiol Clin North Am* 16:309, 1978.
7. Dudley JP, Mancuso AA, Tonkalsrud EW: Arytenoid dislocation and computed tomography, *Arch Otolaryngol* 110:483, 1984.
8. Schaefer SD, Brown OE: Selective application of CT in the management of laryngeal trauma. *Laryngoscope* 93:1473, 1983.
9. Ogura JH, Heeneman H, Spector GJ: Laryngo-tracheal trauma: Diagnosis and treatment. *Can J Otolaryngol* 2:112, 1973.

Chapter 4

CT in the Evaluation of Spine Trauma

ROBERT DeLaPAZ, M.D.
MICHAEL BRANT-ZAWADZKI, M.D.
HIDEYO MINAGI, M.D.

INTRODUCTION

The introduction and rapid development of body computed tomography gave birth to a new perspective on imaging of the spinal canal and its derangements, including those caused by trauma (1, 2). Failure to recognize significant injury to the spine can result in disastrous and irreversible neurologic sequelae. CT has become a welcome addition to the diagnostic armamentarium used in evaluating patients with spinal injury, since the accurate diagnosis of spinal trauma is one of the most difficult challenges the radiologist must face. Plain film evaluation of the injured spine is often difficult for a variety of reasons. First, the radiographic anatomy of the spine is relatively complicated. The radiographic appearance of the vertebral bodies and their appendages changes from level to level, as does the interrelationship of their articulations. Knowledge of this anatomy must be combined with an understanding of the dynamic pathology produced by various vectors of force affecting the spine in a given situation. Second, the spine trauma patient is often in severe pain, may be agitated, and may, therefore, be uncooperative. Third, proper positioning for the radiographs is compromised by the reluctance to move a patient with possibly unstable injuries. All of these factors combine to make the radiologic diagnosis of the patient with an acute spinal injury a sometimes difficult and often time-consuming experience.

The rapidly rising rate of vehicular accidents in this country has helped to increase the incidence of spinal injury in our population. Not only is there a high incidence of spinal fracture, but approximately 10,000 new spinal cord injuries occur in the United States each year (3). Unfortunately, the majority of such injuries involve people under the age of 40. Such statistics emphasize the need for accurate early diagnosis and appropriate therapy of the spine injury pa-

tient. The capability and efficiency of computed tomography in the evaluation of spine trauma render it the prime diagnostic modality in guiding the management of these patients.

INDICATIONS

The place of computed tomography in the diagnostic sequence employed in the evaluation of spine trauma patients is dictated by the clinical assessment and plain radiographs initially obtained in the emergency room. An initial set of anteroposterior and lateral plain films of the region involved continues to be the mainstay of radiographic screening in spinal injury. The alignment of the spinal column and gross bony integrity of its components can be quickly evaluated, and any major disruption can often be depicted. In the absence of bony injury, disruption of the ligamentous structures, which supply significant stability, can be subsequently assessed with flexion-extension views or cinefluorography if the clinical setting allows.

Nevertheless, conventional radiographs underestimate the degree of injury in a significant number of patients with spine trauma. The introduction of thin-section tomography utilizing complex tube motions for high spatial resolution led to a more complete diagnosis and actually was shown to have a direct influence on management in up to 35% of cases (4, 5).

Recently, the continued refinements in the technology of computed tomography—including digital radiographic localization, high spatial resolution, multiplanar image reformation, and rapid-sequence scanning—have increased the value and applicability of this technique to the point that the advantages of this modality have allowed it to supplant conventional tomography in the evaluation of spine trauma (6–8). The geometry of CT scanning permits visualization of the bony spinal canal in the axial plane. Very thin beam collimation not only allows high spatial resolution, but permits reformation of the axial images into a multiplanar format not previously possible. Therefore, multiple imaging planes can be selected without additional patient manipulation or radiation exposure. An accurate, rapid, and safe evaluation of the spinal canal, as well as the spine's complex bony architecture, may thus be achieved. Neural structures within the canal may be further assessed by introduction of water-soluble contrast material into the subarachnoid space. Finally, most CT spine studies can be performed with far less radiation as compared to conventional multidirectional tomographic studies, an important factor particularly if repeated examinations are necessary in young patients (9, 10).

Because of these advantages, we recommend CT when plain films are equivocal or when further evaluation of a known, complex fracture is desirable. If neurologic signs or symptoms accompany the bony disruption, we introduce metrizamide into the subarachnoid space in order to visualize directly any compromise of the cord or nerve roots which might be potentially reversible. If no fracture is found, but instability due to a ligamentous disruption is suspected, a dynamic study such as cinefluorography is carefully performed with the surgeon in attendance.

Postoperative CT scans may also be useful. Evaluating the realignment obtained following surgical stabilization is relatively easy on sagittal reformations, as is detection of residual bone fragments or foreign bodies. Follow-up studies may also be useful in detecting bone fusion in treated patients and in searching for causes of persistent radiculopathy, such as traumatic disc herniation and unsuspected fragments. In patients with previous spinal cord injury, CT may aid the detection of post-traumatic syrinx as a cause of progression in symptomatology. However, magnetic resonance imaging is more sensitive than CT for detection of syrinx and, if available, should be the procedure of choice for initial evaluation of progressive post-traumatic neurologic deficit (11).

Not surprisingly, computed tomography does have certain limitations. Patient motion during the study will degrade image quality, as with conventional radiography, and is especially damaging when image reformation is important in the diagnosis. The volume averaging inherent in a voxel matrix imaging technique is troublesome in the spatial resolution of ultrathin, nondisplaced fractures within thick bone. This is especially true when the fracture lies in the plane of the CT section. Subtle, horizontal fractures (such as at the base of the dens) may be difficult to detect if no displacement is present. Newer reconstruction algorithms, using decreased voxel size in a target area, combined with expansion of the CT number range have offset this difficulty in current generation equipment (Fig. 4.1).

Other limitations include the relatively limited area amenable to study with computed tomography, especially when thin-section technique is employed. Study of more than four vertebral levels is generally impractical but fortunately is rarely needed. Finally, the cost of computed tomography is higher than that of conventional techniques in absolute terms. Nevertheless, when the quality of information produced, the technician and physician time savings, and the ability to study other organs at the same sitting are considered, the cost differential would seem less significant.

TECHNIQUE

Sufficient personnel are required to transfer the spine injury patient carefully onto the scanner couch. Special devices for maintaining traction can be attached to the scanner, or a simple pulley arrangement attached to an IV pole can be utilized (12). The importance of maintaining traction during the scan is illustrated in Figure 4.2; the effectiveness of mechanical traction in achieving and maintaining decompression can thus be illustrated. A localizing digital radiography is then obtained and slice sequence annotated. Since patient comfort and immobilization are important, even in rapid-sequence scanning, sedation and general anesthesia should be used if necessary. Adequate immobilization ensures high-quality images and allows high-detail multiplanar image reformation.

Because of the volume averaging problem mentioned above, slice thickness should not exceed 5 mm. Overlapping 5 mm thick cuts, obtained by moving the table only 3 mm at a time, allow high resolution of reformatted images. Newer scanners allow acquisition of contiguous 3-mm sections. Such technique is sufficient in the relatively large vertebral bodies below the C2 level, but 1.5-mm cuts are optimal at the occipitoatlantoaxial junction due to the intricate and detailed anatomy in this region, as well as in any instance when hairline fracture is a consideration.

The radiographic exposure factors can be quite low, especially since both bone and metrizamide offer sufficiently high attenuation of the X-ray beam to yield high contrast-to-background ratios. Such high contrast allows optimal spatial resolution even at low exposure techniques (approximately 160 to 200 mAs). These low techniques minimize tube heat load, allowing almost continuous scanning and automatic table incrementation. With such technique, up to 45 slices may be obtained in less than 10 minutes of patient time on the G.E. 8800 (13).

The ability to image the spine in multiple planes is a distinct advantage of computed tomography. On first thought, it may appear that since image reformation only manipulates the information present on axial slices, no additional information can be obtained. However, the relationship of adjacent vertebrae is vertically oriented, and disturbances in this relationship are difficult to appreciate on axial images. Subluxation of the vertebral bodies or the facets is much easier

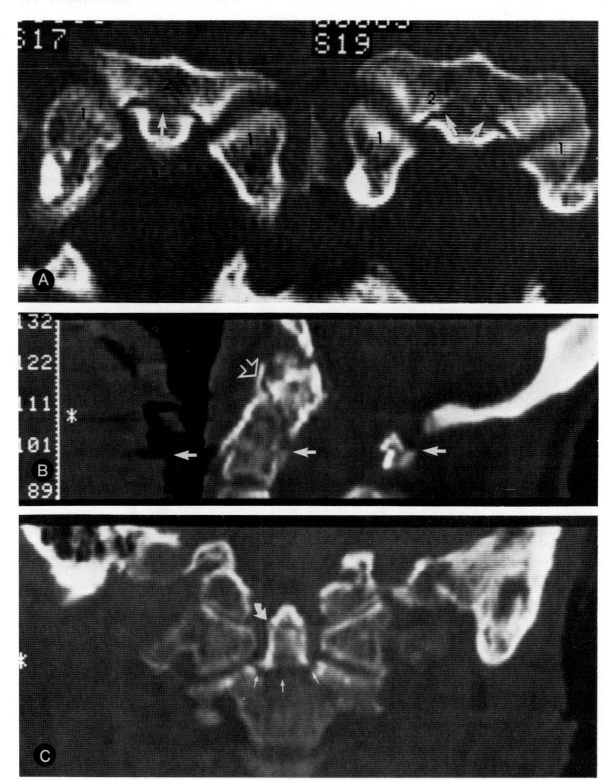

Figure 4.1. Fracture of the odontoid process—target reconstruction algorithm using diminished pixel size and extended CT number range.
A. Axial sections at the C2 plateau level show a fracture line (*arrows*). Note the C1 lateral masses are also in the plane of section due to the angulation of the patient's neck (see **B**).
B. Sagittal reformation localizes the fracture line in **A** to the odontoid base (*open arrow*). Incidentally seen is a misregistration artifact caused by patient movement between axial sections (*bold arrows*). Such an artifact may simulate fracture, but it continues through the entire reformatted image.
C. Coronal reformation verifies the base of dens fracture (*small arrows*) and, in addition, reveals an oblique fracture through its tip (*curved arrow*), where the alar ligament attaches (see the text).

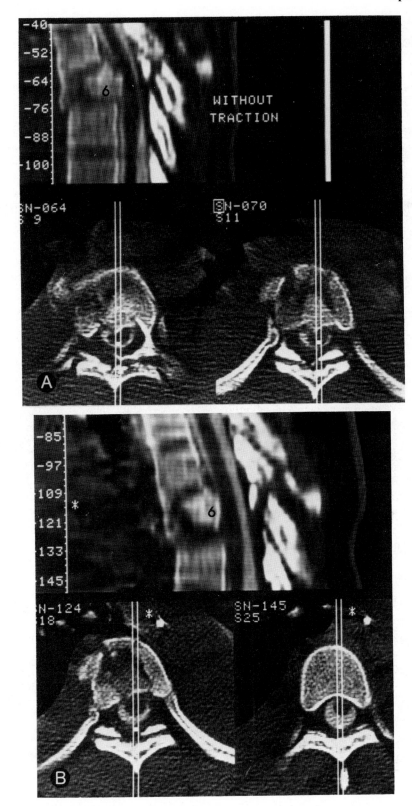

Figure 4.2.   Midthoracic fracture—importance of traction during CT.
A. Midsagittal image reformation of CT in patient with incomplete neurologic deficit following a T6 fracture-dislocation. Persistent cord compression is evidenced as effacement of the metrizamide-filled subarachnoid space caused by posterior displacement of the fragmented vertebrae. Surgical decompression was contemplated until it was realized that traction had been inadvertently suspended during the scan.
B. A repeat study done after traction was reinstituted showed improved alignment and decompression of the cord. Note the increased width of the subarachnoid space filled with metrizamide (same patient as Fig. 4.18).

to detect on sagittal reformations and, indeed, may be missed without the use of such reformations (Fig. 4.3). Such reformations also help to display loss of vertebral body heighth, or horizontally oriented fractures (Fig. 4.1).

In those patients with neurologic deficits, especially when the deficits are not complete, intrathecal metrizamide offers the ability to visualize potentially reversible compression of neural structures directly. Due to the high contrast sensitivity of CT, small doses of the intrathecal contrast agent are sufficient. In most cases, 5 ml of 170 to 190 mg/dl suffice to opacify the subarachnoid space completely and to demonstrate its compromise (Fig. 4.2). The agent can be introduced in the lumbar region; however, when patient immobilization is vital, a C1-C2 puncture should be performed with the patient supine. The patient can then be tilted to distribute the contrast agent into the region in question. All of the images are examined at multiple window and density settings for optimal visualization of bones and soft tissues.

Having discussed the indications and technique, the applicability of computed tomography in evaluating spinal trauma at various levels will now be illustrated.

CERVICAL SPINE TRAUMA

Four basic vectors of force may operate alone or in combination to induce injury to the spine during trauma. The type of fracture, dislocation, or both will depend upon the orientation and combination of these vectors: (*a*) flexion, (*b*) extension, (*c*) axial compression, (*d*) rotation. The level of injury is also of importance. The unique anatomy of the occipitoatlantoaxial region predisposes it to different types of injury than those seen in the lower cervical segment. The major-

ity of patients with significant cervical spine fracture and/or dislocation have two or more injuries. Posterior element (arch) fractures are associated with vertebral body injuries in at least half the cases. The majority of the posterior element injuries are found in the lateral mass and/or lamina. Although multiple injuries are usually seen at contiguous levels, occasionally an upper cervical injury may be combined with a lower cervical one (Fig. 4.4) or even a thoracic or lumbar injury. Neurologic damage is more often produced by trauma in the lower cervical segment than that in the craniocervical junction region (14–17).

The unique anatomy of the occipitoatlantoaxial region is beyond the scope of this discussion, and the interested reader is referred to discussions of the embryology and functional anatomy of this area for a more thorough understanding of its traumatic disruption (18). Probably the most common fracture of the atlas occurs in its posterior arch during forced hyperextension, when the C1 arch is compressed between the occipital bone and the sturdier posterior arch of the axis. However, the most well-known fracture of the atlas is the classical burst fracture originally described by Jefferson (9). It follows a vertical compression force which usually disrupts the atlas ring in two anterior points in addition to the posterior arch fractures. CT shows the multiple points of fracture well, since the fracture lines are generally perpendicular or oblique to the axial plane of the arch and, therefore, to the plane of the section. Associated fractures of C2 may occur but are unusual (Fig. 4.4). Spinal cord damage is uncommon with this fracture. Burst fracture of the atlas may be mimicked by "pseudospread" of the atlas on plain films in children under 5 years old. CT may be used to document this normal variant in childhood trauma (20).

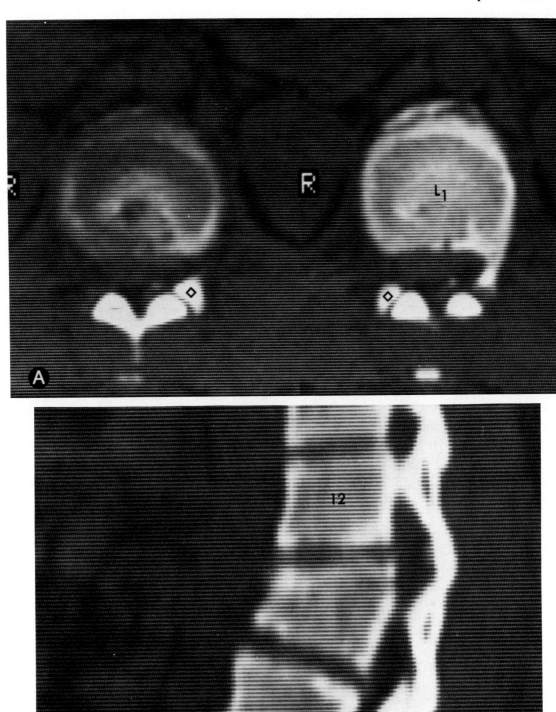

Figure 4.3.   Facet subluxation on image reformation.
A. Adjacent axial sections at the T12-L1 level show an apparently normal relationship between the superior facets of L1 (*diamond*) and the inferior facets of T12.
B. Sagittal reformation discloses that the T12 inferior facet is actually subluxed and "perched" on the superior facet of L1. Note the normal facet relationship at L1-L2. Also seen is a compression fracture of L1, which was difficult to appreciate on the axial sections in **A**.

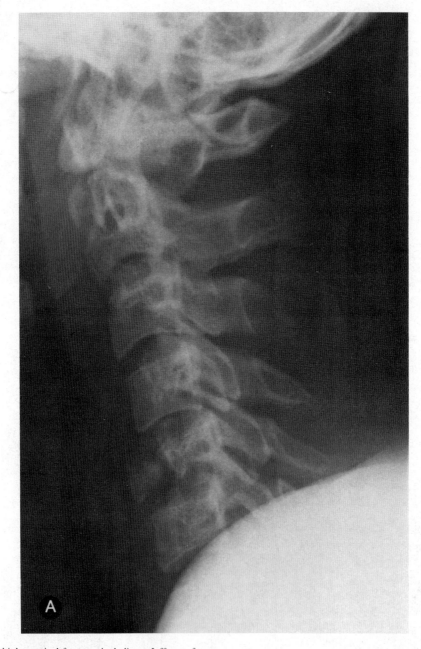

Figure 4.4.   Multiple cervical fractures including a Jefferson fracture.
A. Lateral C-spine film in a patient following a motorcycle accident shows fractures in the posterior arch of C1 and the anterior bodies of C2 and C5.

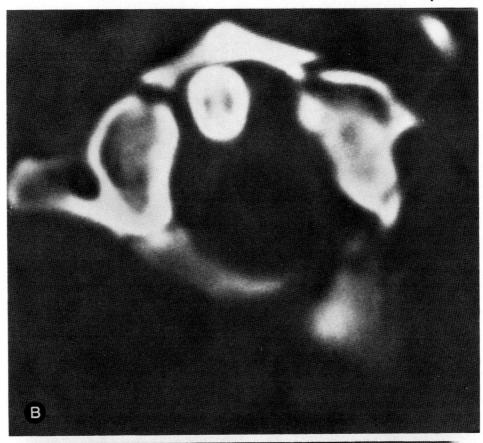

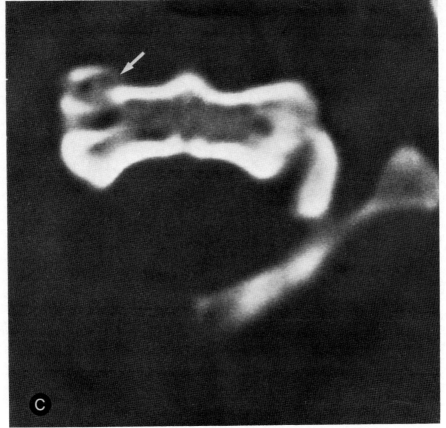

Figure 4.4.
B. Axial CT section reveals a Jefferson fracture at the C1 level.
C. The C2 fracture is localized to the right anterior aspect (*arrow*).

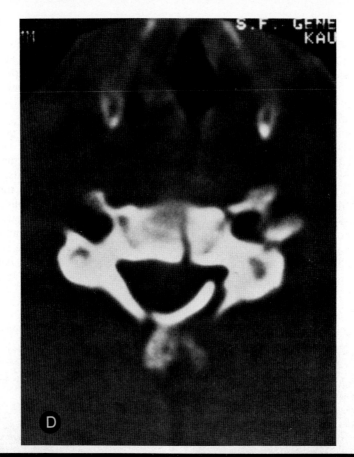

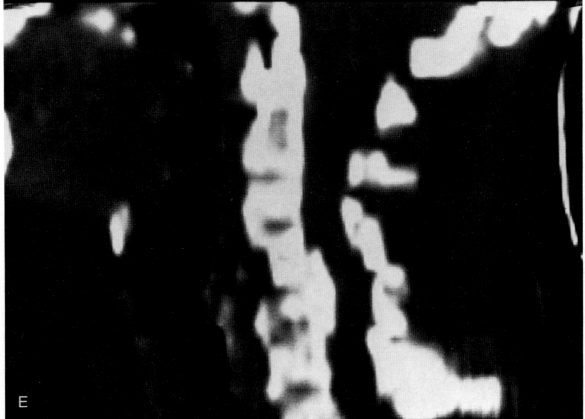

Figure 4.4.
D. The C5 fracture included posterior arch damage shown by CT.
E. A midsagittal reformation shows angulation but no significant compromise of the spinal canal. The patient's only neurologic deficit was a C6 radiculopathy.

The axis is also the site of several well-described fracture types. Wood-Jones first described the classical fracture of C2 produced by judicial hanging (21). Numerous authors have since used the term "hangman fracture" in patients who suffered hyperextension trauma through a variety of mechanisms (22–24). This fracture is characterized by bilateral fractures of the pedicles of the axis with subsequent distraction. Anterior subluxation of C2 on C3 occurs especially when the associated hyperextension also disrupts the anterior longitudinal ligament. The body of C2 is thus allowed to slip forward from its avulsed posterior arch which remains anchored by its articulation with C3 (Fig. 4.5). Despite the origin of the name, neurologic sequelae are uncommon when this type of fracture is caused by mechanisms other than hanging (15). Occasionally, the plain films may suggest a hangman frac-

ture but the CT shows the injury to be a minor variation on the theme (Figs. 4.6 and 4.7).

Another category of C2 fracture is that involving the odontoid process. Fractures of the dens are generally caused by sudden forward or backward movement of the head, with the neck rigidly erect and articulations locked. Variable degree of fracture and displacement of the dens with respect to the CT vetebral body occurs. The dens may be fractured obliquely at its tip, where the alar ligament inserts. More commonly, the base of the dens is fractured transversely, and nonunion here is a frequent complication. Occasionally, a lower horizontal fracture follows the embryologic line of union between the dens and the body of the axis, but fusion of this last fracture is the rule (25, 26). As discussed above, horizontal dens fractures may be difficult to see on axial sections unless significant

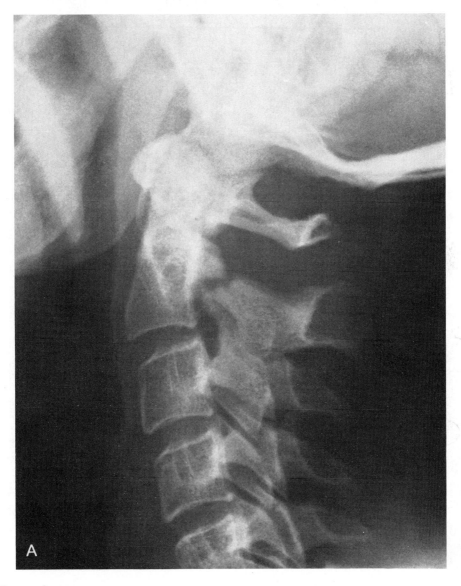

Figure 4.5. Hangman fracture.
A. Lateral C-spine film of a passenger involved in a motor vehicle accident shows the classic pedicle fractures first described in victims of judicial hanging. The lack of soft tissue swelling suggests absence of injury to the anterior longitudinal ligament, and this may explain why no anterior displacement of C2 on C3 is present.

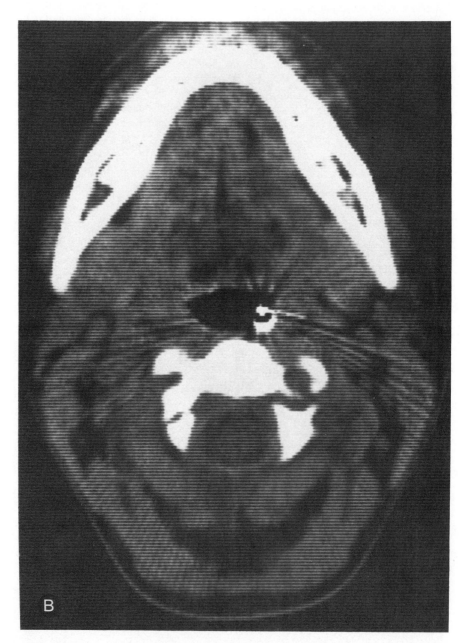

Figure 4.5.
B. Axial CT section of the fractured pedicles also shows the spinal cord outlined by cererospinal fluid.

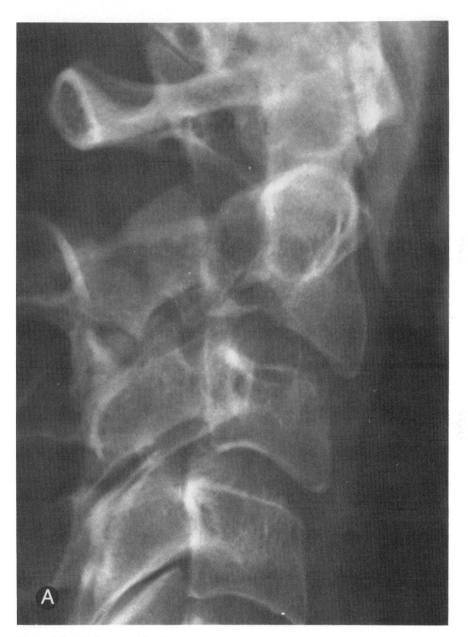

Figure 4.6.   C2 fracture-subluxation.
A. Plain film suggests a hangman fracture in this patient with anterior displacement of C2 on C3.

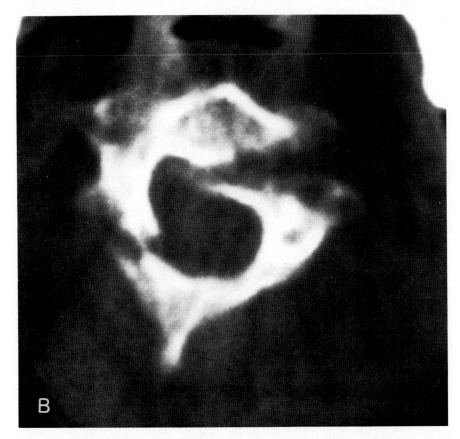

Figure 4.6.
B. Axial CT section of C2 shows a fractured right lamina and an oblique fracture through the back of the vertebral body.

distraction occurs. Therefore, optimal CT evaluation of this injury rests on the thinnest possible axial sections, sagittal or coronal image reformations, and special reconstruction algorithms, if available (Fig. 4.1). Because the initial diagnosis may be clinically or radiographically difficult, patients with an unfused dens fracture may present for evaluation days or weeks after the injury with symptoms of a painful neck or fluctuating long track signs.

Atlantoaxial dislocation may occur following trauma due to disruption of the transverse ligament which binds the dens to the anterior arch of the atlas. Such dislocation may occur rarely without the presence of an associated osseous disruption. Other predisposing factors to C1-C2 subluxation include inflammation (e.g., tonsillitis, pharyngitis). Since the lymphatic drainage of the joints is ultimately into the retropharyngeal and deep cervical glands, this drainage provides a retrograde pathway for the spread of infection to the C1-C2 junction (27). Inflammatory arthritides and Down's syndrome can also weaken the transverse ligament and result in such a subluxation (28). The diagnosis is generally easily ascertained on plain films, while CT shows an abnormal relationship between the anterior arch of C1 and the dens (Fig. 4.8).

A very unusual form of atlantoaxial dislocation is the so-called rotatory subluxation. The atlanto-oc-cipital joint allows only extension and flexion; therefore, most of the rotation between the head and the cervical spine occurs at the C1-C2 articulation. The atlantoaxial facets simulate a ball-and-socket joint and are oriented horizontally. This allows maximum rotation at the cost of stability. Rotation is generally limited to 58° (27). However, complete unilateral dislocation can occur at 45° of rotation, whereas bilateral dislocation of the articular processes can occur at 65° of rotation. The latter situation can narrow the spinal canal sufficiently to compromise the cord at this level (29). The role of trauma versus an idiopathic cause of such a rotatory fixation is debatable. Down's syndrome seems to be a predisposing factor in some of the reported cases. The patient generally exhibits torticollis. Computed tomography is useful in the diagnosis of this entity (30). Adjacent axial sections reveal the degree of atlantoaxial rotation. They also reveal an abnormal relationship between the dens and the arch of C1 (Fig. 4.9). However, many patients with rotatory fixation need not show separation between the dens and the atlas. As a result, dynamic evaluation of this region with cinefluorography or simply fluoroscopy may be needed for full evaluation, since mere rotation due to muscle spasm can simulate rotatory fixation. However, if the posterior arches of the atlas and axis move in unison during rotation, the diagnosis of atlantoaxial rotatory fixation can be made.

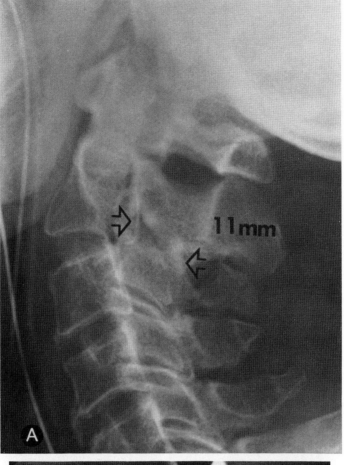

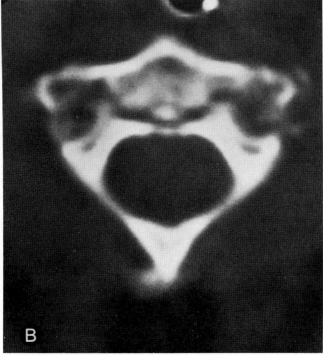

Figure 4.7. C2 fracture causing quadriplegia.
A. Lateral C-spine film in an elderly male rendered quadriplegic by a fall shows a vertical fracture through the back of C2 with posterior displacement of the fracture fragment. The canal, as measured from the back of the fragment to the laminar line of C3 (*open arrows*), is limited to 11 mm.

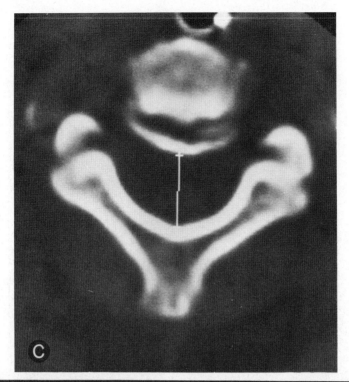

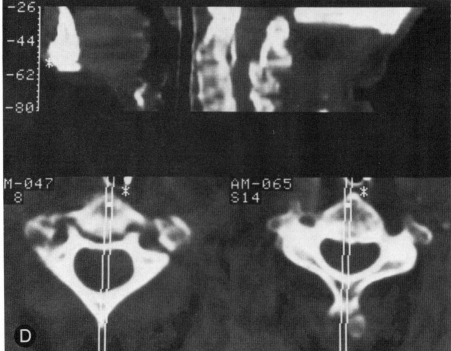

Figure 4.7.
B, C. Sequential axial sections at the upper and lower (respectively) C2 levels verify the fracture of the body, with the posterior elements intact and attached to the posteriorly displaced fragment. Measurement of the canal diameter at the lower level correlated with that of the plain film.
D. Sagittal reformation illustrates the posterior displacement of the C2 fragment and arch with respect to C3.

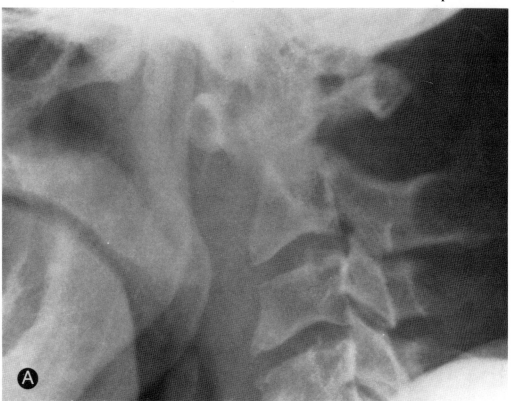

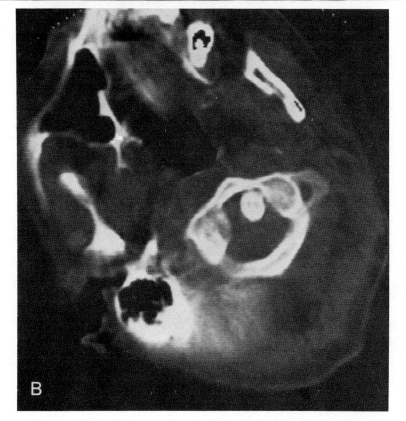

Figure 4.8.   C1-C2 subluxation.
A. Plain film of the upper cervical spine shows prevertebral soft tissue swelling and abnormal atlantodental interval, indicating anterior displacement of C1 on C2. No obvious fracture is noted. The patient was complaining of neck pain radiating down to his legs following a car accident.
B. CT section at the level of the C1 arch shows the dens eccentrically placed in relation to the anterior ring of C1. No fracture was seen on the lower sections.

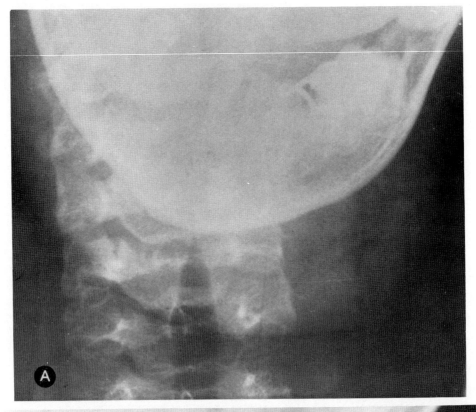

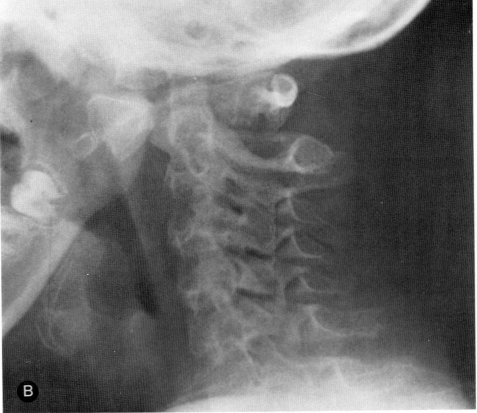

Figure 4.9.   C1-C2 rotatory subluxation.
A, B. Anteroposterior and lateral cervical spine films in this 13-year-old child with Down's syndrome who developed an abnormal head tilt reveal a rotatory abnormality at the C1-C2 level.

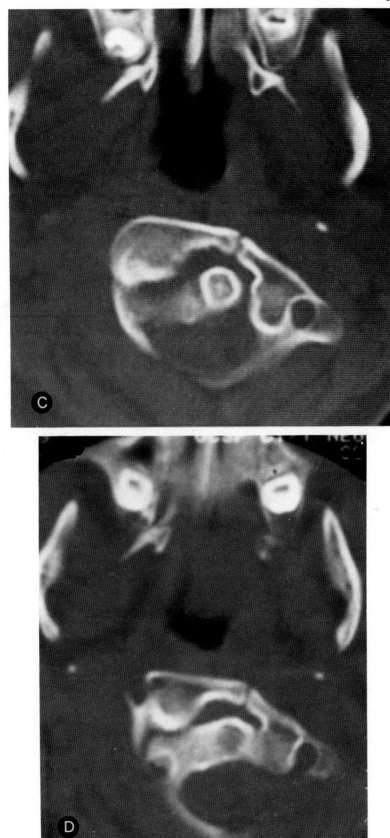

Figure 4.9.
C, D. Adjacent CT sections show the ring of C1 to be rotated off the C2 vertebral body. Note the separation of the dens away from the as yet unfused anterior arch of C1.

LOWER CERVICAL FRACTURES

A brief review of the lower cervical vertebral anatomy serves to clarify subsequent discussion regarding traumatic disruption in this region. The articular processes of the cervical vertebral bodies are small and flat, pointing downward and backward. The articular surfaces are in a relationship that is almost horizonal, and the overlap of the articular surfaces is not great. Motion is relatively limited to flexion and extension, with a small amount of rotation and lateral flexion as well. Fractures may occur with excessive displacement in any of these directions or as a result of axial compression.

Ligaments play a key role in the stability of the cervical region. Isolated ligamentous rupture may lead to significant subluxation in the absence of fracture (31). The ligamentous complex consists of the anterior and posterior longitudinal ligaments bridging the front and back of successive vertebral bodies, respectively. In addition, facet joints are bounded by the capsular ligaments, the laminae are joined by the ligamentum flavum, and the spinous processes are attached via the interspinous ligamentous complex. The posterior ligamentous complex is much more likely to rupture when the spine is subjected to excessive rotational force, rather than simple flexion or extension violence. The posterior ligamentous complex serves to immobilize the posterior elements in the cervical spine; therefore, if it remains intact in the face of flexion violence, the force of flexion is expended upon the vertebral body and a wedge compression fracture results with no significant instability introduced unless the arch also fractures due to an associated axial load (Fig. 4.4). In a flexion-rotation injury, the posterior ligaments are more likely to tear, and disengagement of the articular processes with dislocation may result, with relatively little or no bony damage (Fig. 4.10). Such a pure dislocation is more likely to occur in the cervical spine as opposed to the lower vertebral levels, due to the relatively minor degree of flexion required to disengage the articular processes (32).

The CT appearance of facet subluxation may be subtle when seen on axial views. The key finding is a bony structure posterior to the inferior facet at the involved level. Since the superior facet of the vertebral body below, with its flat posterior border, is normally in front of the upper vertebrae's inferior facet with its flat anterior border when viewed on axial sections, the finding of a bony structure with a flat posterior edge in back of the inferior facet indicates facet subluxation and "locking" (Figs. 4.10–4.12). Posterior element fracture may accompany such facet dislocation, especially if hyperextension occurs in association with a flexion force, as in the so-called "whiplash" event. Such a posterior element fracture is easy to appreciate on axial views, while the facet dislocation may be better delineated on image reformations in the parasagittal plane (Fig. 4.12).

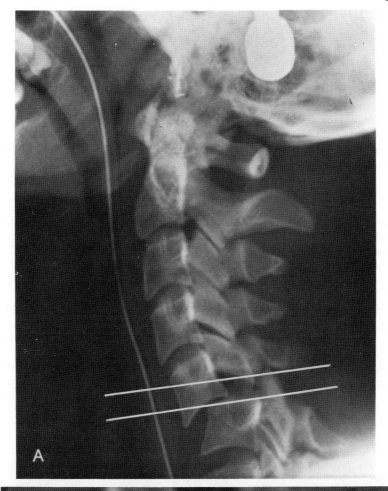

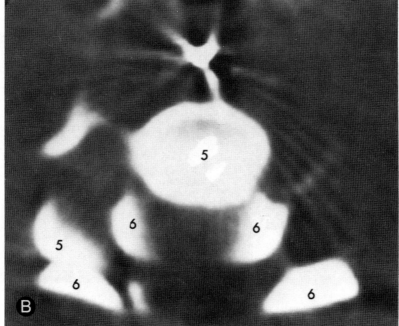

Figure 4.10. Facet subluxation.
A. Lateral cervical spine radiograph in a young female following a car accident shows anterior subluxation of C5 on C6 with bilateral locked facets. *Solid lines* indicate plane of CT section shown in **B**.
B. Axial section at the level of subluxation shows the vertebral body of C5 anterior to that of C6, with displacement of the inferior facets of C5 anterior to those of C6 (seen on the patient's right in this section). (Courtesy of Dr. R. Koch, Ross, CA.)

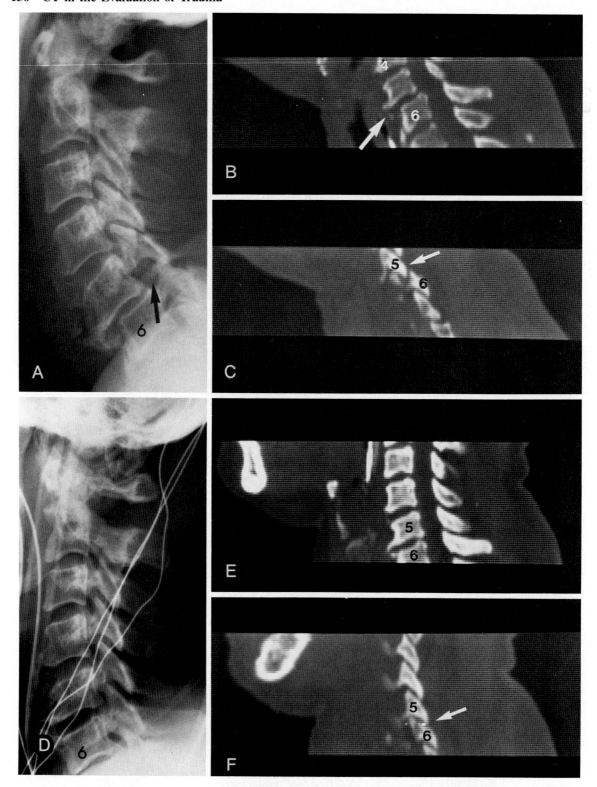

Figure 4.11.   Unilateral facet subluxation and reduction with traction.
A. Lateral radiograph shows a dislocated inferior articular process of C5 (*arrow*) barely visible within the foramen lying anterior to the superior articular process of C6. Anterior displacement of the C5 vertebral body on C6 is present.
B. Sagittal CT reformation in the midline shows the anterior displacement of C5 on C6 (*arrow*).
C. Sagittal CT reformation in the plane of the right-sided facets shows the anterior dislocation of the C5 facet in reference to that of C6 (*arrow*).
D. Lateral radiograph following cervical traction shows restoration of normal vertebral and facet alignment at C5-C6.
E. Sagittal CT reformation in the midline shows restoration of normal vertebral alignment at C5-C6.
F. Sagittal CT reformation in the plane of the right-sided facets shows restoration of normal facet alignment at C5-C6 (*arrow*).

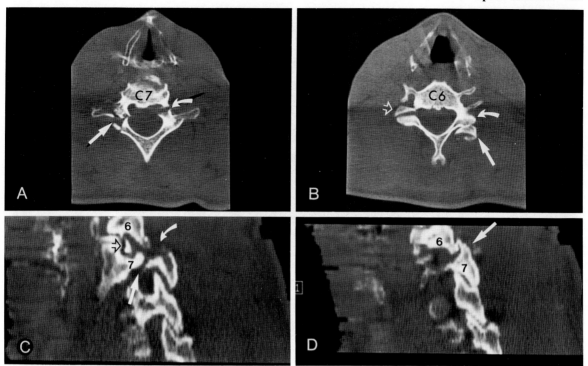

Figure 4.12.   Posterior arch fractures with facet subluxation.
A. Axial sections through the posterior elements of C7 show a fracture through the lamina on the right (*arrow*) and pedicle on the left (*curved arrow*).
B. Axial sections through C6 show the posterior position of the superior articular process of C7 (*arrow*) behind the inferior articular process of C6 (*curved arrow*). A triangular bone fragment appears to lie in the right neural foramen (*open arrow*).
C. Sagittal CT reformation on the right shows disruption of the lamina (*arrow*) and superior articular surface (*curved arrow*) at C7. A bone fragment is clearly present within the neural foramen at C6-C7 (*open arrow*).
D. Sagittal CT reformation on the left shows posterior displacement of the superior articular process of C7 (*arrow*) behind the inferior articular process of C6.

Whereas pure flexion violence generally damages the vertebral body, pure extension violence results in damage of posterior elements (Fig. 4.13). Of course, the two mechanisms can be combined in a flexion-extension type process, such as occurs with a whiplash injury, and both the vertebral body and arch may be involved (Fig. 4.14).

Lateral mass fractures can be difficult to appreciate on plain films but appear with some frequency, since they are the commonest fracture in the cervical spine seen in combination with other injuries (15). A typical mechanism for such articular pillar compression is a blow applied to the anterolateral surface of the head, causing it to move in an arc. As the head and neck move into lateral extension, the force is on the downward segment of the arc and stress is applied to the articular processes (Fig. 4.15).

Hyperextension sprain (momentary dislocation) may produce significant neurologic deficits without any bony or ligamentous injury in those patients who have a congenitally narrowed cervical spinal canal or in patients in whom degenerative changes have caused a developmental narrowing. Image reformations are helpful in such cases in identifying the degree of spinal canal compromise and in assessing facet relationships (Fig. 4.16). The computer software also allows direct measurements of the anteroposterior diameter within the spinal canal.

A final common type of injury seen in the lower cervical spine is the vertical compression injury, classically described in divers (33). The fracture produced is either a sagittal or coronal cleavage of the vertebral body or a burst of the body into multiple fragments with varying degrees of canal compromise (Figs. 4.4 and 4.17). If sufficient extension or axial loading is associated with the trauma, posterior elements may likewise be injured. The mild form of this injury is simply a superoanterior wedge compression of the vertebral body caused by a combination of axial load and mild flexion.

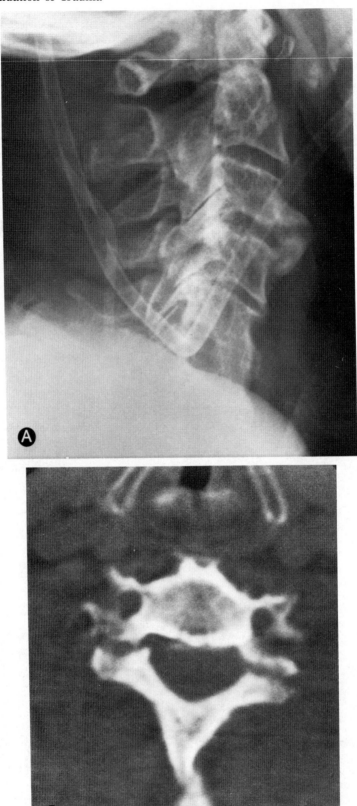

Figure 4.13. Posterior element fracture due to hyperextension.
A. Lateral cervical spine film in an elderly paraplegic shows inadequate visualization at the C6-C7 level. Incidentally noted are extensive degenerative changes.
B. Axial section at the C7 vertebral body shows fractures through both lateral masses, as well as an oblique fracture through the spinous process tip.

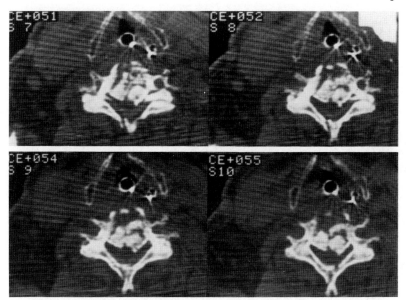

Figure 4.14. "Whiplash" flexion-extension injury. Consecutive axial sections of the C5 vertebral body in this patient seen in the emergency room following a rear-end collision reveal fragmentation of the vertebral body with posterior arch fracture.

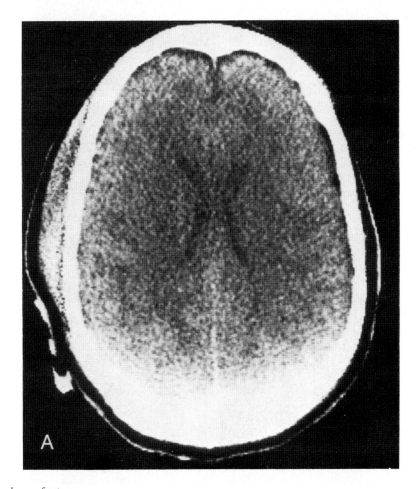

Figure 4.15. Lateral mass fracture.
A. CT brain scan of this young female complaining of neck pain following head trauma sustained in a car accident shows a soft tissue contusion on the right lateral aspect of the skull.

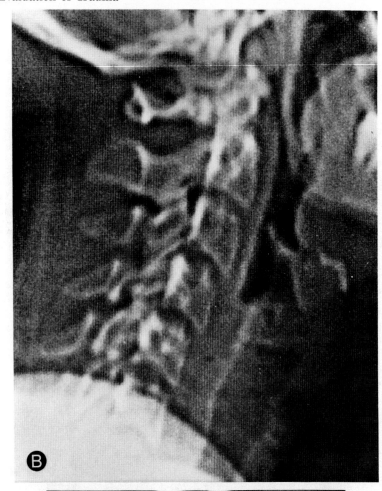

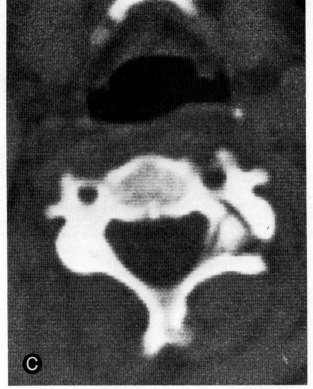

Figure 4.15.
B. Digital scout radiograph prior to spine CT scan shows a slight subluxation at C3-C4 and an obvious one of C4 on C5.
C. Axial section at the C4 level depicts a comminuted fracture of the left lateral mass.

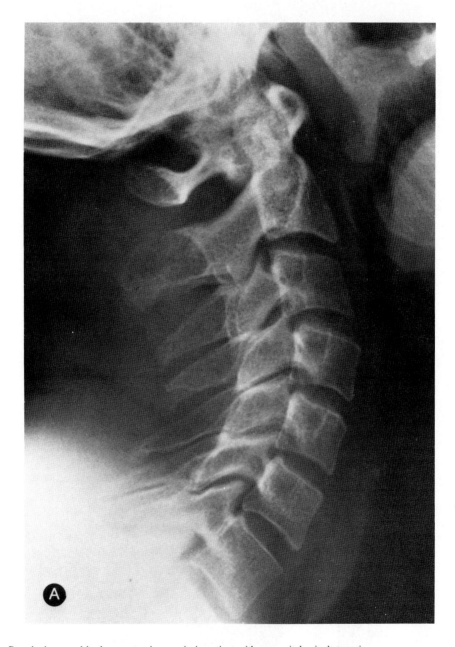

Figure 4.16.   Paraplegia caused by hyperextension sprain in patient with congenital spinal stenosis.
A. Lateral C-spine film in a patient rendered paraplegic after a 20-foot fall shows minimal posterior displacement of C3 on C4 and the presence of congenital spinal stenosis, as suggested by the observation that the lateral masses fill the entire anteroposterior dimension of the spinal canal (measurement bore this out). No evidence of fracture is seen.

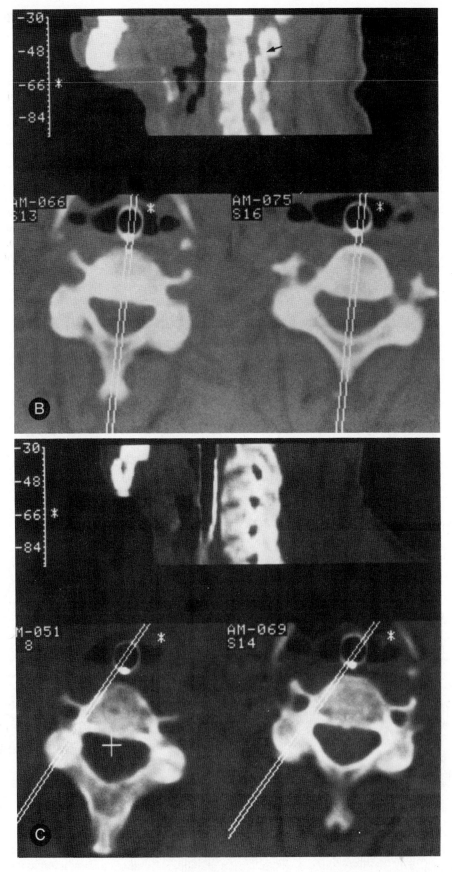

Figure 4.16.
B. Sagittal reformation verifies the narrow canal and minor displacement at the C3-C4 level (*arrow*).
C. Para-axial reformations through the pedicles reveal normal facet relationships and no evidence of other abnormality. The patient had partial recovery of his neurologic deficit, and he subsequently offered a history of previous episodes of electrical sensation radiating from his neck to his lower extremities with hyperextension of his head.

In patients with cervical spinal cord injury who have incomplete or progressive neurologic deficits, CT with metrizamide via C1-C2 puncture may be indicated. When done in the supine position, metrizamide tends to flow away from the midcervical region into the posterior fossa. With the patient supine and semi-upright, a small volume (5 ml) of metrizamide (190 mg of I/ml, following seizure prophylaxis of 130 mg of phenobarbital intravenously or intramuscularly will achieve sufficient opacification of cerebrospinal fluid in the midcervical region. A common finding in this clinical setting is compression of the cord by bony fragments or swelling of the cord which may obliterate the subarachnoid space and block the flow of metrizamide. Other acute lesions for which metrizamide CT is useful in the cervical region include lacerated spinal cord (metrizamide enters the cord), herniated disc, epidural hematoma, and dural tears (34, 35). As magnetic resonance imaging becomes more available, it is likely to replace metrizamide CT for evaluation of spinal cord injuries (11). CT will remain the procedure of choice for evaluation of bony injuries.

THORACIC SPINE FRACTURES

Traumatic fractures in the upper and midthoracic spine are not seen with the frequency of those in the cervical and thoracolumbar junction regions, because of the sturdiness of the thoracic vertebral structure and the additional structural stability provided by the rib cage and its costovertebral articulations. The gentle kyphosis in the thoracic spine and the extension stresses; thus most violent force is translated into a flexion vector. This generally produces anterior wedging of the vertebral bodies, while preserving the posterior elements and ligaments. When severe extension does occur in this region, neurologic deficit almost always results (36, 37). Computed tomography offers exquisite delineation of complex thoracic spine fractures, since the vertebral bodies and their associated appendages are relatively large and easily depicted (Figs. 4.2 and 4.18). In addition to the bony damage, cord compromise, when present, can be well depicted with the use of metrizamide. Occasionally, cord damage is caused not by bony compression, but by an intrinsic hematoma induced by the trauma (Fig. 4.19).

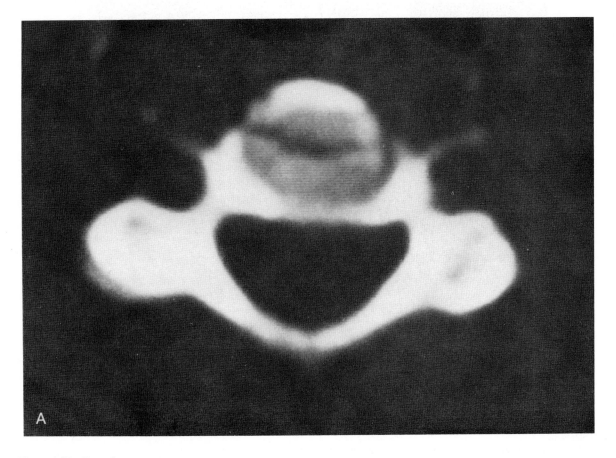

Figure 4.17. Burst fracture.
A. Axial section at the C6 level of a young patient following a dive into a swimming pool and subsequent paraplegia shows a coronal cleavage of the superior aspect of the vertebral body.

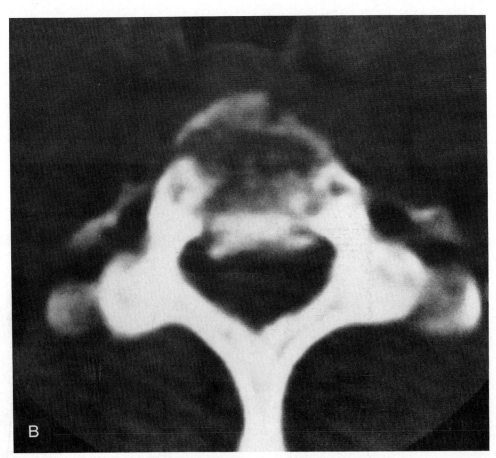

Figure 4.17.
B. Lower section in the same vertebral body shows its comminution and posteriorly displaced bony fragments compromising the spinal canal.

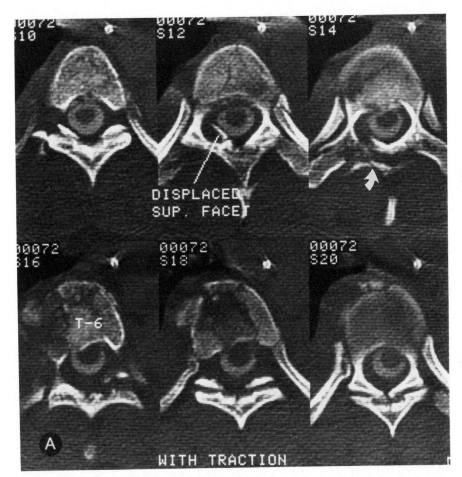

Figure 4.18. Complex midthoracic fracture with posterior element injury.
A. Sequential axial sections at the T5-T7 level in this young female with incomplete paraplegia show a marked comminution of the T6 vertebral body. A portion of the right superior facet is seen displaced medially into the spinal canal, since it is attached to the fractured posterior ring fragment shown by the *bold curved arrow* in slice 14 (*upper right*). This same section shows a right transverse process fracture. Metrizamide outlines the spinal cord.

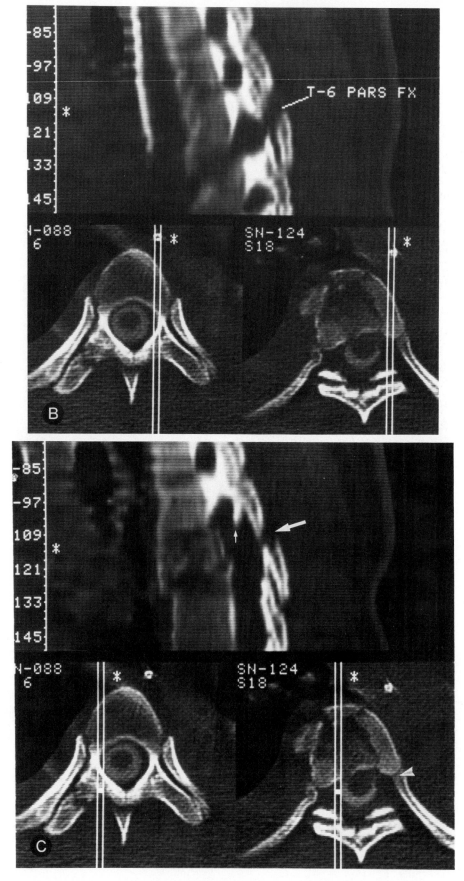

Figure 4.18.
B. Parasagittal reformation through the left pedicle disclosed an unsuspected pars fracture on this side as well (same patient as Fig. 4.2).
C. Sagittal section through the right pedicle nicely delineates the disrupted posterior elements on the right, showing the displaced superior facet (*small arrow*) and a pars fracture (*bold arrow*).

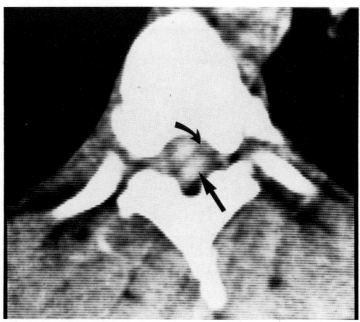

Figure 4.19.   Thoracic cord hematoma. The central high attenuation within the spinal canal (*arrow*) represents an intramedullary hematoma superior to a midthoracic fracture. Beam hardening artifact (*curved arrow*) partially obscures the lesion.

The use of seat belts has recently introduced a previously rare form of hyperflexion injury seen in the lower thoracic spine following vehicular trauma. The lap belt anchors the spine below the level of injury, allowing the force of forward acceleration and flexion to disrupt the posterior ligamentous complex. Further flexion results in vertical distraction to such a degree that disarticulation of the facets occurs, allowing the vertebrae above the involved level to dislocate anteriorly (Fig. 4.20) (38). Occasionally, a seemingly inexplicable dissociation occurs between the gross disruption evidenced by CT and the patient's clinical status (Fig. 4.21). This serves to remind us that imaging is not sufficient by itself for thorough diagnosis.

FRACTURES OF THE SPINE IN THE THORACOLUMBAR JUNCTION AND LUMBAR REGION

Although the forces that act upon the thoracolumbar and lumbar spine during trauma are the same as those previously described when discussing trauma in the cervical region, the structural and mechanical factors are quite different. The transition from the thoracic to the lumbar region is characterized by loss of the stablizing influence of the ribs, by the change in curvature from a kyphotic to a lordotic one, and also by a notable change in the facet relationships of the adjacent vertebral bodies. The facets of the thoracic spine are sturdy and overlap markedly in a plane close to the coronal. This facet relationship changes at the

T12-L1 level to one with a more sagittal orientation. The superior facets, being anterolateral, wrap around the inferior facets of the vertebral body above. These factors just mentioned increase the mobility of the spine in the thoracolumbar junction and lumbar region, while its mechanical pivotal location (with approximately half the body's weight above and half below) exaggerates the traumatic stresses placed upon it.

Perhaps the most common fracture suffered in this region is consequent to an axial load placed upon the vertebral bodies due to a vertical fall, causing anterior wedging of the vertebral body (39). Although plain films are adequate in many mild injuries of this type, falls from significant heights may produce burst fractures of the vertebral body with varying degrees of fragment retropulsion into the spinal canal. Plain films can underestimate the degree of canal compromise (40). CT evaluates the degree of such encroachment with accuracy and allows more direct evaluation of any posterior element injury. Image reformations are especially helpful in the latter instance (Figs. 4.22 and 4.23). In addition, reformations may delineate significant soft tissue injury, causing instability even when the bony derangement is minimal (Fig. 4.3).

A severe compression force on the lumbar region when it is rigid or minimally extended may produce a dural tear in addition to bony fracture (7, 40). Such dural tears are significant, since nerve roots may become entrapped within bony fragments once they herniate beyond the dural confines. This finding is es-

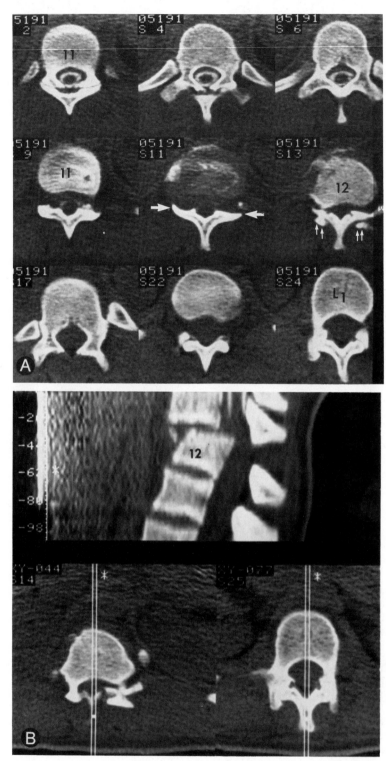

Figure 4.20. Seat belt injury.
A. This young male was paraplegic after being involved in a car accident while wearing a lap belt. Sequential axial sections from the T11 through the L1 level show a normal articulation of the inferior facets of T10 with the superior facets of T11 (*upper left-hand corner*). Progressive sections show loss of the metrizamide within the subarachnoid space. In the middle section, the inferior facets of T11 are seen isolated (*bold arrows*). The superior facets of T12 are not seen in their usual location, anterior to the inferior facets of T11. In fact, the superior facets are displaced behind the inferior facets of T11 (*small arrows*), as seen on the next section. Incidentally noted is a rib dislocation at the T12 level of the left (*lower left-hand corner*).
B. Midsagittal reformation verifies the anterior subluxation of T11 and T12. The metrizamide column can be seen totally blocked by the angulation of the spinal canal at this level.

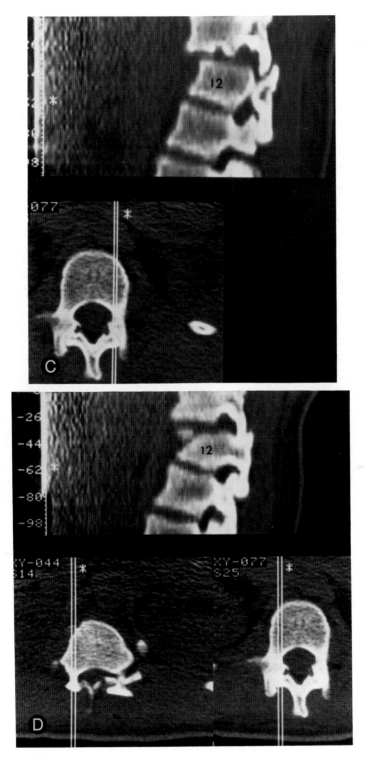

Figure 4.20.
C, D. Parasagittal sections through both the left and right facets nicely delineate the anterior subluxation of the inferior facets of T11 with respect to the superior facets of T12.

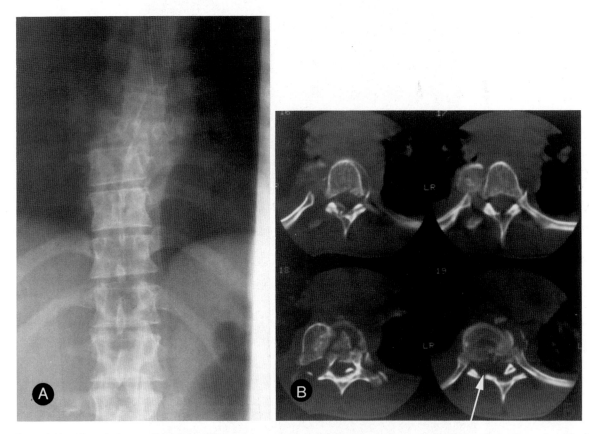

Figure 4.21.   Thoracic fracture-dislocation without major neurologic deficit. Patient was treated conservatively with traction and remained stable.

A. Anteroposterior radiograph of the thoracic spine shows a severe fracture dislocation at T8-T9. The degree of compromise of the spinal canal could not be accurately assessed on plain films alone.

B. The axial CT images show that the subluxation of T8 on T9 is directly lateral with preservation of a nearly normal anteroposterior canal diameter under the right pedicle of T8 (*arrow*). Several bone fragments are present which do not significantly compromise the canal along the course of the thecal sac and cord. (Case courtesy of Dr. Leon Kaseff, Peninsula Hospital, Burlingame, CA.)

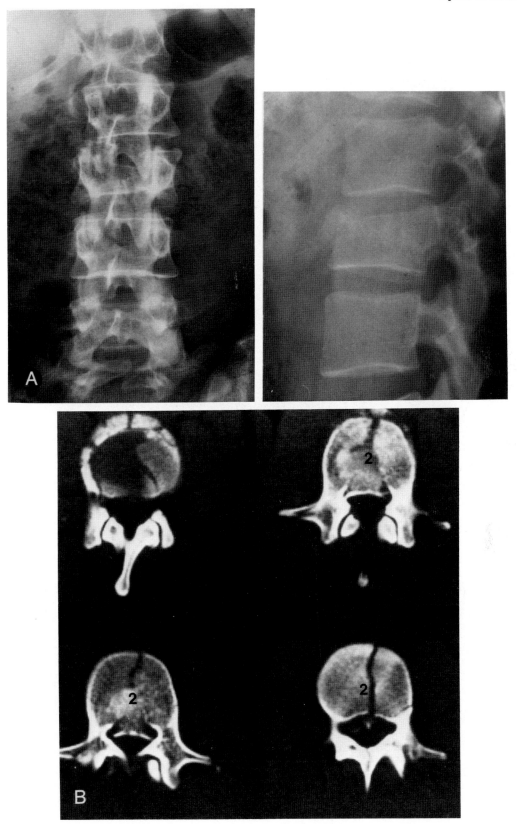

Figure 4.22. L2 fracture.
A. Anteroposterior and lateral plain films obtained in the emergency room on this young male with back pain following a 20-foot jump showed an L2 compression fracture, with widened interpediculate distance of that level.
B. Selected sequential axial CT sections reveal a burst fracture of the L2 vertebral body, with significant compromise of the spinal canal due to a displaced bony fragment. The lowest cut (*lower right*) shows a linear fracture through the posterior arch.

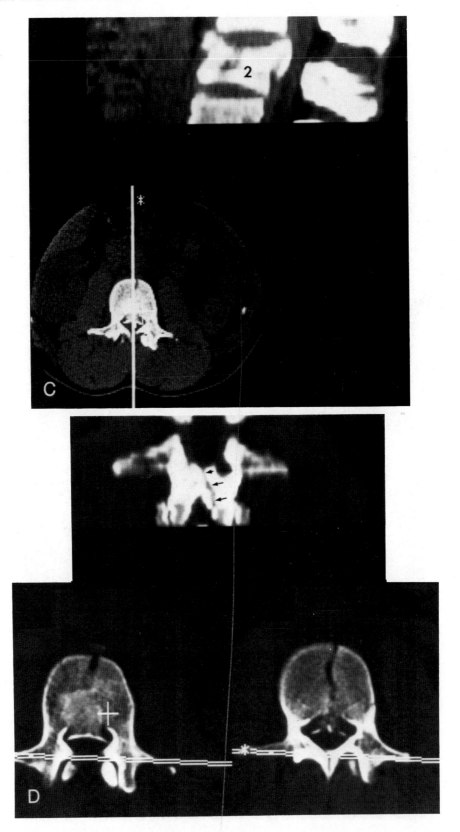

Figure 4.22.
C. Midsagittal plane reformation shows loss of height of the L2 vertebral body, with better delineation of the canal compromise caused by retropulsion of a bony fragment at this level.
D. Coronal reformation through the posterior arch better defines the vertical fracture, extending from right to left (*arrows*).

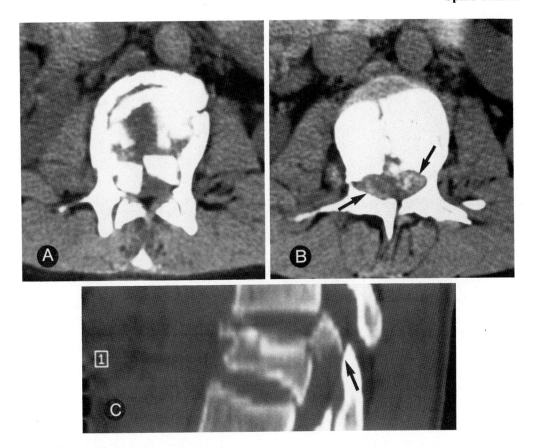

Figure 4.23.   L2 fracture with epidural hemorrhage.
A,B. Axial sections through L2 show the comminuted fracture of the vertebral body with multiple retropulsed fragments. High-attenuation tissue within the canal and outside the thecal sac (**B**, *arrows*) represents epidural hemorrhage which replaces normal epidural fat density.
C. Sagittal reformation through the fracture shows the position of a retropulsed bone fragment within the spinal canal (*arrow*).

pecially important to recognize if emergency surgery for decompression and/or stabilization is contemplated, since the unwary surgeon may transect nerve roots herniated beyond the spinal canal confines. The diagnosis of dural tear is made possible on CT with instillation of a small dose of intrathecal metrizamide. Leakage of the contrast agent into the paraspinal soft tissues at the site of fracture indicates such a dural rupture (Fig. 2.24).

Metrizamide is also helpful in other cases of thoracolumbar trauma in which neurologic symptoms and/or signs accompany the injury. Direct compression of the conus medullaris and/or cauda equina nerve roots can be demonstrated and may indicate the need for emergency surgical decompression if the symptoms or signs are incomplete but progressing. However, conservative decompression via traction may accomplish therapeutic relief (Figs. 4.25 and 4.26). Indeed, considerable controversy exists regarding the treatment of neurologic deficits associated with thoracolumbar fractures. Incomplete neurologic deficits can be produced simply by contusion and may, therefore, be spontaneously reversible. Persistent compression of the conus or nerve root en-

trapment will not resolve without surgical intervention in many cases. Therefore, therapeutic decisions are somewhat subjective. Hence, CT demonstration of such post-traumatic features as compromise of the cord or neural foramen by fragments (Fig. 4.27) or post-traumatic disc herniation (Fig. 4.28) is important in guiding appropriate patient management.

A second controversy regarding management of these patients involves the proper stabilization of unstable injuries. Conservative opinion opts for postural reduction in extension and prolonged bed rest, or possibly plaster bracing (41, 42). However, the introduction of Harrington rods for surgical immobilization has allowed good reduction and stabilization, while permitting earlier mobilization of patients and also more rapid rehabilitation (43). As we have seen, unstable injuries may be difficult to diagnose completely without dynamic studies; however, computed tomography can strongly suggest instability when it reveals posterior element fracture, facet subluxation, or even unusual angulation. CT may provide a new diagnostic insight into the controversies regarding proper patient management following severe thoracolumbar trauma resulting in instability.

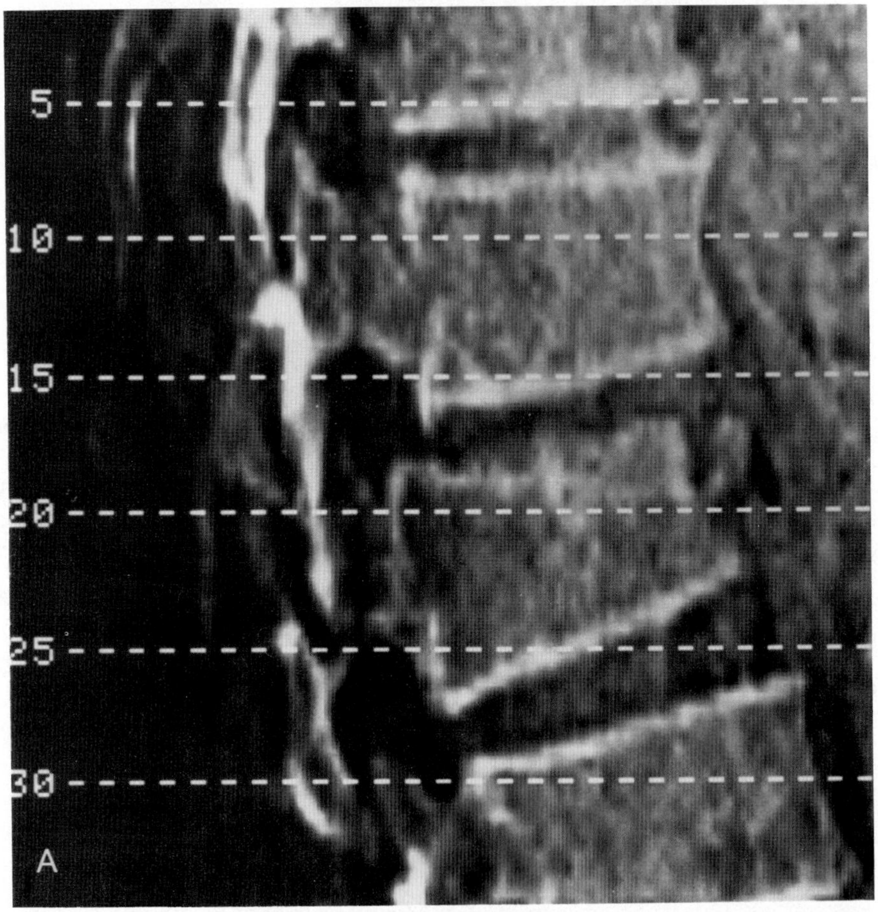

Figure 4.24. Lumbar fracture-dislocation, with dural tear.
A. Digital scout radiograph of a 36-year-old-male who fell 15 feet shows a compression fracture of the L1 vertebral body with anterior displacement of T12 on L1. Numbers at the left represent actual slice locations, with every fifth section annotated.

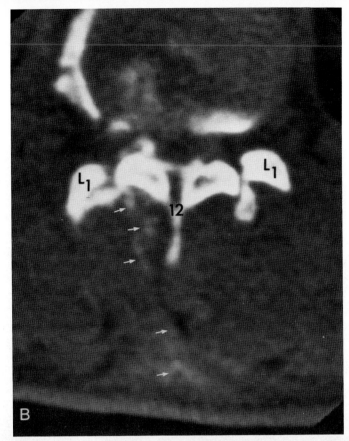

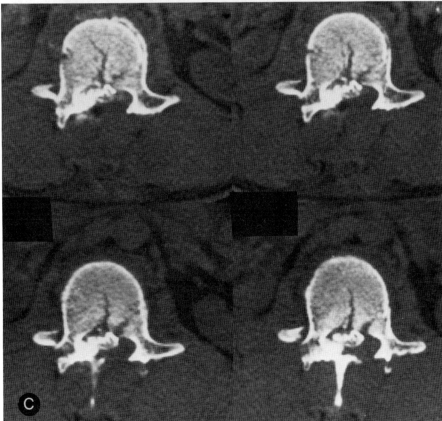

Figure 4.24.
B. Axial section at the T12-L1 level shows anterior dislocation of the inferior facets of T12 with respect to the superior facets of L1 (see the normal lu.nbar facet relationship in Fig. 4.19**B**). Metrizamide was introduced into the subarachnoid space prior to the CT, is effaced at the level of this subluxation, and can be seen leaking into the posterior paraspinal muscles (*arrows*).
C. Sequential sections lower in the L1 vertebral body reveal multiple fractures through the body, disruption of the posterior arch, and compression of the metrizamide-filled subarachnoid space with its nerve root contents, seen on multiple sections.

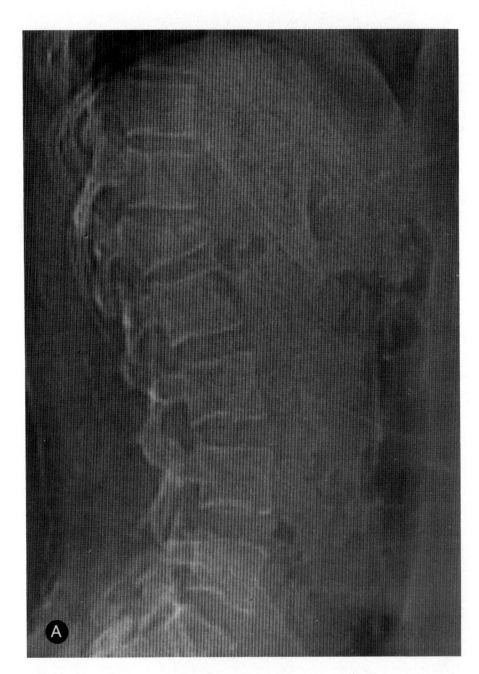

Figure 4.25.   L1 fracture with conus medullaris compression.
A. Digital scout radiograph shows a compressed L1 vertebral body in this middle-aged male who jumped from a height of 30 feet.

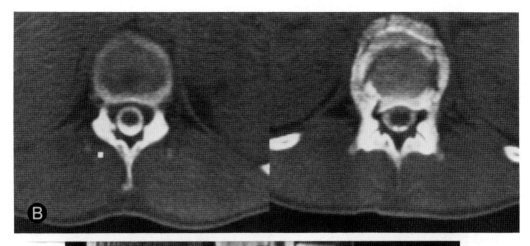

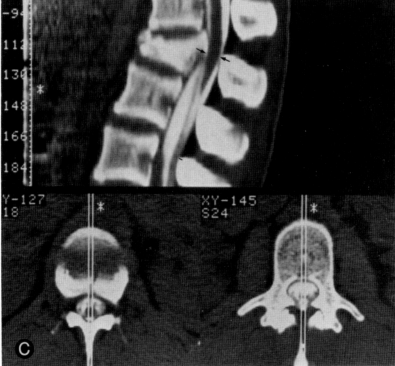

Figure 4.25.
B. Selected axial sections at the T11-T12 interspace (*left*) and the T12-L1 interspace (*right*) are shown. Note the comminution of the L1 vertebral body with posterior displacement of a fragment mildly effacing the metrizamide-filled subarachnoid space. The conus medullaris can be seen surrounded by the metrizamide posterolaterally.
C. Midsagittal reconstruction verifies the severe compression of L1 and indicates a more ominous compromise of the spinal canal, possibly explaining this patient's L3 radiculopathy. This compromise is in an oblique plane (*arrows*), one inaccessible to axial sections. Mechanical traction was instituted, and the patient's radiculopathy resolved.

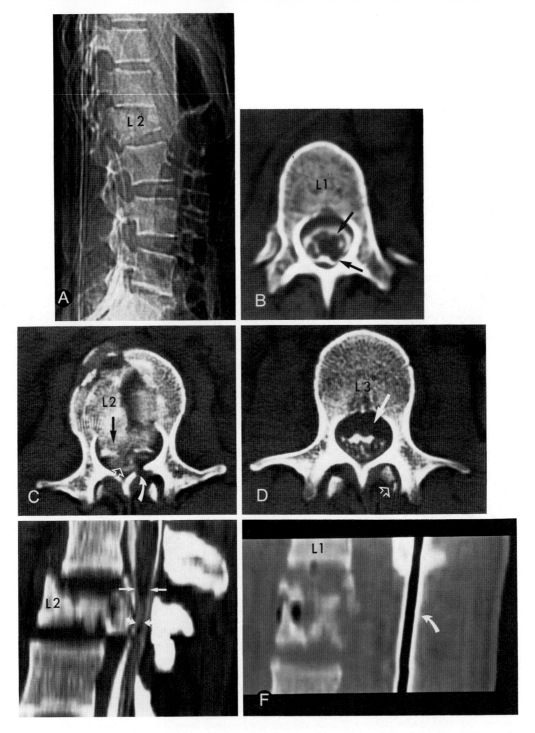

Figure 4.26. L2 fracture producing conus medullaris tip and cauda equina compression. Twenty-four-year-old woman with symptoms of conus medullaris compression following a motor vehicle accident.

A. Digital scout radiograph shows an L2 compression fracture with compromise of the spinal canal.

B. Axial section through L1 shows asymmetric enlargement of the conus medullaris outlined by metrizamide, probably due to swelling of the conus and proximal nerve roots on the left (*arrows*).

C. Axial section through L2 shows a comminuted fracture with a retropulsed fragment (*arrow*) producing severe compromise of the spinal canal and compression of the thecal sac (*open arrow*). Metrizamide is present in the compressed thecal sac. Laminar fracture on the left is also present (*curved arrow*).

D. Axial section through L3 shows an epidural hematoma (*arrow*) compressing the thecal sac. The multiple roots of the cauda equina are outlined by metrizamide. A small fracture of the inferior articular process of L2 is also present on the left (*open arrow*).

E. Sagittal CT reformation shows the compression of the tip of the conus medullaris (*arrows*) and proximal cauda equina (*curved arrows*) at L2 by the retropulsed fracture fragment.

F. Sagittal CT reformation through L2 following stabilization with Harrington rods shows resolution of the spinal canal compromise. Current image reconstruction techniques minimize the artifact (*curved arrow*) from dense metal appliances and allow adequate visualization of the adjacent spinal canal.

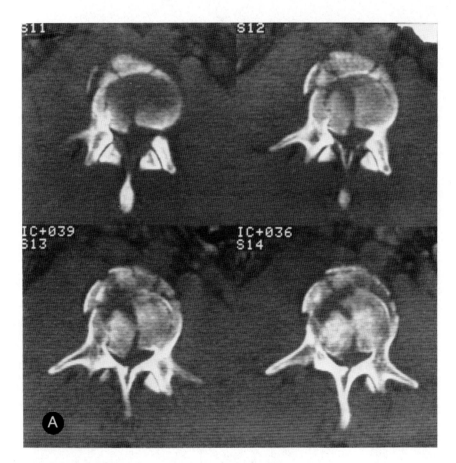

Figure 4.27.   L3 fracture with radiculopathy.
A. Sequential axial CT sections through the L3 vertebral level demonstrate severe comminution of the vertebral body with compromise of the spinal canal.

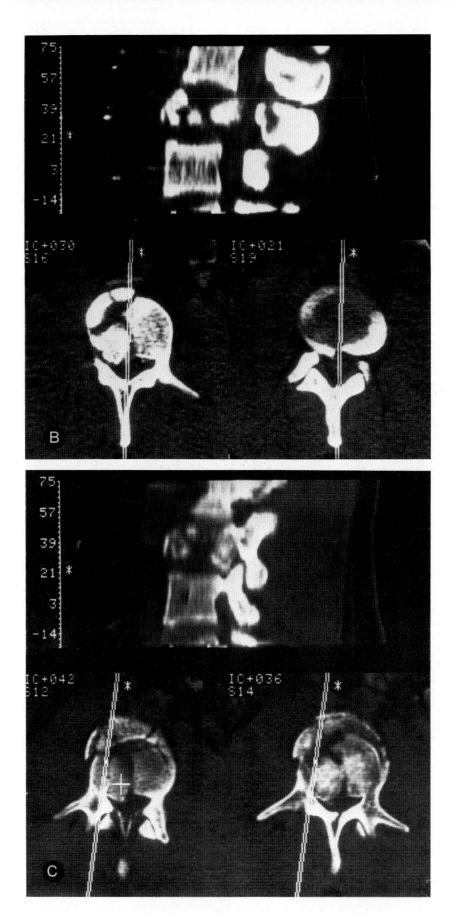

Figure 4.27.
B. Midsagittal plane reformations delineate the fragmentation of the L3 vertebral body to better advantage.
C. Para-axial reformations through the plane of the neural foramen depict marked compromise of the neural foramen due to the fracture. Surgical decompression relieved the right L3 radiculopathy.

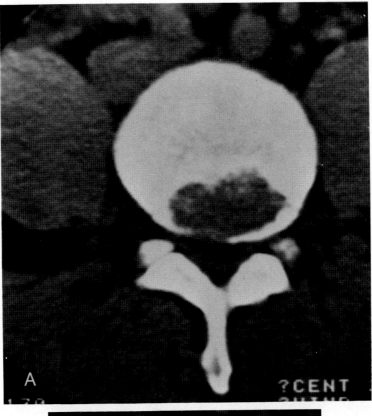

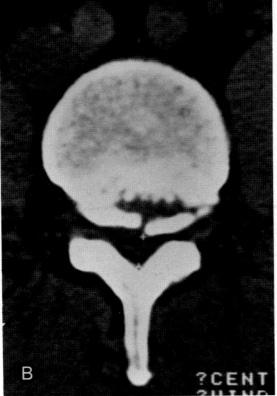

Figure 4.28. Persistent radiculopathy and low back pain following mild trauma were evaluated with a CT scan in this young patient. Consecutive axial sections (**A, B**) showed herniation of the nucleus pulposus into the L4 end plate, with displacement of bony fragments into the spinal canal. Surgical decompression of the disc and bone fragments relieved the symptoms. (Courtesy of Dr. Robert Jahnke, Albuquerque, NM.)

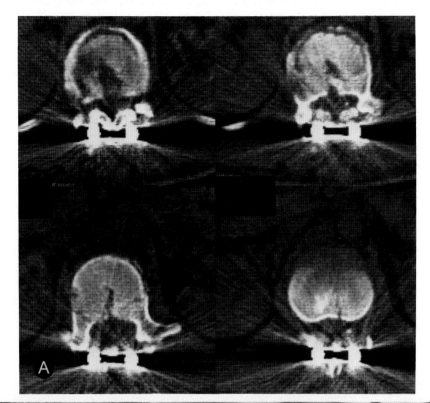

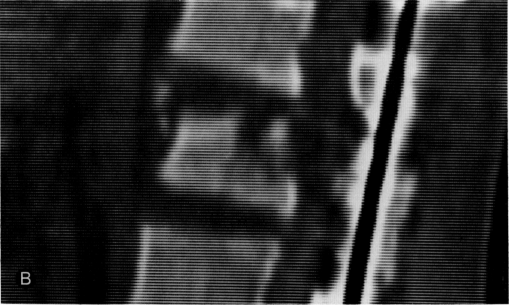

Figure 4.29.   CT of T12-L1 fracture-dislocation following stabilization with Harrington rods.
A. Sequential axial sections at the T12-L1 level show the Harrington rods with marked streak artifacts. Nevertheless, the relationships of the inferior-superior facet junction can be evaluated, as can the bony fragmentation of the vertebral body.
B. Sagittal reformation nicely delineates the relative realignment of the spinal canal at this level. The streak artifacts are seen as a black column on this reformation (same patient as Fig. 4.24).

Incidentally, follow-up CT studies following internal fixation with metallic rods can be performed despite the considerable streak artifacts produced by such devices. Sagittal reconstructions will adequately reveal the degree of spinal realignment obtained (Figs. 4.26 and 4.29). This is because streak artifacts, although degrading the quality of imaging within soft tissue, rarely affect the visualization of bony detail. For similar reasons, gunshot injury to the spine is likewise easily evaluated with computed tomography (Fig. 4.29). The location of bullet fragment disruption of the bony structures and the compromise of important neural or vascular structures can be ascertained (Figs. 4.30 and 4.31).

SUMMARY

The introduction of computed tomography has had a major impact on the diagnostic approach to the spine trauma patient. The high resolution of new generation CT equipment allows definitive evaluation of bony disruption within the spinal column. Multiplanar image reformation permits three-dimensional assessment of the injury, optimizes patient comfort and safety, and minimizes the time necessary for the diagnosis. Water-soluble contrast can be used to expand greatly the utility of computed tomography. Utilizing the cervical puncture approach, small doses of contrast can be instilled in the subarachnoid space with the patient supine and semi-upright on a tiltable gurney. Such contrast enhancement can provide additional information in acutely traumatized patients with neurologic deficits. Dynamic sequence scanning with automatic table incrementation permits thorough evaluation of severe spinal trauma in less than 15 minutes following patient transfer onto the scanning couch. Because of its many advantages, CT has become the diagnostic procedure of choice in the evaluation of spinal injury when plain films and/or clinical data indicate the need for further diagnostic measures.

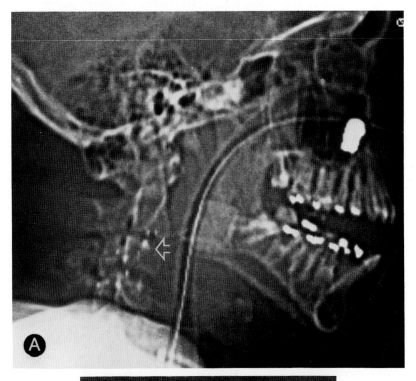

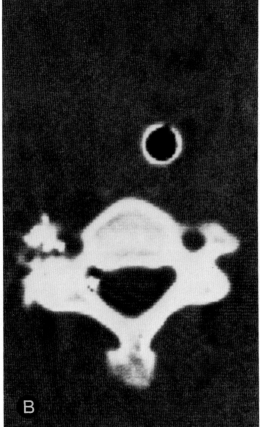

Figure 4.30.   Gunshot injury of the cervical spine.
A. Lateral scout radiograph of the upper cervical spine and face reveals a bullet superimposed on the maxillary sinus. Bullet fragments can be noted at the C3 level (*open arrow*).
B. Axial CT section at the C3 level shows fragments disrupting the vertebral artery canal on the right, and fragment is also seen within the spinal canal itself. Incidentally, note the severe prevertebral swelling; the airway had to be maintained with a nasotracheal tube.

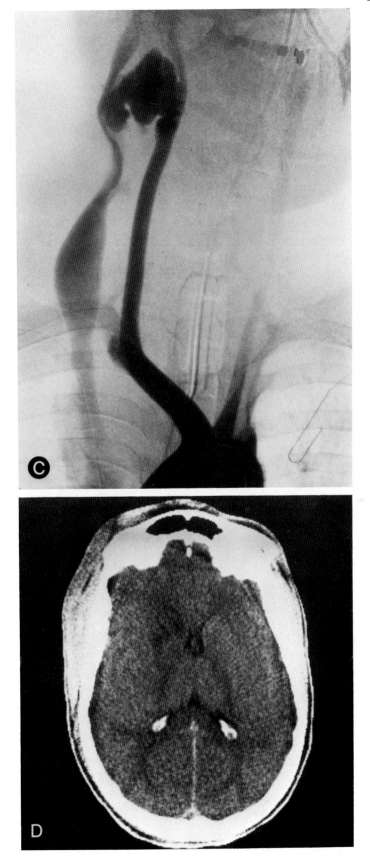

Figure 4.30.
C. An aortic arch study revealed a traumatic carotid-jugular fistula.
D. Brain CT scan obtained on this patient following repair of the fistula depicted an early infarction in the region of the right caudate nucleus and anterior capsule.

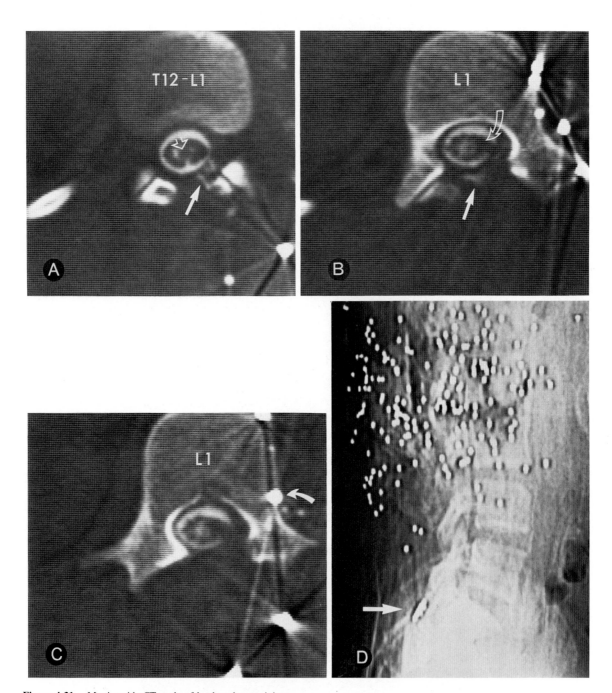

Figure 4.31. Metrizamide CT study of lumbar shotgun injury.

A–C. Metrizamide in the thecal sac outlines the cauda equina and tip of the conus medullaris (**A**, *open arrow*). Enlargement of the nerve roots on the left (**B**, *open curved arrow*) may represent intrathecal hematoma or traumatic swelling or both. It is not clear whether the multiple epidural high densities in the posterolateral spinal canal (**A, B**, *arrows*) are due to metrizamide leakage or bone fragments. High-density shotgun pellets are seen in the paraspinous soft tissues (**C**, *curved arrow*).

D. The scout view is helpful in clarifying the ambiguity of the axial images. A dural tear is suggested by the presence of pellets lined up in the region of the distal thecal sac (*arrow*).

REFERENCES

1. Lee BCP, Kazam E, Newman AD: Computed tomography of the spine and spinal cord. *Radiology* 128:95, 1978.
2. Roub, LW, Drayer BP: Spinal computed tomography: Limitations and applications. *AJR* 133:267, 1979.
3. Green BA, Callahan RA, Klose KJ, De La Torre J: Acute spinal cord injury: Current concepts. *Clin Orthop* 154:125, 1981.
4. Binet F, Moro JJ, Marangola JP, Hodge CT: Cervical spine tomography in trauma. *Spine* 2:162, 1977.
5. Maravilla KR, Cooper PR, Sklar FH: The influence of thin-section tomography on the treatment of cervical spine injuries. *Radiology* 127:131, 1978.
6. Brant-Zawadzki M, Miller EM, Federle MP: CT in the evaluation of spine trauma. *AJR* 136:369, 1981.
7. Brant-Zawadzki M, Jeffrey RB, Minagi H, Pitts LM: High-resolution CT of thoracolumbar fractures. *AJNR* 3:69, 1982.
8. Handel SF, Lee Y: Computed tomography of spinal fractures. *Radiol Clin North Am* 19:69, 1981.
9. Maue-Dickson W, Trefler M, Dickson DR: Comparison of dosimetry and image quality in computed tomography and conventional tomography. *Radiology* 131:509, 1979.
10. Pentlow KS: Dosimetry in computed tomography. In Newton TH, Potts DC (eds): *Radiology of the Skull and Brain: Technical Aspects of Computed Tomography.* St Louis, CV Mosby, 1981, pp 3918–3940.
11. Norman D, Mills CM, Brant-Zawadzki M, et al: Magnetic resonance imaging of the spinal cord and canal: Potentials and limitations. *AJR* 141:1147, 1983.
12. Deeb ZL, Drayer BP, Rosenbaum AE: A simple traction device for use in the radiology department. *Radiology* 125:826, 1977.
13. Brown BM, Brant-Zawadzki M, Cann CE: Dynamic CT scanning of spinal column trauma. *AJR* 139:1177–1181, 1982.
14. Miller MD, Gehweiler JA, Martinez S, Charlton OP, Daffner RH: Significant new observations on cervical spine trauma. *AJR* 130:659, 1978.
15. Gehweiler JA Jr, Clark WM, Schaaf RE, Powers B, Miller MD: Cervical spine trauma: The common combined conditions. *Radiology* 130:77, 1979.
16. Calenoff L, Chessare JW, Rogers LF, Toerge J, Rosen JS: Multiple level spinal injuries: Importance of early recognition. *AJR* 130:665, 1978.
17. Jefferson G: Discussion of spinal injuries. *Proc R Soc Med* 8:625, 1927.
18. Penning L: *Functional Pathology of the Cervical Spine.* Baltimore, Williams & Wilkins, 1968.
19. Jefferson G: Fractures of the atlas vertebra. *Br J Surg* 7:407, 1920.
20. Suss RA, Zimmerman RD, Leeds NE: Pseudospread of the atlas: False Jefferson fracture. *AJR* 140:1079, 1983.
21. Wood-Jones F: The ideal lesion produced by judicial hanging. *Lancet* 1:53, 1913.
22. Elliott JM Jr, Rogers LF, Wissinger JP, et al: The hangman's fracture: Fractures of the neural arch of the axis. *Radiology* 104:303, 1972.
23. Brashear HR Jr, Venters GC, Preston ET: Fractures of the neural arch of the axis: A report of 29 cases. *J Bone Joint Surg* 57A:879, 1975.
24. Seljeskog EL, Chou SN: Spectrum of the hangman's fracture. *J Neurosurg* 45:3, 1976.
25. Amyes EW, Anderson FM: Fracture of the odontoid process (report of 63 cases). *Arch Surg* 72:377, 1956.
26. Harris JH: Acute injuries of the spine. *Semin Roentgenol* 13:53, 1978.
27. Shapiro R, Youngberg AS, Rothman SLG: The differential diagnosis of traumatic lesions of the occipito-atlanto-axial segment. *Radiol Clin North Am* 11:505, 1973.
28. Martel W: The occipito-atlanto-axial joints in rheumatoid arthritis and ankylosing spondylitis. *AJR* 86:223, 1961.
29. Fielding JW, Hawkins RJ: Atlanto-axial rotatory fixation. *J Bone Joint Surg* 59A:37, 1977.
30. Fielding JW, Stillwell WT, Chynn KY, Spropoulos EC: Use of computed tomography for the diagnosis of atlanto-axial rotatory fixation. *J Bone Joint Surg* 60A:1102, 1978.
31. Green JD, Harle TS, Harris JH: Anterior subluxation of the cervical spine: Hyperflexion sprain. *AJNR* 2:243, 1981.
32. Holdsworth FW: Fractures, dislocations, and fracture-dislocations of the spine. *J Bone Joint Surg* 45B:6, 1963.
33. Coin CG, Pennink M, Ahmad WD, Keranen V: Diving-type injury of the cervical spine: Contribution of computed tomography to management. *J Comput Assist Tomogr* 3:362, 1979.
34. Cooper PR, Cohen W: Evaluation of cervical spinal cord injuries with metrizamide myelography-CT scanning. *J Neurosurg* 61:281, 1984.
35. Morris RE, Hasso AN, Thompson JR, Hinshaw DB Jr, Vu H: Traumatic dural tears: CT diagnosis using metrizamide. *Radiology* 152:443–446, 1984.
36. Griffith HB, Gleave JRW, Taylor RG: Changing patterns of fracture in the dorsal and lumbar spine. *Br Med J* 1:891, 1966.
37. Rogers LF, Thayer C, Winberg PE, Kim KS: Acute injuries of the upper thoracic spine associated with paraplegia. *AJNR* 1:89, 1980.
38. Rogers LF: The roentgenographic appearance of transverse or change fractures of the spine: The seat belt fracture. *AJR* 111:844, 1971.
39. Smith, GR, Northrop CH, Loop JW: Jumpers' fractures: Patterns of thoracolumbar spine injuries associated with vertical plunges. *Radiology* 12:657, 1977.
40. Miller CA, Dewey RC, Hunt WE: Impaction fracture of the lumbar vertebrae with dural tear. *J Neurosurg* 53:765, 1980.
41. Guttman L: Surgical aspects of the treatment of traumatic paraplegia. *J Bone Joint Surg* 31B:399, 1949.
42. Burke DC, Murray DD: The management of thoracic and thoracolumbar injuries of the spine with neurological involvement. *J Bone Joint Surg* 58B:72, 1976.
43. Jacobs RR, Asher MA, Snider RK: Thoracolumbar spinal injuries: A comparative study of recumbent and operative treatment in 100 patients. *Spine* 5:463, 1980.

Chapter 5

CT of Chest Trauma

PHILIP C. GOODMAN, M.D.

INTRODUCTION

There appears to be a limited role for computed tomography in the evaluation of chest trauma. The literature contains few papers specifically addressing the use of CT in the setting of chest trauma (1–3). Another series of articles relates anecdotal experiences in this regard (4–12). This paucity of reports attests to the remarkable amount of information present on conventional chest radiographs as well as the lack of clear indications for CT in the setting of chest trauma.

In this chapter traumatic lesions of various areas of the thorax are discussed. The conventional radiographic findings are briefly described and the potential or proven application of CT is addressed.

INDICATIONS AND TECHNIQUE

In stable patients with confusing findings on conventional chest films, CT may provide information beneficial to the patient's management. In particular, within a day or two of the traumatic event, CT may permit differentiation of pleural from parenchymal abnormalities. The diagnosis of diaphragmatic rupture, difficult to make on plain films, may be aided by CT. Incidental findings of fractures, pneumomediastinum, pneumopericardium, pneumothorax, contusion, or traumatic lung cysts have been demonstrated by CT. However, no reported or personal experience would suggest that these entities be specifically investigated by CT. Tracheal and esophageal injuries are rare and correctly diagnosed by initial endoscopy or contrast studies. CT with the administration of oral contrast may be useful if esophageal perforation is being considered. If one suspects trauma to the aorta or great vessels angiography is the appropriate procedure. CT is not indicated in this setting and in fact may delay diagnosis while adding to the patient's contrast load.

Thoracic CT scans are obtained as 10 mm sections made at 10- to 20-mm intervals at the appropriate thoracic level depending upon the nature of the injury, clinical setting, and chest film findings. Abdominal scanning may be indicated if lower thoracic trauma

has been sustained. Intravenous iodinated contrast medium is usually not helpful.

Soft Tissues

A significant contrast difference between air and soft tissues allows an exquisite demonstration of subcutaneous emphysema by CT. If skin lacerations are absent, air in the soft tissues suggests the presence of an underlying pneumomediastinum or pneumothorax (Fig. 5.1).

Soft tissue hematomas or contusions may similarly be shown by CT. In general these are clinically insignificant, but one paper describes the use of CT scanning to differentiate a chest wall hematoma from what was considered to be a pleural fluid collection on radiographs made at the bedside (4). Findings of mottled subcutaneous air and/or soft tissue swelling seen days or weeks following trauma may represent an abscess. Clinical signs and symptoms, physical examination, or conventional chest radiography will usually suggest this diagnosis, but the extent of involvement prior to surgical drainage (if indicated) might be well delineated by CT. In the evaluation of poststernotomy wound infections, CT may afford excellent visualization of soft tissue, bone, and mediastinum (13).

Bony Thorax

The majority of traumatic rib fractures occur in adults, involve the midportion of the bony thorax, and are usually of little clinical significance. Flail chest, fractures of the first and second ribs, or tenth through twelfth ribs may be accompanied by severe intrathoracic or intra-abdominal injury and warrant further radiographic investigation (e.g., abdominal CT, aortography) (14–16).

Although CT of the bony thorax has been advocated for benign and malignant processes (17), its use for the evaluation of traumatic thoracic bone injury is most often pre-empted by the excellent demonstration of bone provided by conventional radiography (12, 18). Nevertheless, we have been able to clarify the etiology of an extrapleural mass (hematoma) by CT demonstration of an underlying rib fracture not visualized on chest films or on a limited rib series (Fig. 5.2). It has also been our experience that unsuspected scapular (Fig. 5.3) and sternal fractures (Fig. 5.4) may be better imaged on CT scans than on supine chest radiographs.

Posterior dislocation of the clavicle relative to the sternum is another injury perhaps best visualized by CT (19). Posterior displacement of the clavicle and sternal fracture fragments are also clearly depicted by this modality (Fig. 5.5). Extrinsic impingement upon the great vessels (e.g., superior vena cava) should be reliably demonstrated.

Pleural Space

Pneumo- and hemothorax represent two of the most common post-traumatic chest injuries. Depending on the amount of air or blood in the pleural space, treatment may be conservative (observation) or aggressive (thoracotomy or thoracostomy). Treatment of sizable hemothorax is best accomplished by tube thoracostomy, because late complications of empyema and restrictive pleural peel may otherwise occur.

In most instances of thoracic trauma, plain chest radiographs will provide adequate information regarding the presence of clinically important hemo- or pneumothorax. However, many post-traumatic pleural

fluid collections and some small pneumothoraces are missed on plain film radiography but are easily detected by CT (1). The incidental discovery of pneumothorax while performing post-traumatic abdominal CT has been described (20) (Figs. 5.6 and 5.7). Sections through the upper abdomen (lower thorax) should be viewed with wide window widths in these cases. The clinical significance of these otherwise unsuspected findings is variable. In general they do not influence the clinical course of the patient. However, in some instances, as with tension pneumothorax, or in individuals being ventilated with positive pressure or those undergoing anesthesia with nitrous oxide administration, chest tube therapy may be initiated (21).

CT is especially beneficial in evaluating post-traumatic pleural space complications. Various series have shown that the incidence of loculated hemothorax (Fig. 5.8) or empyema following penetrating chest trauma may approach 5 to 10% (22). CT demonstrates not only these pleural abnormalities but also permits accurate assessment of proper chest tube placement (Fig. 5.9). Finally, CT scanning may allow differentiation between hydro- and hemothorax, one report suggests (1), and may be useful in distinguishing the rare case of chylothorax.

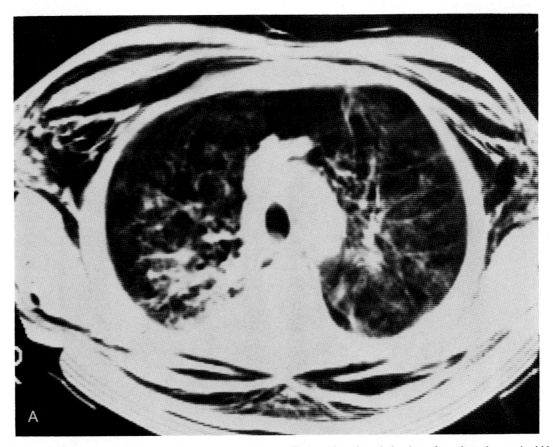

Figure 5.1. Subcutaneous emphysema and bilateral pneumothoraces. Three sections through the chest of a patient who sustained blunt chest trauma demonstrate a significant amount of subcutaneous emphysema in the anterior and lateral thoracic wall (**A**) as well as air in the leaves of the diaphragm (**B**, *arrows*). A right-sided pneumothorax is poorly imaged at this level (**B**, *circle*) but is better seen (along with a left pneumothorax) on a more caudal section (**C**, *circles*).

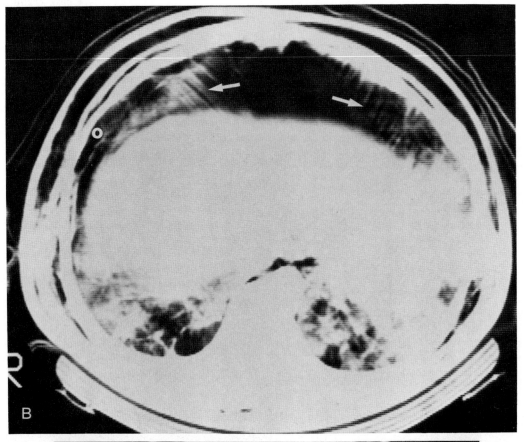

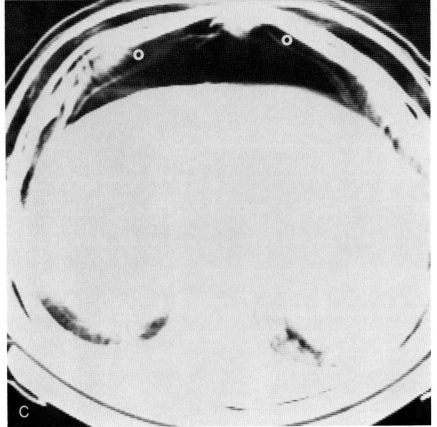

Figure 5.1.   B, C.

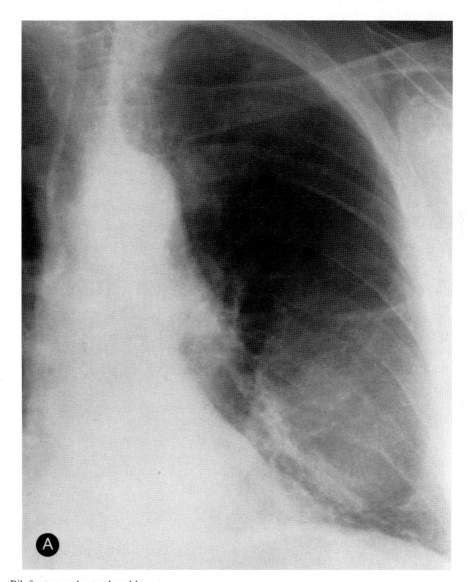

Figure 5.2.   Rib fracture and extrapleural hematoma.
A, B. Posteroanterior and lateral radiographs demonstrate posterior pleural or extrapleural soft tissue mass. Patient was unreliable historian who recalled no episode of trauma. Conventional films failed to reveal bony abnormality.
C. CT sections through the mass demonstrate an adjacent acute rib fracture.

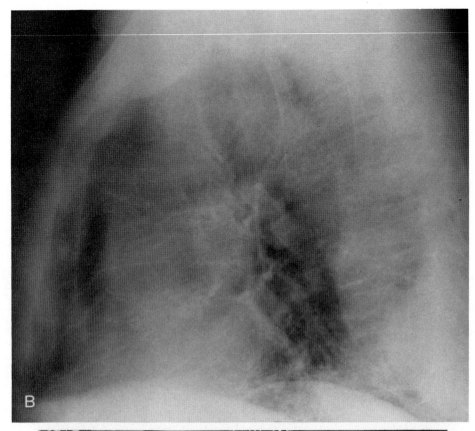

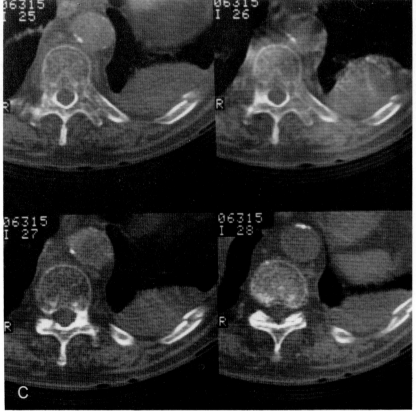

Figure 5.2.   B. C.

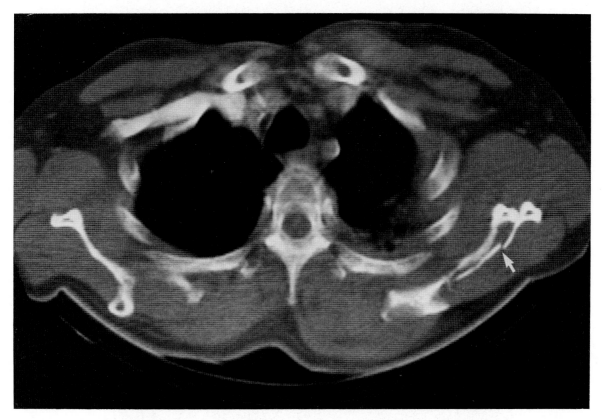

Figure 5.3. Scapular fracture. A CT section through the area of trauma reveals a scapular fracture (*arrow*) not appreciated on the chest radiograph. Incidentally revealed are an underlying hemothorax and lung contusion.

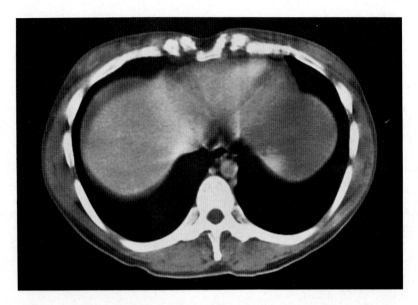

Figure 5.4.   Fracture of the sternum. The patient was struck in the upper abdomen. A section from the CT scan reveals a depressed lower sternal fracture not appreciated on plain films.

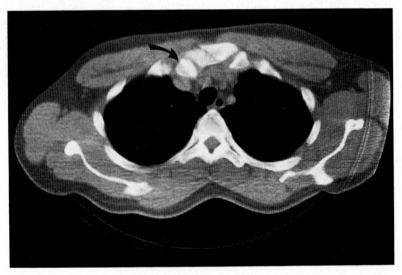

Figure 5.5.   Fracture of the sternum. A section from the CT scan demonstrates posterior displacement of the right clavicle (*arrow*) and right sternal fracture fragment. The clavicular head lies adjacent to but is not compressing the superior vena cava. Unsuspected sternal fracture following a ski accident in which the patient fell on the right shoulder.

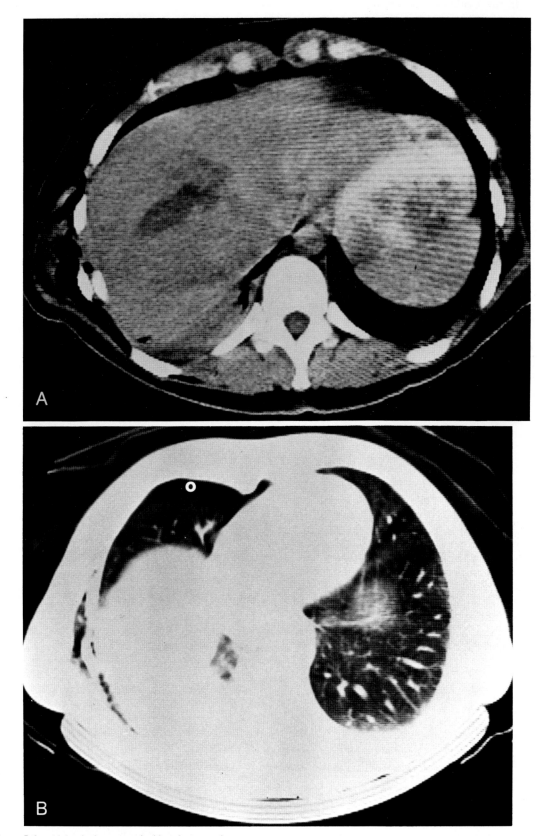

Figure 5.6.   Abdominal trauma—incidental pneumothorax.
A A CT section through the upper abdomen of a patient who sustained blunt trauma reveals a laceration of the right lobe of the liver and a displaced rib fracture.
B. A higher section imaged at a wide window width demonstrates a small, otherwise undetected right pneumothorax (*circle*). Subcutaneous emphysema is seen in the soft tissues of the right hemithorax.

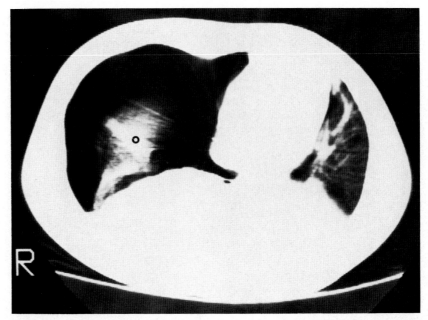

Figure 5.7. Tension pneumothorax. A CT section of the lower thorax was obtained during abdominal scanning. The right lower lobe is compressed (*circle*), and the heart is shifted to the left because of a large right tension pneumothorax. This was not detected in the emergency room and may have occurred on route to or in the CT area.

Pericardium

The diagnosis of life-threatening pericardial tamponade is suggested by clinical findings. There is no time for radiography, as without immediate pericardiocentesis or thoracotomy the patient will likely die (23). Less critical injury may result in pneumopericardium or a slowly acquired and better tolerated hemopericardium. On conventional chest radiographs pneumopericardium appears as a thin radiolucent line that parallels the heart border and root of the aorta or main pulmonary artery. Hemopericardium is seen as nonspecific cardiac enlargement. On CT, air or small fluid collections in the pericardium are readily demonstrated (Fig. 5.10) (24). Both conditions are generally benign and resolve in a period of days to weeks. Standard chest films and echocardiography are recommended for follow-up if clinically indicated.

Heart

Injury to the heart is reported in 16 to 76% of patients following blunt chest trauma and may be manifested by cardiac contusion, rupture, infarction, or, rarely, septal disruption (25). Patients may present with varied clinical complaints, nonspecific ECG findings, or elevated serum enzyme levels. The standard chest radiograph is rarely diagnostic. Heart size may be normal or enlarged; nonspecific pulmonary edema may or may not be present.

Unless sophisticated CT techniques (26, 27) are utilized, acute cardiac abnormalities will not be demonstrated on the initial scan. The value of these special scanning modalities in cardiac trauma diagnosis is not known.

Ventricular aneurysm may occur as a sequel to cardiac contusion or trauma-induced myocardial infarction. This has been noted from 3 weeks to 18 years after trauma (28) and can be detected on CT or conventional chest films by a change in heart contour, as well as calcium within the wall of the aneurysm (Fig. 5.11).

Lung

Pulmonary contusion is probably the most commonly suffered traumatic chest injury (29). Shearing of alveolar and capillary walls is the result of a force or shock wave transmitted from the site of impact through the lung. The initial chest roentgenogram usually reveals a nonsegmental interstitial or alveolar pattern which resolves significantly within 3 to 5 days. Persistent abnormalities should raise the possibility of superimposed pneumonia, a not infrequent occurrence (30). Pulmonary lacerations result in hematomas or traumatic lung cysts (31), which on chest radiography appear as spherical or elliptical soft tissue densities and round cavitary lesions, respectively (Fig. 5.12). The initial appearance of traumatic lung cysts may be obscured by surrounding contusion and/ or hemorrhage. Resolution time for these abnormalities is usually 1½ to 4 months. In general, the diagnosis and follow-up of contusion, hematoma, traumatic lung cyst, bullet tracts, and lung herniation, as well as potential complications such as atelectasis

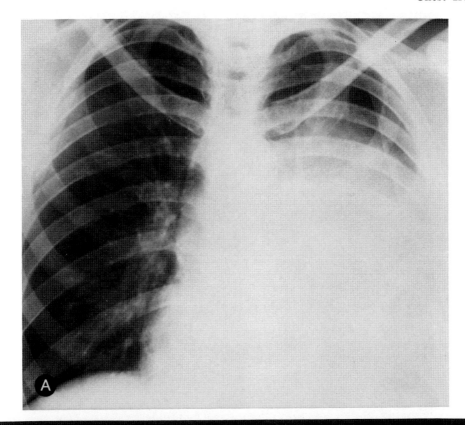

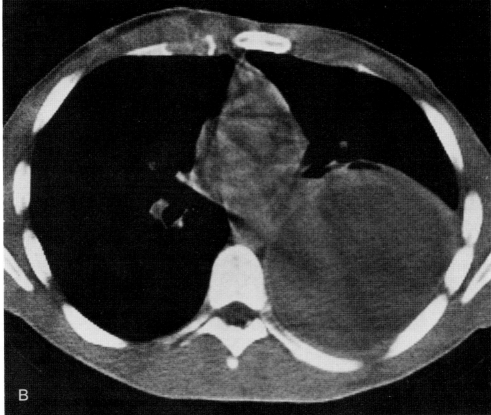

Figure 5.8.   Loculated hemothorax. The patient had been stabbed in the left chest 1 week earlier.
A. Posteroanterior chest radiograph demonstrates poorly marginated homogeneous opacification of lower left hemithorax.
B. CT scan of the thorax reveals a large, well-defined, low-density mass with a higher density rim. Chest tube placement resulted in drainage of a large amount of old blood.

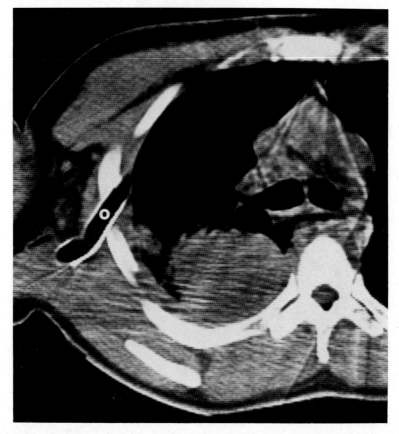

Figure 5.9.   Malpositioned chest tube. A CT scan reveals a previously diagnosed loculated empyema in a patient who had been stabbed 2 weeks earlier. Chest tube drainage had stopped, yet the patient continued to be febrile. The CT section demonstrates that the chest tube (*circle*) is well anterior to the fluid collection. Subsequent repositioning of the tube resulted in resolution of the patient's symptoms.

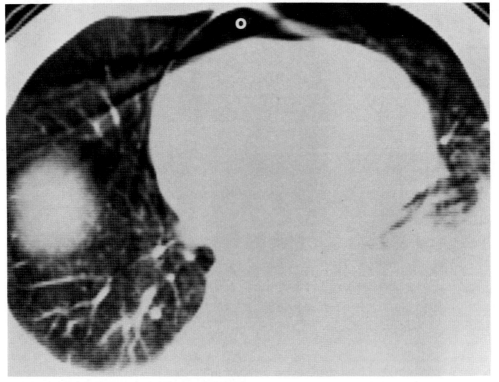

Figure 5.10.   Pneumopericardium. A CT section through the heart photographed at a wide window width reveals air in the anterior pericardial space (*circle*). The patient had sustained blunt chest trauma 10 hours earlier.

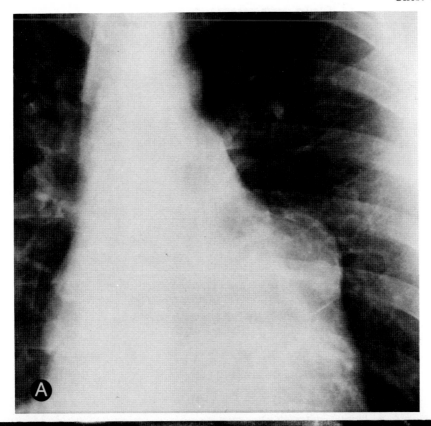

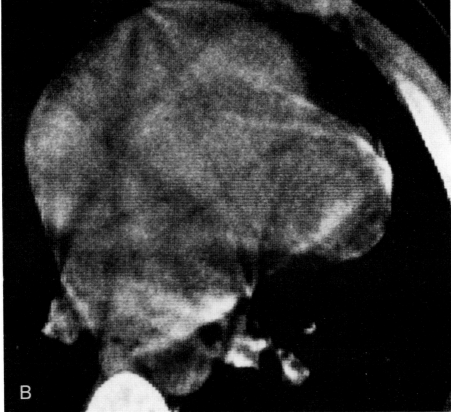

Figure 5.11.   Ventricular aneurysm. The patient suffered blunt chest trauma 1 year prior to admission.
A. A routine posteroanterior chest radiograph reveals a focal bulge in the left ventricular margin. A calcified rim is barely discernible around this aneurysm.
B. A CT section through the heart demonstrates the same focal aneurysm and calcified rim.

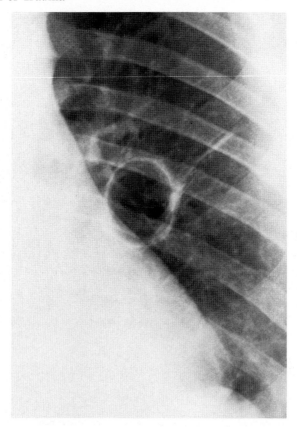

Figure 5.12.   Traumatic lung cyst. A magnified section of a posteroanterior chest film demonstrates a thin-walled, air-containing cavity that developed in the superior segment of the left lower lobe following a stabbing.

and pneumonia, are easily and inexpensively made on initial and follow-up chest films.

As compared to conventional chest radiography, CT may be more accurate in determining the extent of lung contusion. On CT, as on chest films, contusion is often depicted as a peripherally situated heterogeneous or homogeneous opacification of nonsegmental distribution (Figs. 5.13–5.15). Areas that appear normal on chest film may be abnormal on CT. Pulmonary hematomas (1), bullet tracts (1), possible post-traumatic atelectasis (1), and traumatic lung cysts (Figs. 5.16 and 5.17) have also been shown by CT.

In conclusion, although CT may provide some additional information regarding pulmonary contusion, it does not appear that the cost and effort of obtaining this information are warranted. Therapy is directed at the clinical status of the patient (respiratory symptoms, blood gases, ventilatory requirements, etc.) and is unlikely to be altered by the demonstration of slightly more lung damage than depicted on plain films. Although there may be a role for CT in the evaluation of patients with infectious complications of trauma (demonstration of an otherwise undetectable lung abscess or localized empyema), the standard chest film remains the primary radiographic modality for the investigation of traumatic pulmonary disease.

Aorta and Great Vessels

The significance of trauma to the thoracic aorta and great vessels cannot be overemphasized. Up to 90% of patients with this injury die immediately. Of the untreated survivors, 50% will die within 24 hours (6). Only 2 to 5% of untreated patients will live, and they subsequently develop chronic aortic aneurysms which may rupture at any time over the next several years (32).

Although it is obvious that early diagnosis is mandatory to preserve life, this is often hindered by the nonspecific presentation of the victims, who have generally sustained multiple injuries.

The initial chest film usually provides the first clue to the diagnosis. Typical findings include widening of the mediastinum, left apical pleural cap, or rightward displacement of the trachea or esophagus (33, 34, 35). Aortography must be performed to confirm the presence of aortic trauma. This modality not only permits demonstration of aortic pseudoaneurysms and initimal tears, but also defines injuries to the great vessels of the aortic arch (36–38).

CT has not been proven to be of benefit in the diagnosis of aortic trauma. In one report, five trauma victims had CT to assess the aorta. The authors used the appearance of surrounding hematomas or medi-

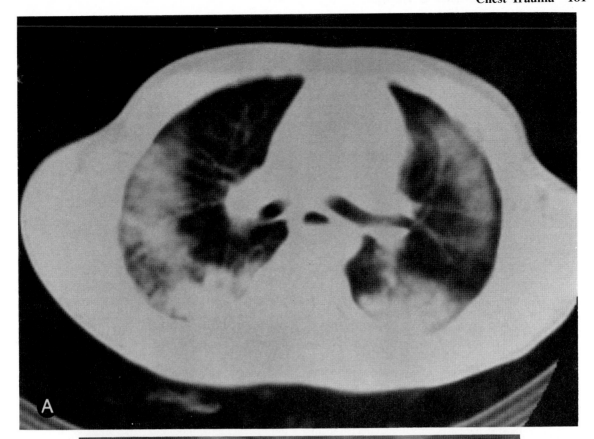

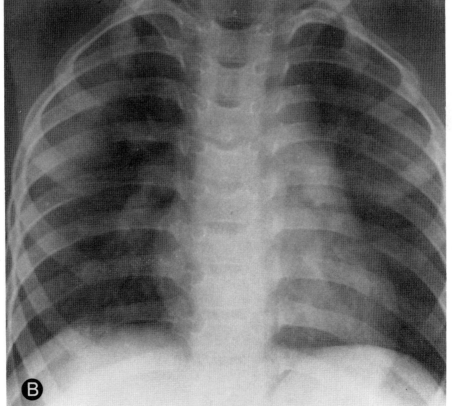

Figure 5.13.   Pulmonary contusion—child struck by an automobile.
A. A CT section of the thorax reveals bilateral, peripheral, nonsegmental areas of increased density.
B. These findings correlated well with similar chest film abnormalities which resolved within 3 days, thus supporting the diagnosis of pulmonary contusion.

astinal widening to suggest the presence of aortic injury. Subsequent aortography was then performed and was normal in all cases. In one patient without mediastinal widening the authors predicted that the aortogram would be negative; in three patients they believed the aortogram would be negative but could not be sure; and in one case they thought the aortogram should be positive (39). This study emphasizes an important consideration—that although mediastinal widening, indeed mediastinal hemorrhage, is common in thoracic trauma, in up to two-thirds of patients the bleeding occurs from small arteries or veins not amenable to radiographic demonstration or surgical intervention. Thus, although CT may demonstrate blood in the mediastinum, this finding in no way implicates the aorta as the source of bleeding. Conversely, absence of mediastinal hemorrhage cannot exclude the presence of an aortic intimal tear.

Another article listed the CT findings of aortic rupture in four patients. Those observed were false aneurysm, linear lucency in the opacified aortic lumen, irregularity of the aorta, periaortic or intramural aortic hematoma, and dissections (Fig. 5.18). Their cases were performed in stable patients after indicated CT head scans. All instances of rupture (four) were detected in 10 patients. No false negatives were recorded (3). They concluded that, although CT was sensitive in their selected and small population, it could not be used as the basis for surgical decisions in all patients and that its sensitivity for small tears was unknown.

I and others (40) do not feel that CT has a role in this setting. The findings of aortic rupture on CT may be subtle or indeterminate (39), and, given the explosive nature of this injury, there is no time to spare in proceeding to angiography, the time-tested procedure of choice. Furthermore, these patients are difficult to examine by CT as they are very often critically ill with other injuries, and patient movement, artifact-producing body parts (e.g., shoulders), and life support apparatus may cause degradation of the CT image (Fig. 5.18). Finally, CT will probably not prove sensitive in detecting trauma to the innominate or subclavian vessels and could thus miss a potentially life-threatening lesion.

In conclusion, it is best assumed that CT is not applicable to the evaluation of aortic arch injuries. Aortography remains the appropriate technique for diagnosis.

Trachea and Bronchi

Rupture of the tracheobronchial tree is an uncommon result of chest trauma. Fractures of the trachea and bronchi usually occur within 2½ cm of the carina (7) and thus are easily visualized by either rigid or flexible bronchoscopy. The diagnosis is usually suggested by certain clinical circumstances including a setting of severe chest trauma, significant mediastinal and subcutaneous emphysema, persistent pneumothorax or air leak, and atelectasis of a lobe or lung (41).

Chest film findings include pneumothorax, pneumomediastinum, subcutaneous emphysema, "bayonet" deformity of the interrupted bronchus, rib fractures, and the "falling lung sign" where, in the presence of pneumothorax, the lung on the side of bronchial disruption falls to the dependent portion of the hemithorax (42).

CT has not been reported to be beneficial in diagnosing tracheobronchial injuries. Although this modality would certainly detect the abnormalities incurred from trauma (Fig. 5.19), the standard chest radiograph and appropriate clinical findings are usually enough to suggest bronchoscopy for definite diagnosis.

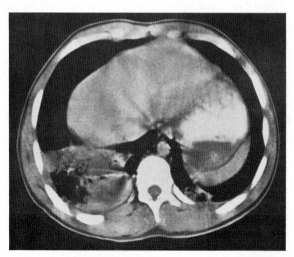

Figure 5.14. Pulmonary contusion. A CT section through the lower thorax demonstrates a large area of increased density in the right lower lobe. A large, irregular, lucent zone within the contusion may represent the early appearance of a traumatic lung cyst.

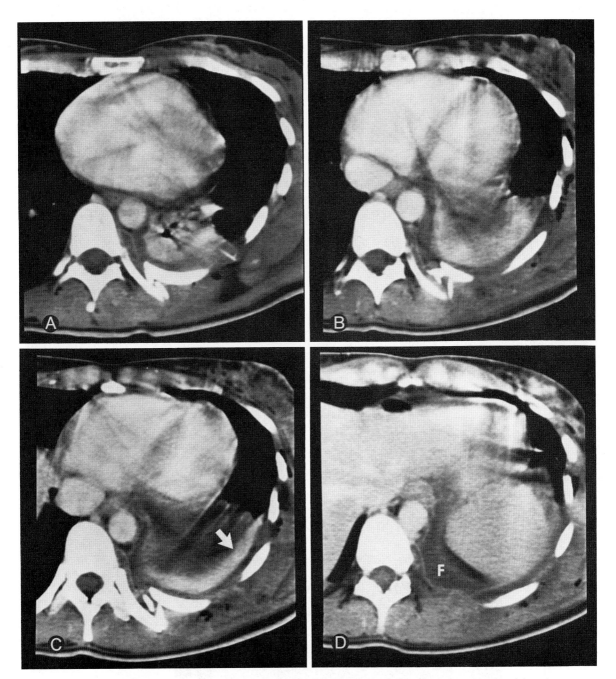

Figure 5.15.   Lung contusion. Four sections reveal a left lower lobe contusion. In the superior aspect of the contusion air bronchograms are noted (**A**). On a lower section a more dense and homogeneous appearance is evident (**B**). This is due to contrast enhancement in the injured, airless lung. The next lower section (**C**) reveals a crescent shape to the enhancing lower lobe (*arrow*). This may simulate clotted blood in the pleural space. On a more caudal section (**D**) near water density pleural fluid (*F*) is seen in the paravertebral pleural space.

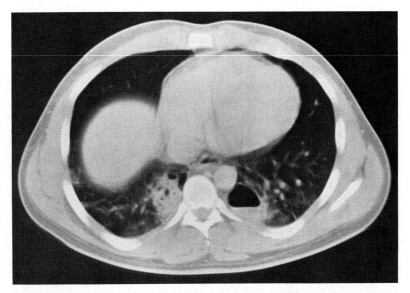

Figure 5.16.   Traumatic lung cyst. A CT section through the lower thorax reveals bilateral lower lobe contusions. In addition, a thin-walled cavity containing an air-fluid level is present on the left. The patient had fallen from a ladder hours before the CT scan.

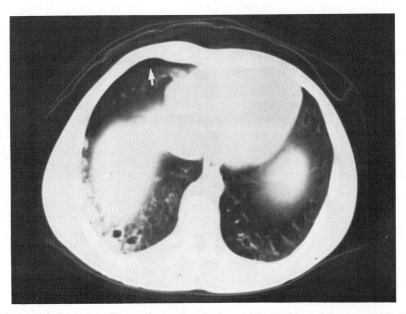

Figure 5.17.   Multiple traumatic lung cysts. Two poorly margined, air-containing cavities are demonstrated in the right lower lobe. Peripheral contusion is noted just anterolateral to the cavities, one of which contains an air-fluid level. A small right pneumothorax is incidentally seen (*arrow*). The patient was struck by an automobile.

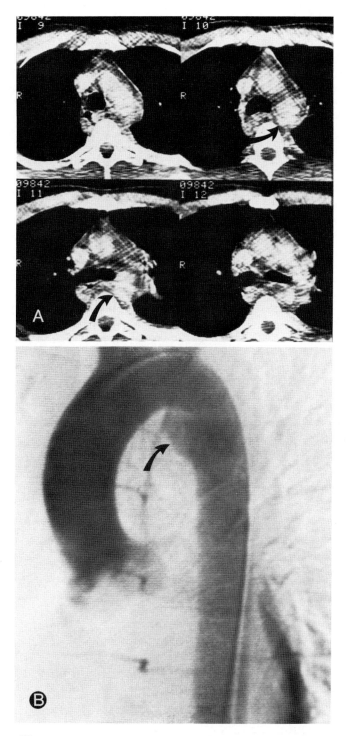

Figure 5.18. Aortic rupture—CT.
A. Four sections of a dynamic sequence reveal irregularity of the proximal descending thoracic aorta (*arrows*). Note degradation of the image due to artifacts emanating from the bony thorax. The patient initially underwent a head scan. The chest CT was then performed because of a widened mediastinum. Instead the patient should have been taken directly to angiography.
B. Aortic rupture—intra-arterial digital subtraction aortography. A right posterior oblique view of the aortic arch reveals a traumatic rupture at the aortic isthmus (*arrow*).

Esophagus

Because of its central location and the protective nature of the bony thorax, the esophagus is rarely injured following chest trauma. When rupture occurs it is usually secondary to severe chest and/or abdominal compression. Death due to fulminant mediastinitis may occur in 80 to 90% of patients (30, 43). Iatrogenic penetrating injuries account for the vast majority of traumatic esophageal perforations. Tracheoesophageal fistulas may be formed following either blunt or penetrating trauma and may, in fact, protect the patient from mediastinitis by providing a drainage route for esophageal contents (43).

Clinically these patients present with fever, chest pain, tachycardia, dyspnea, dysphagia, and shock. The chest radiograph may reveal pneumomediastinum, widened mediastinum, pneumothorax, and pleural fluid. Both barium and water-soluble contrast agents have been used to demonstrate the site of perforation in up to 75% of patients (42), and this remains the procedure of choice if esophageal injury is suspected.

CT may be useful in assessing mediastinitis from an unsuspected or delayed esophageal perforation (44). This modality is particularly useful in demonstrating the air and fluid collections seen with mediastinal inflammation. The site of tracheoesophageal fistula or communication between the esophagus and a mediastinal air-fluid collection might also be imaged on CT scan (Fig. 5.20) (44).

Diaphragm

Approximately 3 to 5% of patients suffering blunt chest trauma will incur a diaphragmatic rupture (11, 45, 46). Seventy-five to 90% of these occur on the left, creating a potential for herniation of colon, stomach, small bowel, omentum, or spleen. Recognition of diaphragmatic tears may be delayed for days, months, or years; they are often only discovered when the patient presents with herniated intra-abdominal contents.

The difficulty in the diagnosis of ruptured diaphragm is well appreciated. Clinical findings are often masked by signs and symptoms of concomitantly suffered injuries. Chest radiographic findings may range from nonspecific diaphragmatic irregularity to definite evidence of a hollow viscus in the left hemithorax (47). Nuclear medicine and ultrasound have been used to diagnose right-sided ruptures with liver herniation (12, 48, 49). Fluoroscopy, diagnostic pneumoperitoneum, arteriography, and emergency thoracoscopy have also been advanced as approaches to this difficult problem.

Several cases of CT diagnosis of traumatic diaphragmatic hernia have been reported (1, 8, 10, 11, 50). Most have involved the left hemidiaphragm or central tendon of the diaphragm with herniation of stomach, omentum, small bowel, spleen, or large bowel into the thorax or pericardium (Fig. 5.21). If the diaphragm is clearly demonstrated with intra-abdominal contents lateral to it, then discontinuity of the

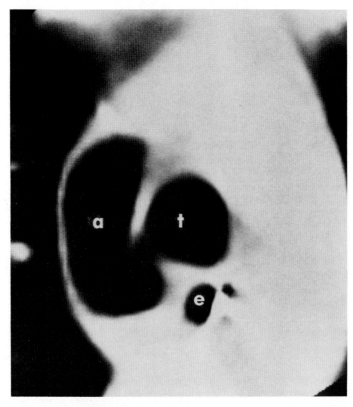

Figure 5.19. Tracheomediastinal communication. This patient developed mediastinitis following esophageal instrumentation. Several days into his hospital course, a CT scan was obtained to define the mediastinal anatomy better. A section through the upper mediastinum reveals a perforation in the right posterior wall of the trachea (*t*) with communication to a large abscess cavity (*a*). (*e*, esophagus.)

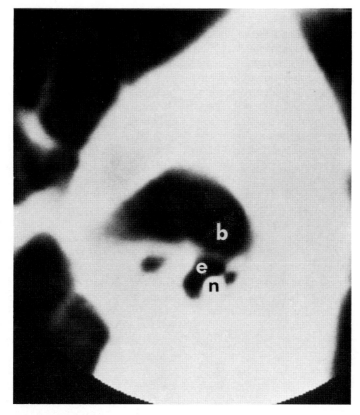

Figure 5.20.   Bronchoesophageal fistula—same patient as in Figure 5.19. A CT section at the level of the carina reveals a communication between the proximal left mainstem bronchus (*b*) and the esophagus (*e*). (*n*, nasogastric tube.)

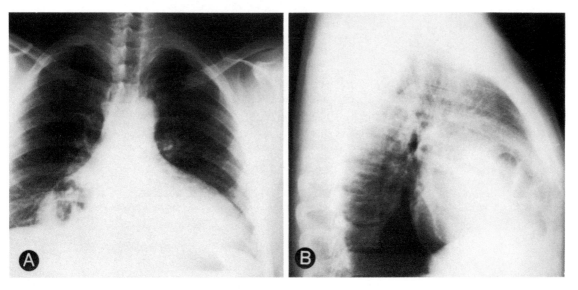

Figure 5.21.   Diaphragmatic hernia.
A, B. Posteroanterior and lateral chest radiographs reveal an air-containing structure overlying the right anterior hemithorax.

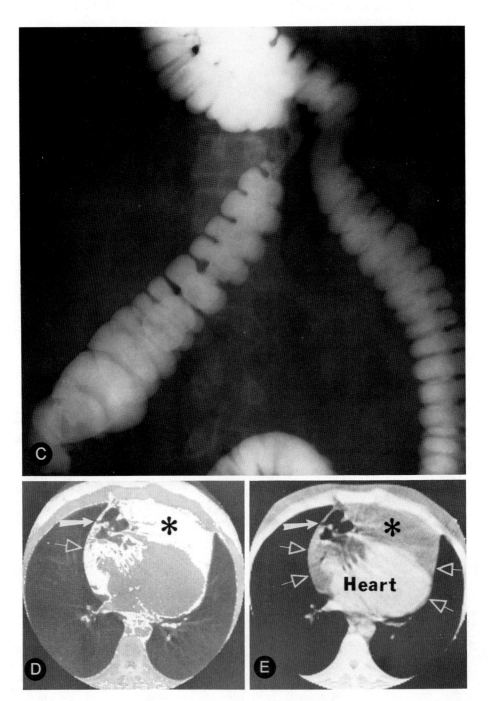

Figure 5.21.
C. A subsequent barium enema demonstrates a portion of large bowel herniated above the diaphragm.
D, E. CT scan of the thorax reveals both herniated bowel (*white arrow*) and fat (*) within the pericardium (*open arrows*). (From Fagan CJ, Schreiber MH, Amparo EG, Wysong CB: Traumatic diaphragmatic hernia into the pericardium: Verification of diagnosis by computed tomography. *J Comput Assist Tomogr* 3:405, 1979.)

diaphragm with herniation must be present (Fig. 5.22). However, without this clear definition of diaphragm, apparent intrathoracic herniation of abdominal structures may actually represent an eventration or high position of an intact diaphragm.

As there is a fairly high incidence of intra-abdominal organ damage seen in association with diaphragmatic rupture or with lower thoracic penetrating or blunt trauma (9), CT should be directed toward examination of the abdomen in such situations.

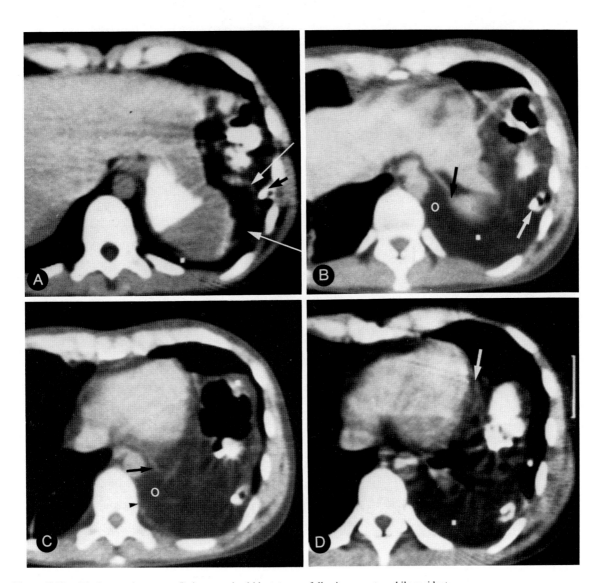

Figure 5.22.   Diaphragmatic rupture. Patient sustained blunt trauma following an automobile accident.
A. A CT section through the lower thorax demonstrates a contrast- and air-filled loop of bowel (*black arrow*) lateral to diaphragm (*white arrows*).
B. A section done 2 cm higher reveals fat (*circle*) posterior to the diaphragm, where it is contiguous with the spleen tip or gastric fundus (*black arrow*). Bowel loops (*white arrow*) are seen lateral to the expected position of the diaphragm, thus indicating their intrathoracic location.
C. Another section 1.4 cm above demonstrates loops of bowel in the chest lateral to the pleural-pericardial reflection (*arrow*).
D. A CT section done 1.4 cm above the previous slice demonstrates loops of bowel in the chest lateral to the pleural-pericardial reflection (*arrow*). (From Heiberg E, Wolverson MK, Hurd RN, et al: CT recognition of traumatic rupture of the diaphragm. *AJR* 135:369, 1980.)

REFERENCES

1. Toombs BD, Sandler CM, Lester RG: Computed tomography of chest trauma. *Radiology* 140:733, 1981.
2. Hagemann J, Gurtler K-F: Thoraxverletzungen. In *Fortschritte auf dem Gebiete der Rontgenstrahlen und der Nuklearmedizin. Diagnostik, Physik, Biologie, Therapie,* suppl 119. Stuttgart, Georg Thieme Verlag, 1984. chap. 6.
3. Heiberg E, Wolverson MK, Sundaram M, Shields JB: CT in aortic trauma. *AJR* 140:1119, 1983.
4. Roddy LH, Unger KM, Miller WC: Thoracic computed tomography in the critically ill patient. *Crit Care Med* 9:515, 1981.
5. Toombs BD, Lester RG, Ben-Menachem Y, Sandler CM: Computed tomography in blunt trauma. *Radiol Clin North Am* 19:17, 1981.
6. Fishbone G, Robbins DI, Osborn DJ, et al: Trauma to the thoracic aorta and great vessels. *Radiol Clin North Am* 11:543, 1973.
7. Krish MM, Orringer MB, Behrendt DM, et al: Management of tracheobronchial disruption secondary to nonpenetrating trauma. *Ann Thorac Surg* 22:93, 1976.
8. Fagan CJ, Schreiber MH, Amparo EG, Wysong CB: Traumatic diaphragmatic hernia into the pericardium: Verification of diagnosis by computed tomography. *J Comput Assist Tomogr* 3:405, 1979.
9. Moore JB, Moore EE, Thompson JS: Abdominal injuries associated with penetrating trauma in the lower chest. *Am J Surg* 140:724, 1980.
10. Adamthwaite DN, Snyders DC, Mirwis J: Traumatic pericardiophrenic hernia: A report of 3 cases. *Br J Surg* 70:117, 1983.
11. Adamthwaite DN: Traumatic diaphragmatic hernia. *Surg Ann* XX:vol. 15 73, 1983.
12. Kim EE, McConnell BJ, McConnell RW, et al: Radionuclide diagnosis of diaphragmatic rupture with hepatic herniation. *Surgery* 94:36, 1983.
13. Kay HR, Goodman LR, Teplick SK, Mundth ED: Use of computed tomography to assess mediastinal complications after median sternotomy. *Ann Thorac Surg* 36:706, 1983.
14. Wilson JM, Thomas AN, Goodman PC, Lewis FR: Severe chest trauma: Morbidity implication of first and second rib fracture in 120 patients. *Arch Surg* 113:846, 178.
15. Yee ES, Thomas AN, Goodman PC: Isolated first rib fracture: Clinical significance after blunt chest trauma. *Ann Thorac Surg* 32:278, 1981.
16. Goodman PC: Blunt chest trauma. In Margulis AR, Gooding CA (eds): *Diagnostic Radiology.* San Francisco, University of California Press, 1978, pp 599–607.
17. deGautard R, Dussault RG, Chahlaoui J, et al: Contribution of CT in thoracic bony lesions. *J Can Assoc Radiol* 32:39, 1981.
18. DeLuca SA, Rhea JT, O'Malley T: Radiographic evaluation of rib fractures. *AJR* 138:91, 1982.
19. Levinsohn EM, Bunnell WP, Yuan HA: Computed tomography in the diagnosis of dislocation of the sternoclavicular joint. *Clin Orthop* 140:12, 1979.
20. Wall S, Federle MF, Jeffrey RB, Brett CM: CT diagnosis of unsuspected pneumothorax after blunt abdominal trauma. *AJR* 141:919, 1983.
21. Cohn R: Nonpenetrating wounds of the lungs and bronchi. *Surg Clin North Am* 52:585, 1972.
22. Grover FL, Richardson DJ, Fewel JG, et al: Prophylactic antibiotics in the treatment of penetrating chest wounds. *J Thorac Cardiovasc Surg* 74:528, 1977.
23. Trunkey DD, Lewis FR: Chest trauma. *Surg Clin North Am* 60:1541, 1980.
24. Houang MTW, Arozena X, Shaw DG: Demonstration of pericardium and pericardial effusion by computed tomography. *J Comput Assist Tomogr* 3:601, 1979.

25. Symbas P: *Trauma to the Heart and Great Vessels.* New York, Grune & Stratton, 1978.
26. Lipton MJ, Higgins CB, Farmer D, Boyd DP: Cardiac imaging with a high-speed cine-CT scanner: Preliminary results. *Radiology* 152:579, 1984.
27. Oyama Y, Uji, T, Hirayama T, et al: Gated cardiac imaging using a continuously rotating CT scanner: Clinical evaluation of 91 patients. *AJR* 141:865, 1984.
28. Silver GN, Spampinato N, Favolara R, et al: Ventricular aneurysms and blunt chest trauma. *Chest* 63:628, 1973.
29. Williams JR, Bonte FJ: *The Roentgenological Aspect of Nonpenetrating Chest Injuries.* Springfield, IL, Charles C Thomas, 1961.
30. Jones KW: Thoracic trauma. *Surg Clin North Am* 60:957, 1980.
31. Ganske JG, Dennis DL, Vanderveer JB Jr: Traumatic lung cyst: Case report and literature review. *J Trauma* 21:493, 1981.
32. Parmley LF, Mattingly TW, Manion WC, et al: Nonpenetrating traumatic injury of the aorta. *Circulation* 17:1086, 1958.
33. Simeone JF, Minagi H, Putman CE: Traumatic disruption of the thoracic aorta: Significance of the left apical extrapleural cap. *Radiology* 17:265, 1975.
34. Tisnado J, Tsai FY, Als A, Roach JF: A new radiographic sign of acute traumatic rupture of the thoracic aorta: Displacement of the nasogastric tube to the right. *Radiology* 125:603, 1977.
35. Stark P: Traumatic rupture of the thoracic aorta: A review. *CRC Crit Rev Diagn Imaging* 21:229, 1984.
36. Baldwin JC, Oyer PE, Guthaner DF, Stinston EB: Combined azygous vein and subclavian artery injury in blunt chest trauma. *J Trauma* 24:170, 1984.
37. Dula DJ, Hughes HG, Majernick T: Traumatic disruption of the brachiocephalic artery. *Ann Emerg Med* 12:639, 1983.
38. Faro RS, Monson DO, Weinberg M, Javid H: Disruption of aortic arch branches due to nonpenetrating chest trauma. *Arch Surg* 118:1333, 1983.
39. Egan TJ, Neiman HL, Herman RJ, et al: Computed tomography in the diagnosis of aortic aneurysm, dissection or traumatic injury. *Radiology* 136:141, 1980.
40. Godwin JD, Korobkin M: Acute disease of the aorta. Diagnosis by computed tomography and ultrasonography. *Radiol Clin North Am* 21:551, 1983.
41. Maltby JD: The post-trauma chest film. *CRC Crit Rev Diagn Imaging* 14:1, 1980.
42. Moore AV, Putnam CE, Ravin CE: The radiology of thoracic trauma. *Bull NY Acad Med* 57:272, 1981.
43. Worman LW, Hurley JD, Pemberton AH, Narodick BG: Rupture of the esophagus from external blunt trauma. *Arch Surg* 85:173, 1962.
44. Faling LJ, Pugatch RD, Robbins AH: The diagnosis of unsuspected esophageal perforation by computed tomography. *Am J Med Sci* 281:31, 1981.
45. Brooks JW: Blunt traumatic rupture of the diaphragm. *Ann Thorac Surg* 26:199, 1978.
46. Orringer MG, Kirsch MM: Traumatic rupture of the diaphragm. In Kirsch MM, Sloan H (eds): *Blunt Chest Trauma, General Principles of Management.* Boston, Little, Brown and Co, 1977.
47. Minagi H, Brody WR, Laing FC: The variable roentgen appearance of traumatic diaphragmatic hernia. *J Can Assoc Radiol* 28:124, 1977.
48. Harman PK, Mentzer RM Jr, Weinberg AC, et al: Early diagnosis by liver scan of a right-sided traumatic diaphragmatic hernia. *J Trauma* 21:489, 1981.
49. Rao KG, Woodlief RM: Grey scale ultrasonic demonstration of ruptured right hemidiaphragm. *Br J Radiol* 53:812, 1980.
50. Heiberg E, Wolverson MK, Hurd RN, et al: CT recognition of traumatic rupture of the diaphragm. *AJR* 135:369, 1980.

Chapter 6

CT of Abdominal Trauma

MICHAEL P. FEDERLE, M.D.

INTRODUCTION

In the United States, accidents rank fourth as the cause of death, and approximately 10% of the annual 160,000 trauma-related deaths in the United States are due to abdominal injury (1, 2). Abdominal trauma may cause injury to multiple intra-abdominal and retroperitoneal viscera, and it is frequently difficult accurately to evaluate the site and extent of suspected internal injuries in the abdomen. There have been numerous reports on the efficacy of various imaging modalities—such as plain radiography, radionuclide scanning, and angiography—in diagnosing specific types of injuries, such as splenic or renal lacerations. However, in the comprehensive evaluation of patients with abdominal trauma, these tests have been of limited value. As a result of diagnostic uncertainty, patients frequently undergo nontherapeutic exploratory laparotomy or suffer from delayed diagnosis of significant traumatic injuries.

Soon after it became available for clinical use, cranial CT became the method of choice for evaluating head trauma. Only relatively recently have newer generation full-body scanners been installed at major trauma centers, but experience is rapidly being gained in the utilization of CT for abdominal trauma. CT has proved highly accurate in diagnosing a wide variety of injuries to both intra- and retroperitoneal organs in pediatric and adult patient populations (3–9). The impact has been evident not only in decreasing utilization of other diagnostic tests, such as angiography, but also in practical management decisions, such as whether to perform exploratory laparotomy. This chapter details our approach to evaluation of abdominal trauma by CT.

INDICATIONS

The type and extent of injury help to dictate the nature of the radiographic evaluation. Cases of life-threatening injuries accompanied by unstable vital signs permit only the most cursory radiologic evaluation. In less threatening circumstances, clinical and laboratory findings should be considered in selecting the most appropriate diagnostic studies. Referring physicians should be consulted as to the mechanism of injury and the presence or absence of physical findings, such as ecchymosis or focal tenderness, and relevant laboratory data, such as elevated serum amylase or hematuria. Frequently, there are some signs on preliminary radiographs, such as rib, spine, or pelvic fractures, which suggest a need for close scrutiny of adjacent viscera and which help to direct the choice of further diagnostic evaluation. Patients with penetrating peritoneal trauma, peritonitis, or hypotension unresponsive to volume replacement are *not* candidates for CT scanning. At the opposite end of the injury spectrum, patients with trivial injuries and normal vital signs are usually adequately evaluated clinically and do not require CT scanning.

Two groups of patients are best evaluated by CT. The first is that group with physical and laboratory evidence of substantial abdominal trauma, but relatively stable vital signs. These patients often have a lowered hematocrit, leukocytosis, hyperamylasemia, and rib fractures. While some physicians might consider these adequate criteria for surgical exploration, we find that CT often excludes abdominal injury completely or demonstrates lesions not amenable to surgical repair (e.g., certain retroperitoneal injuries). The second group consists of patients with signs of generalized or abdominal trauma in whom the abdominal physical examination is believed to be unreliable. This includes patients with altered mental status due to intoxication or head trauma and paraplegic or quadriplegic patients, as well as patients with severe pelvic or extremity injuries. Patients suffering head and abdominal trauma are commonly studied by cranial and body CT immediately after emergency department evaluation and resuscitation. As discussed later, CT is now used to evaluate patients who would formerly have been studied by diagnostic peritoneal lavage. Figure 6.1 is a flow diagram illustrating the suggested role of CT in evaluation of blunt abdominal trauma (10).

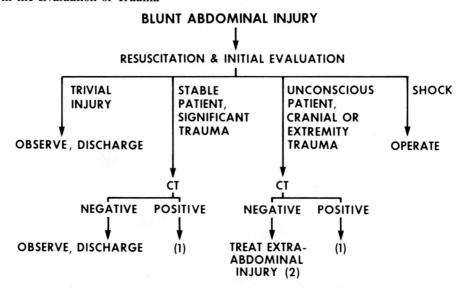

Figure 6.1.   Suggested use of CT in evaluation of blunt abdominal trauma.

TECHNIQUE

CT examinations for abdominal trauma are performed in a fairly standardized manner at our center. All patients receive a dilute solution of Gastrografin (Squibb, meglumine and sodium diatrizoate) either orally or by nasogastric tube, since unopacified bowel may be mistaken for abnormal fluid collections. Ideally, 500 ml of a 2% solution are administered 30 to 45 minutes prior to the CT examination; this can be done in the emergency department during initial evaluation and stabilization. However, many patients have an ileus or must be scanned without waiting for contrast to reach distal bowel. It is optimal to have the stomach and proximal bowel opacified by even more dilute contrast material (240 ml of 1 to 2% Gastrografin), since more concentrated solutions produce streak artifacts due to the air-contrast level within the stomach. At the end of the CT examination, the stomach is emptied via nasogastric suction, especially in obtunded patients or those likely to undergo surgery. In scans of the pelvis, it is occasionally useful to opacify rectosigmoid colon with about 150 ml of 2 to 3% Gastrografin to distinguish colon from pelvic hematomas.

Intravenous contrast medium is also extremely useful for identifying and classifying renal injuries and for improving detectability of other abdominal visceral injuries. As later explained more completely, hematomas and parenchymal lacerations are generally less dense than contract-enhanced liver or spleen. Hematomas are commonly similar in density (attenua-

tion) to nonenhanced parenchyma, but they are rarely similar to enhanced parenchyma. Therefore, contrast-enhanced scans are always obtained unless the patient has a record of severe contrast allergy. If nonenhanced sections through the upper abdomen are obtained, they may demonstrate hematomas as hyperdense relative to viscera, thus improving diagnostic certainty in those cases in which the hematoma is nearly isodense with contrast-enhanced parenchyma.

An adequate volume of contrast medium must be administered to accentuate the difference between hematomas and parenchyma. We usually inject a 50 ml bolus followed by a continuous drip (for a total of 100 to 150 ml) of 60% iothalamate meglumine. Children receive 2 to 3 ml/kg of body weight. Smaller amounts of contrast media increase the likelihood of isodense hematomas and decrease the accuracy of diagnosis.

Proper spacing of CT sections is also important. In our early work, we suggested that sections through the lower abdomen and pelvis were necessary only if bleeding or visceral injuries were evident on higher sections. However, the extent of hemoperitoneum may be seriously underestimated unless sections through the pelvis are obtained. We have seen many cases with a seemingly trivial laceration and a small amount of blood on sections through the upper abdomen, but a large pool of blood in the pelvis. We therefore recommend closely spaced (every 10 or 15 mm) sections 10 mm thick from the diaphragm through the bottom of the kidneys, and sections at 2- or 3-mm intervals through the pelvis (Fig. 6.2).

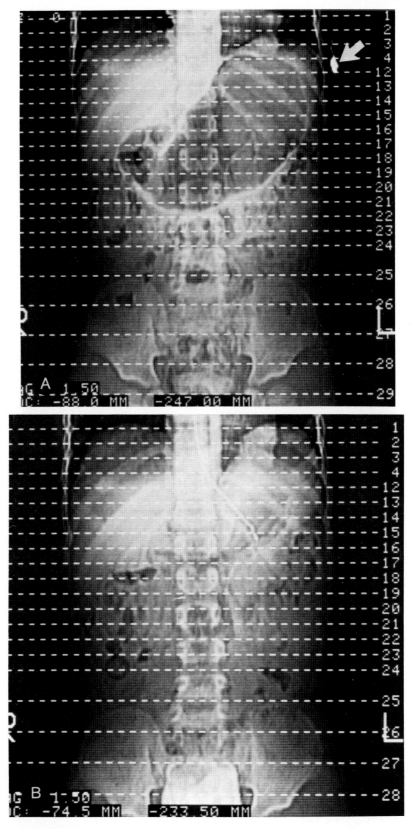

Figure 6.2.   CT scanning technique.

A. Digital radiograph (Scoutview, G.E.) with numbered lines indicating level of CT sections to be obtained at 1-cm intervals from diaphragm to bottom of kidneys, then at 2-cm intervals through the pelvis. Note presence of gastric distention and ECG monitor lead over left upper abdomen (*arrow*). Both would cause streak artifacts.

B. Repeat radiograph following insertion of nasogastric tube to decompress stomach. After instillation of dilute Gastrografin, the tube will be withdrawn into the distal esophagus. The ECG lead has been removed from the scanning field.

In addition to the usual "soft tissue windows" for viewing trauma CT scans, sections through the upper abdomen should be viewed and photographed at "lung windows" (level—700 Hounsfield units (H), width 1000 to 1500 H). A substantial portion of the minus lower thorax is visible on sections taken through the top of the liver and spleen. When viewed at lung window settings, traumatic thoracic lesions that are not detectable on soft tissue windows become evident, including pneumothorax and lung laceration (11) (Fig. 6.3). The importance of these observations is discussed in Chapter 5 (CT of Chest Trauma).

Various artifacts are commonly encountered in trauma CT studies and may seriously degrade images and decrease accuracy. Newer CT scanners with 1- to 3-second scan times have markedly decreased the severity of artifacts, but attention to proper scan technique is always important and can minimize artifacts. Streak artifacts from the gastric air-fluid level are decreased by decompression of the stomach by nasogastric tube prior to installation of contrast medium. The tip of the nasogastric tube should then be withdrawn into the distal esophagus. All extraneous objects should be removed from the scanning field,

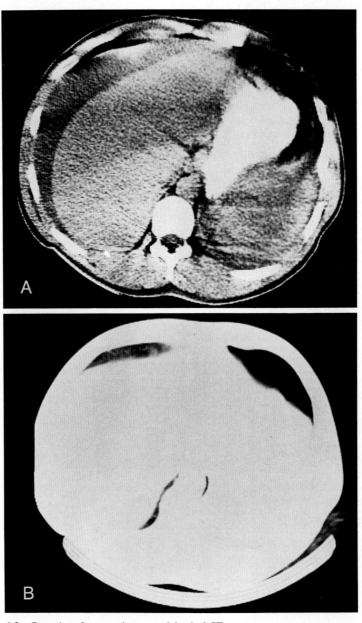

Figure 6.3.   Detection of pneumothorax on abdominal CT scans.
A. Section photographed at "soft tissue window" shows hemoperitoneum and splenic laceration.
B. Same section photographed at "lung window" shows left pneumothorax, clinically unsuspected.

including ECG monitor leads, intravenous tubing, and other support apparatus. The arms should be placed over the chest or above the head whenever possible. If the arms must remain over the abdomen, a large scanning field of view should be utilized to decrease artifacts while a smaller display field of view is selected to improve resolution.

Some artifacts are difficult to avoid but can usually be differentiated from true lesions. Rib artifacts are areas of factitious low attenuation found adjacent to ribs moving with respiration during the scan cycle. As an isolated finding, a low-density parenchymal area that lies immediately beneath a rib should be viewed with caution. A phenomenon that seems peculiar to fourth-generation CT scanners is the "pseudosubcapsular hematoma." A lenticular low-density lesion along the surface of the liver, spleen, or kidney may be simulated by motion of the organ during the scan cycle. The key to proper diagnosis is the recognition of a similar phenomenon bordering the rectus muscles on the same section, and the disappearance of the "lesion" on adjacent or repeat sections (Fig. 6.4).

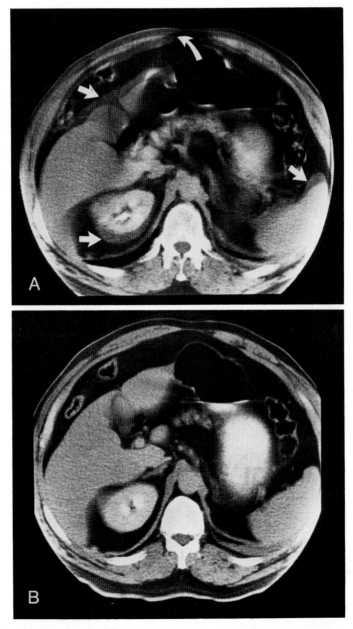

Figure 6.4. "Pseudosubcapsular hematoma" artifact.
A. A lenticular low density lies along the dorsal surface of the left kidney and the ventral surface of the spleen and liver (*straight arrows*), simulating subcapsular hematomas. Note also the double image of the anterior abdominal wall (*curved arrow*).
B. Repeat section moments later shows normal organs and a single image of the abdominal wall. The artifact is due to respiratory motion of the organs during the data acquisition.

With combative adults or young children (less than 4 years old) it may be impossible to perform a diagnostic CT examination without sedation. We use parenteral medication only, usually an intramuscular injection of a mixture of Demerol (25 mg/ml), Phenergan (6.25 mg/ml), and Thorazine (6.25 mg/ml) in a dosage of 0.1 ml/kg. Children receive a maximum of 2 ml. Other useful drugs are intravenous pentobarbital (Nembutal), fentanyl, and morphine, administered in the recommended dosages and given in consultation with the surgical staff.

Patients should never be scanned prior to adequate evaluation and resuscitation, and they must be monitored throughout the CT examination. The patient should be observed directly or via TV monitor by the technologist *and the surgical staff* or nurse. Cardiorespiratory monitoring is recommended, and an emergency "crash cart," oxygen, suction, and ventilation should be immediately available in the scanning room.

HEMOPERITONEUM

The detection and quantitation of intraperitoneal hemorrhage have important clinical implications and are based on two principles: understanding the anatomy of the peritoneal cavity and distinguishing blood from abdominal masses or other abdominal fluids.

Anatomy

It is necessary to understand some basic principles of cross-sectional anatomy of the peritoneal cavity so that collections of intraperitoneal blood can be appropriately sought and recognized. Much of what follows is based on the pioneering work of Meyers (12). The pelvis is the most dependent part of the peritoneal cavity in either the supine or erect position. Large amounts of blood may accumulate in the pelvis following abdominal trauma, first in the central rectovesicle or rectouterine space (pouch of Douglas) and the lateral paravesicle fossae. The pelvis is anatomically continuous with both paracolic gutters, the peritoneal recesses lateral to the ascending and descending colon. The right paracolic gutter is wide and deep and is continuous superiorly with the right subhepatic space and its posterosuperior extension deep to the liver known as Morison's pouch or the hepatorenal fossa (Figs. 6.5 and 6.6). The right subhepatic space is anatomically continuous with the right subphrenic space. In contrast, the left paracolic gutter is narrow and shallow and is interrupted from continuity with the left subphrenic space (perisplenic space) by the phrenicocolic ligament, which extends from the splenic flexure of the colon to the left diaphragm (Fig. 6.7).

Small amounts of blood from right upper quadrant sources tend to accumulate around the liver (subphrenic space) and Morison's pouch, the deepest per-

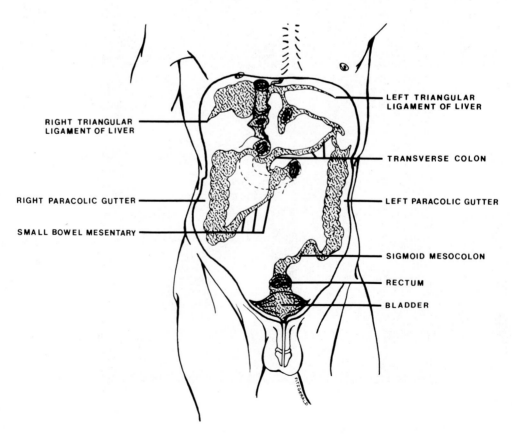

Figure 6.5. Frontal view of the eviscerated abdomen demonstrating the peritoneal attachments that form potential spaces and influence the distribution of peritoneal fluids.

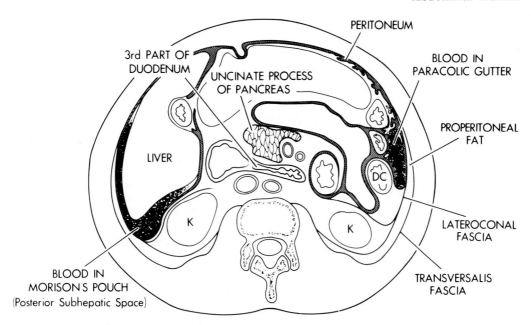

Figure 6.6.   Cross-sectional anatomy—peritoneal recesses. Intraperitoneal hemorrhage collects in the dependent recesses of the peritoneal cavity, including Morison's pouch and the paracolic gutters. Note displacement of descending colon (*DC*) from properitoneal fat, the CT equivalent of the "flank stripe" sign on plain radiographs. (*K*, kidney.)

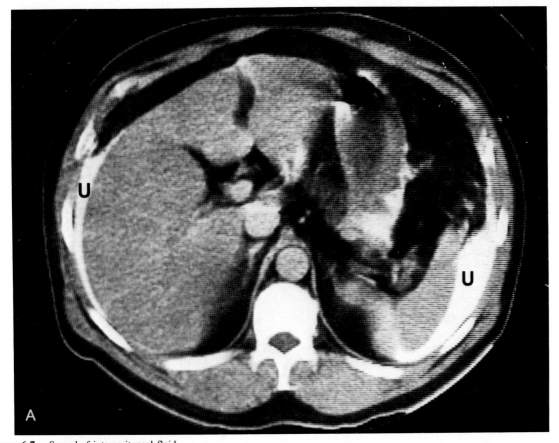

Figure 6.7.   Spread of intraperitoneal fluid.

A, B. Very dense fluid (*U*) fills dependent parts of both subphrenic spaces and both paracolic gutters.

C. Abdominal film following cystogram (preceded CT scan). Intraperitoneal extravasation of opacified urine due to ruptured bladder. Note narrow left paracolic gutter (*LG*), broader right paracolic gutter (*RG*), Morison's pouch (*M*), paravesicle fossae (*PF*). These are the common sites of accumulation of intraperitoneal hemorrhage. (*L*, liver.)

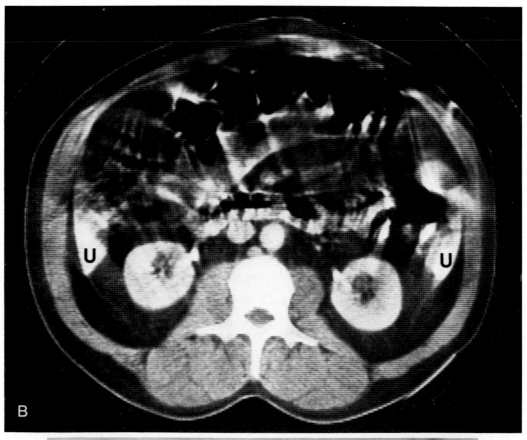

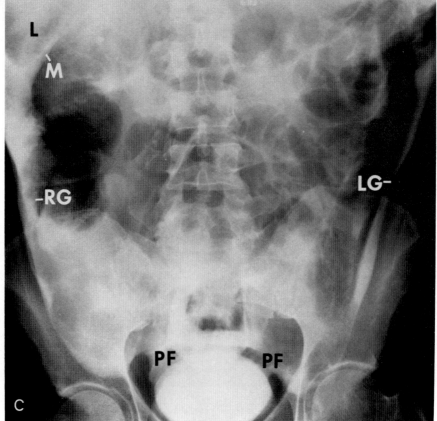

Figure 6.7.   B, C.

itoneal reflection in the upper abdomen. Larger amounts continue down the right paracolic gutter to the pelvis and may then extend into the left paracolic gutter. Splenic hemorrhage, on the other hand, is first confined to the perisplenic space (left subphrenic). It may then overflow the phrenicocolic ligament to flow down the left paracolic gutter, or first seek out Morison's pouch.

CT Appearance of Blood

Those with experience in cranial CT scanning are familiar with the appearance of intracranial hemorrhage. Acute intra- or extra-axial collections of blood are usually obvious and stand out as "white" collections in contrast to the brain parenchyma. Similar findings are uncommonly encountered in abdominal CT scanning for a number of reasons. One factor which alters the appearance of intra-abdominal blood is the convention of photographing abdominal CT scans at a much wider window width than is customary for cranial CT scanning. A wider window is necessary for optimal visualization of the abdominal contents, which have a much wider range of attenuation coefficients than the brain parenchyma. Photographing at a wider window width has the effect of increasing the gray scale and minimizing the density difference between substances of similar attenuation (e.g., splenic parenchyma and hematoma).

Blood may be hypo-, hyper-, or isodense relative to splenic or hepatic parenchyma depending upon the hematocrit and physical state of the blood (clotted or lysed), the use of iodinated contrast media, and the density of the adjacent organ.

Hemoglobin is a major determinant of the CT attenuation of blood, and a linear relationship between attenuation and hematocrit has been established (13–15). The high density of recent hemorrhage results from clot retraction and/or sedimentation of cellular elements in liquid blood (16). Chronic anemia (but not acute blood loss) may result in clots of lower attenuation. Clotted blood is usually nonhomogeneous due to disruption of the collection by tissue barriers, separation of clot from serum, and sedimentation of cellular elements. Intermittent bleeding may result in episodes of clot formation and retraction. Curvilinear peripheral layers of clot reflect the tendency of clot to form in contact with tissue (Fig. 6.8). Fluid-fluid levels occur following liquefaction of clotted blood or in fresh bleeding that fails to coagulate (Fig. 6.9). The later phenomenon is seen in hemophiliacs and those on anticoagulation medication (17).

Densely clotted blood may have a CT attenuation of more than 100 H. Most clots have an attenuation range of 50 to 75 H (Fig. 6.10). Lysed blood flowing freely within the peritoneal cavity has an attenuation range of about 30 to 45 H. Hemoperitoneum should never have an attenuation value less than 20 H, excluding severe chronic anemia, errors due to CT artifacts or poor calibration, or blood more than 48 hours old (18). Therefore, we can usually distinguish hemoperitoneum from pre-existing ascites or retained peritoneal lavage fluid (Fig. 6.11).

Perisplenic blood clot is almost always present in cases of splenic laceration and is usually isodense or hyperdense relative to unenhanced splenic parenchyma (19). Following intravenous administration of contrast medium, however, the spleen generally becomes hyperdense relative to the nonenhancing hematoma, assuming that an adequate volume of contract medium has been given (see "Technique," above). From these observations it follows that using a small volume of contrast medium increases the likelihood of encountering isodense hematomas, by causing the spleen (or liver) to enhance to a density similar to clotted blood. This error in technique is a potential cause of false negative interpretations.

Densely clotted blood may be hyperdense to enhanced liver or spleen, but portions of the blood clot and lysed blood elsewhere in the peritoneal cavity can almost always be identified as lower density fluid collections (Fig. 6.8). Hepatic steatosis (fatty liver) may result in the liver being of lower density (attenuation) than adjacent blood (Fig. 6.12). This represents a potential source of misdiagnosis as discussed further in the section of hepatic trauma.

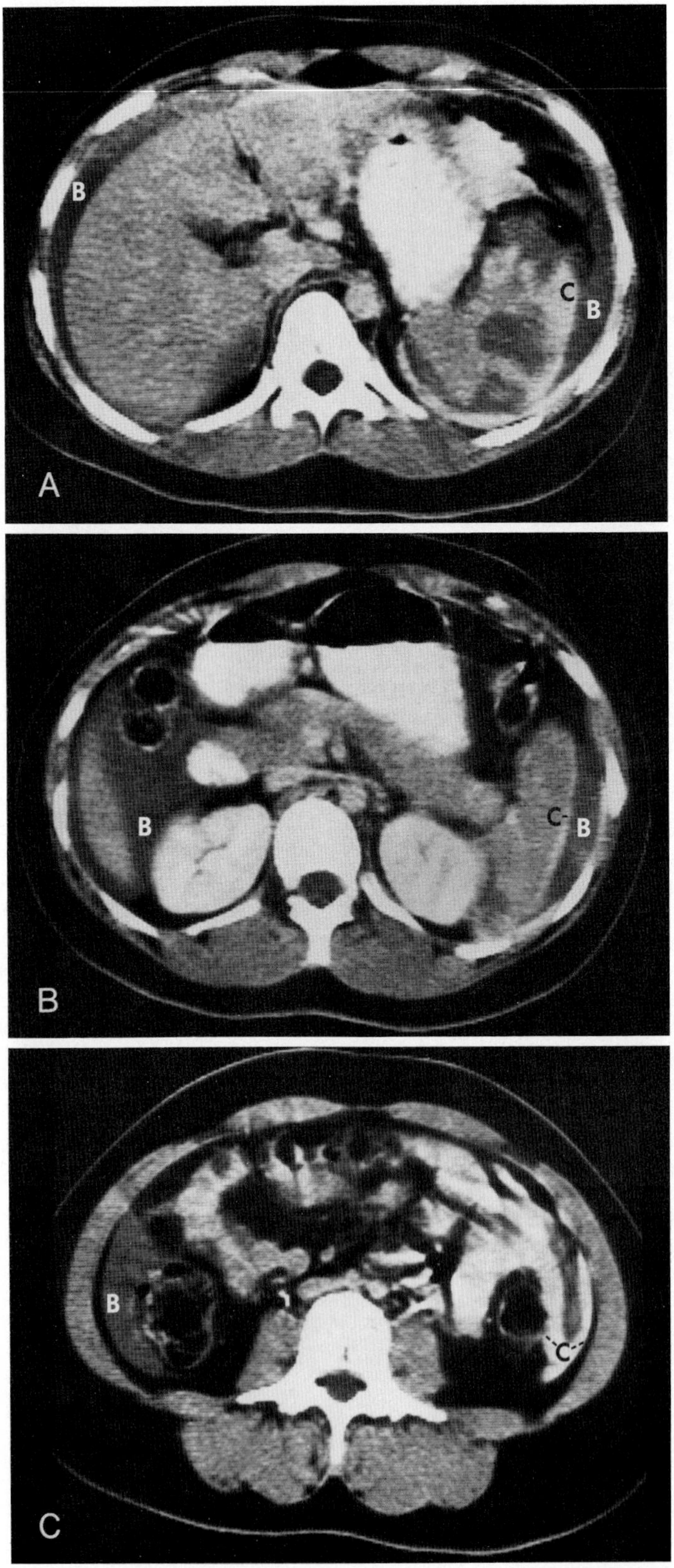

Figure 6.8. Lacerated spleen; hemoperitoneum.
A. Splenic contour is irregular with rounded heterogeneous intrasplenic hematomas. Note dense blood clot (*C*) along the lateral margin of the spleen and blood (*B*) in both subphrenic spaces.
B, C. Layers of highly attenuating dense blood clot (*C*) are apparent in the left paracolic gutter and adjacent to the spleen. Note less dense, free-flowing lysed blood (*B*) in Morison's pouch and the right paracolic gutter.

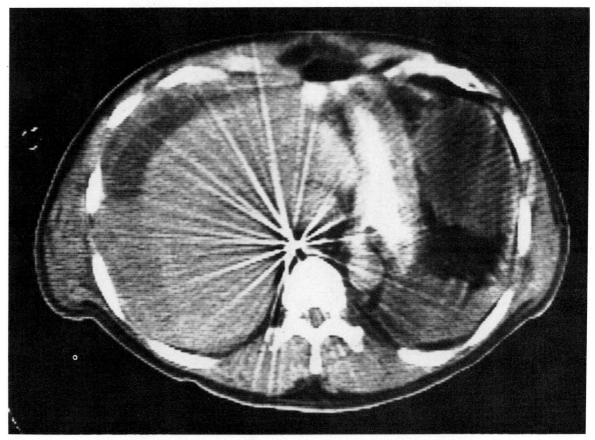

Figure 6.9. Hemoperitoneum with "hematocrit effect." A fluid layer is noted in a blood collection lateral to the liver due to settling of cellular elements of blood and clot. This effect is seen in anticoagulated patients or those with bleeding disorders.

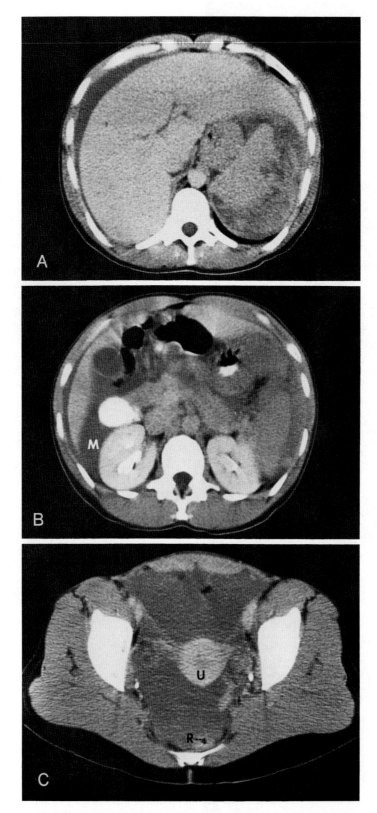

Figure 6.10. Lacerated spleen; hemoperitoneum.
A–C. Heterogeneous clotted blood (50 to 65 H) near the irregular lacerated margin of the spleen. Less dense (35 H) lysed blood is seen in the right subphrenic space, Morison's pouch (M), and pelvis. (U, uterus; R, rectum.)

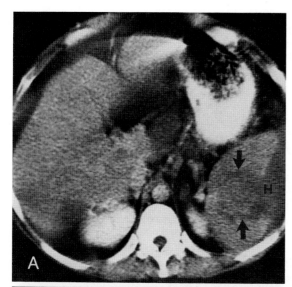

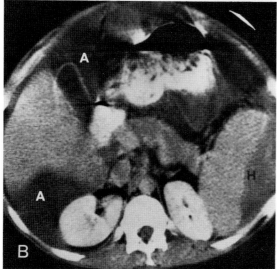

Figure 6.11.   CT was used to differentiate blood from ascites in this chronic alcoholic with a blunt abdominal injury. A high-density (45 H) hematoma (*H*) in the perisplenic fossa, as well as subcapsular distribution, is shown. Note the lacerations (*arrows*) of the splenic parenchyma. A large amount of low-density (0 H) ascites (*A*) is apparent due to cirrhosis. The amount of intraperitoneal hemorrhage was small. This patient recovered without undergoing an operation. (From Federle MP, Jeffrey RB: Hemoperitoneum studied by computed tomography. *Radiology* 148:187, 1983.)

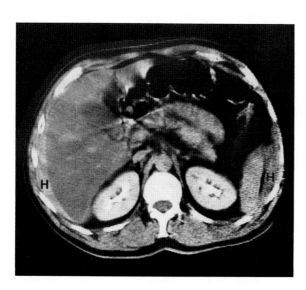

Figure 6.12.   Blood (*H*) adjacent to liver and spleen is of similar attenuation (45 to 55 H), but appears hypodense to the contrast-opacified spleen (the usual relationship) and hyperdense to the liver due to fatty infiltration of the liver.

SPECIFIC INJURIES

Spleen

The spleen is the intraperitoneal organ most frequently injured in blunt trauma. Abdominal injury may cause splenic laceration or it may produce a hematoma that is limited by the splenic capsule.

Subcapsular Hematoma

CT has proved to be a very accurate and simple means of diagnosing subcapsular hematomas (20). Most often, the hematoma has the appearance of a crescentic low-density area along the lateral margin of the spleen, with flattening or indentation of the normally convex lateral margin of the spleen (Fig. 6.13). Occasionally, the hematoma may extend around to the medial surface of the spleen, and there may be an intraparenchymal component as well (Fig. 6.11). True subcapsular hematomas are relatively uncommon, and, by definition, there should be no evidence of free peritoneal blood from the splenic injury (Fig. 6.14).

Splenic subcapsular hematomas or minor lacerations may go undetected on initial clinical evaluation, especially since a history of trauma may be minimal or completely absent. Most cases of "delayed splenic rupture" are, in fact, merely delays in diagnosis, although verified cases of delayed rupture have been reported, including cases in which peritoneal lavage and/or CT had initially been normal (21, 22). Sub-acute or chronic splenic hematomas are usually similar in appearance to acute hematomas, although the attenuation coefficient is less due to lysis of blood clot and resorption of protein. Chronic splenic hematomas may have the same appearance as cysts (23) (Fig. 6.15).

Splenic Lacerations

Several reports have established CT as an excellent method for detecting splenic lacerations (3, 10, 20, 24), although the findings are more subtle and variable than in subcapsular hematoma. The findings include indistinct margins of the spleen (Fig. 6.16), and inhomogeneous splenic parenchyma (Figs. 6.17 and 6.18). Intrasplenic hematomas and lacerations may be linear (Fig. 6.19), stellate (Fig. 6.20), or rounded (Fig. 6.21). On bolus-enhanced scans, densely opacifying areas may represent areas of extravasation of vascular contrast medium (Fig. 6.22). Perisplenic blood clot, interposed between the spleen and the stomach, tail of pancreas, and/or kidney, is seen in virtually every case of splenic laceration. More extensive bleeding which overwhelms the partially closed perisplenic space (left subphrenic space) spills over into the peritoneal cavity. Commonly identified sites of accumulation are the left and right paracolic gutters, the posterior subhepatic space (Morison's pouch), and the pelvis.

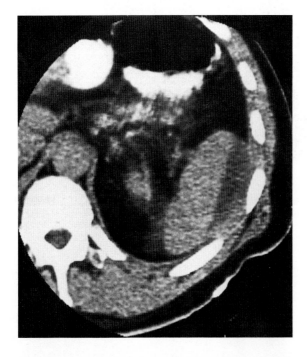

Figure 6.13. Subcapsular hematoma. Typical lenticular collection that flattens the lateral margin of the spleen.

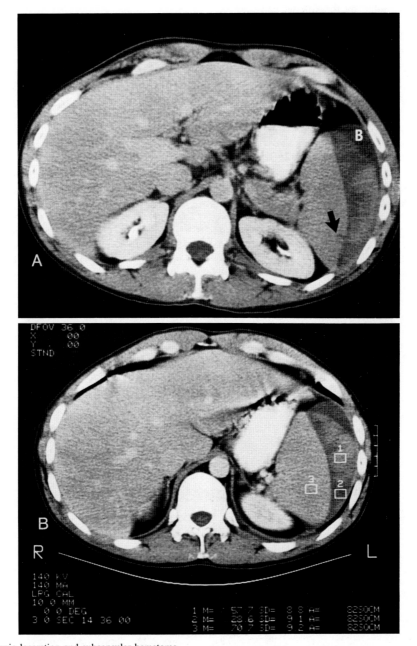

Figure 6.14.   Splenic laceration and subcapsular hematoma.
A, B. A large lenticular subcapsular hematoma is noted with areas of clot (*cursor 1*) measuring 58 H. Lysed blood (*cursor 2*) measures 29 H, and some is found outside the capsule in the left subphrenic space (*B*), indicating capsular disruption. Also note the small parenchymal tear (*arrow*).

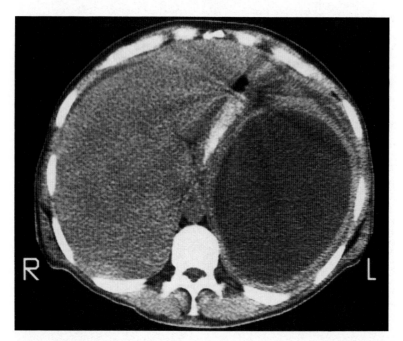

Figure 6.15.   Chronic subcapsular hematoma resembles a splenic cyst (5 H); surgically proved.

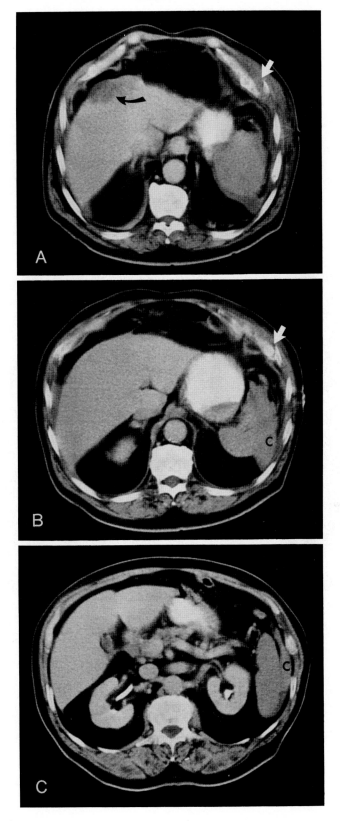

Figure 6.16.   Splenic laceration.
A, B. Displaced rib fractures (*white arrows*) and chest wall hematoma. Splenic injury is primarily detected as an irregular contour and perisplenic blood clot (*C*) that is nearly as dense as the spleen. Subcapsular hepatic hematoma (*curved arrow*), not clinically suspected but proved at surgery.
C. Dense perisplenic clot (*C*) is separated from the spleen by a fat plane.

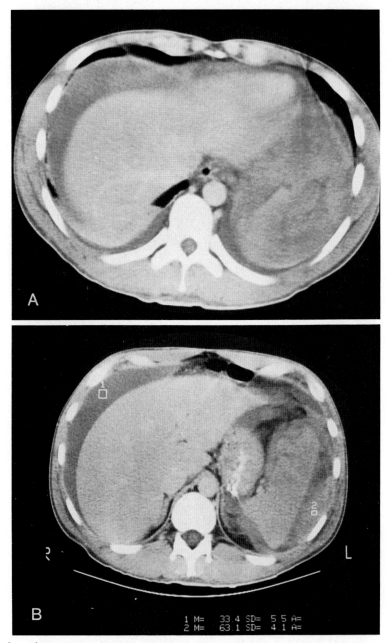

Figure 6.17. Splenic laceration.
A, B. Splenic parenchyma is macerated and inhomogeneous, surrounded by heterogeneous blood clot. Perisplenic clot (*cursor 2*) measures 63.1 H, while free lysed blood (*cursor 1*) measures 33.4 H.

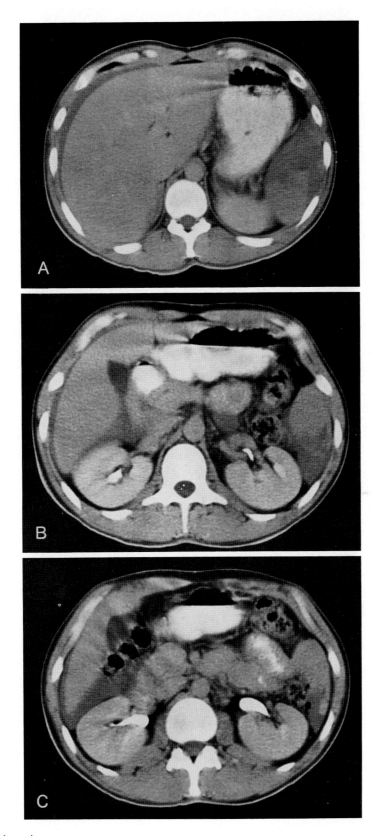

Figure 6.18.   Splenic laceration.
A, B, C. Splenic parenchyma is macerated and surrounded by heterogenous clot. Lysed blood is evident in Morison's pouch, and a large volume was present in the pelvis.

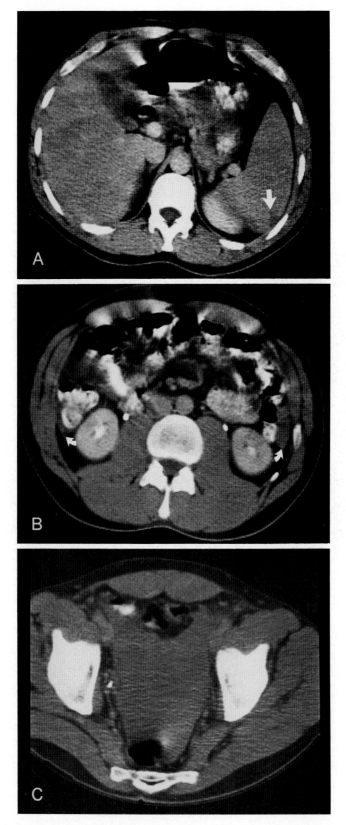

Figure 6.19.   Linear splenic laceration.

A. Splenomegaly with a small peripheral laceration (*arrow*).

B. Only a small amount of blood is present in the paracolic gutters (*arrows*).

C. A large amount of blood is present in the pelvis. At surgery a small splenic laceration was found to be actively bleeding and was repaired. If CT sections through the pelvis had not been obtained, the extent of hemoperitoneum would have been seriously underestimated.

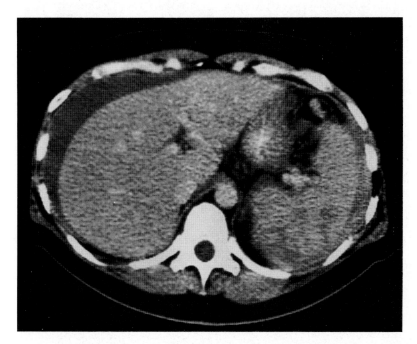

Figure 6.20.   Stellate splenic laceration. Multiple fracture planes, perisplenic clot, and large hemoperitoneum.

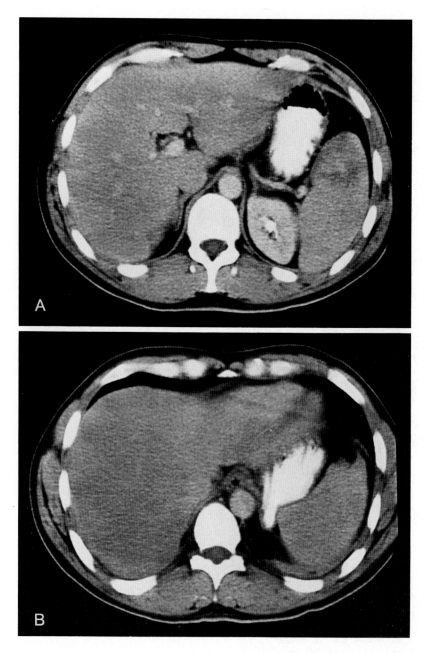

Figure 6.21.
A. Rounded splenic hematoma/laceration.
B. Nearly isodense hematoma obscures the lateral margin of the spleen. A large amount of less dense blood was found on lower sections.

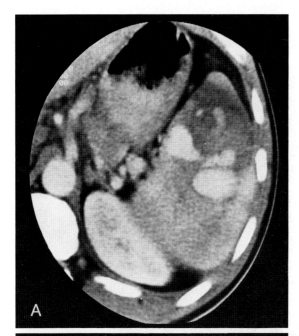

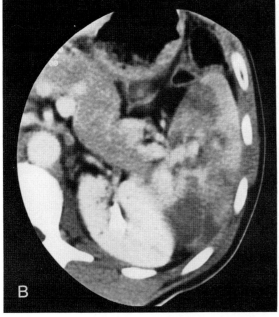

Figure 6.22.
A, B. Splenic laceration. Sections obtained during the rapid bolus administration of contrast medium demonstrate high-density intrasplenic collections that enhance at the same time as abdominal vessels, probably representing extravasation of opacified blood. This is unusual and is only found in cases of very active bleeding. Persistent high-density (>60 H) collections represent clotted blood, not extravasated contrast from bleeding vessels.

A few normal anatomic and physiologic variants are frequently encountered but should be easily recognized. Clefts through the splenic parenchyma are common, especially on axial sections through the upper pole. These are distinguished from lacerations by their smooth contours and especially by the absence of perisplenic hematoma (Fig. 6.23). Similarly, an elongated left lobe of the liver may appear to be part of a lacerated spleen, although close examination of contiguous sections will show continuity with the liver (Fig. 6.24). Mere inhomogeneity of the splenic parenchyma should be interpreted with caution. Because of its unique histology, consisting of red and white pulp, the spleen may enhance inhomogeneously following a bolus infusion of contrast medium (25). In questionable cases, repeat sections should be obtained following equilibration of the contrast agent. In normal cases the spleen will then appear homogeneous

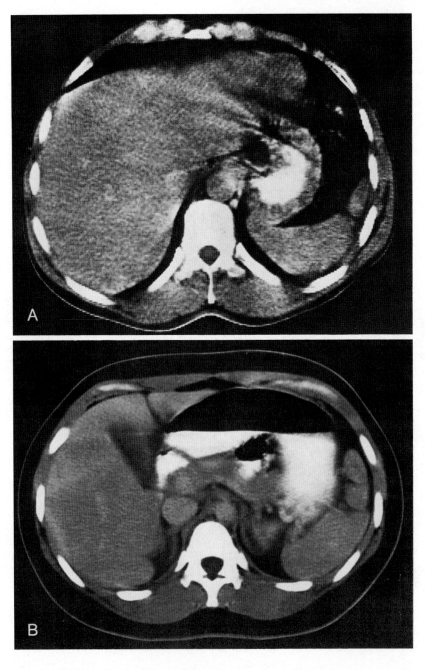

Figure 6.23.
A. Congenital clefts of the spleen are common, especially along the medial margin. This was misinterpreted as a laceration on radionuclide scintigraphy. CT shows absense of any perisplenic blood, ruling out laceration. (From Jeffrey RB, Laing FC, Federle MP, Goodman PC: Computed tomography of splenic trauma. *Radiology* 131:719, 1981.)
B. Another patient with congenital splenic clefts.

with no surrounding hemorrhage. Another anatomic variant that may simulate splenic trauma is a high perisplenic position of jejunal segments. When poorly opacified by oral contrast medium, these may simulate fragments of splenic parenchyma or hematoma. Repeat CT sections or real-time sonography help confirm the bowel origin (Fig. 6.25).

Pathologically enlarged spleens are prone to laceration, but hematomas must be distinguished from other parenchymal lesions. Splenic infarcts occur in patients with splenomegaly and hemoglobinopathies. Infarcts are usually subcapsular or wedge-shaped parenchymal defects and are not commonly associated with perisplenic hemorrhage (Fig. 6.26). Absence of perisplenic hemorrhage is also the key distinguishing feature in evaluating potential splenic trauma in patients with lymphoma, acquired immune deficiency syndrome, and other causes of splenomegaly that may be associated with discrete parenchymal lesions.

The most difficult problem in CT diagnosis of splenic trauma is the isodense hematoma that may obscure an underlying splenic laceration (26). This occurs uncommonly when an adequate volume of vascular contrast medium has been administered. Clotted blood typically has an irregular contour, with an inhomogeneous density (50 to 80 H) (Figs. 6.21 and 6.27). A portion of the normal perisplenic fat plane can often be recognized (Figs. 6.28 and 6.29), and free peritoneal hemorrhage is present in almost all cases (Figs. 6.28–6.30). Even in the absence of a visible parenchymal laceration, splenic trauma should be strongly suspected when there is perisplenic clot and free peritoneal hemorrhage.

Several reports have now established CT as an excellent method for detecting splenic trauma, and the accuracy of CT is being established by large prospective series (7). In the first 50 patients whom we studied for a suspected splenic injury, CT results were correct in 48; 27 of 28 were true negative, and 21 of 22 were true positive (24). We have now studied several hundred cases of suspected splenic trauma, and our accuracy remains very close to 100%.

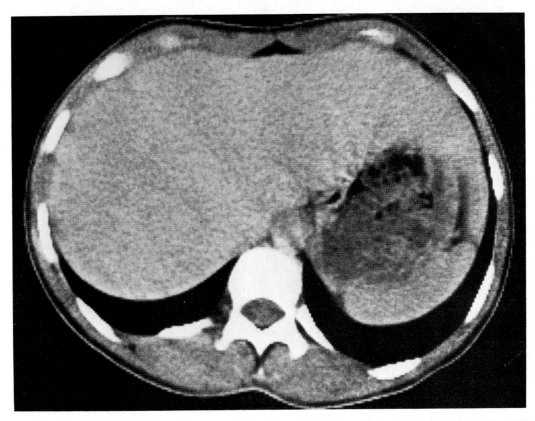

Figure 6.24. Another congenital variation which may result in a false positive radionuclide scan is a long left lobe of liver. CT easily identifies the "laceration" as a normal interface between the adjacent liver and spleen.

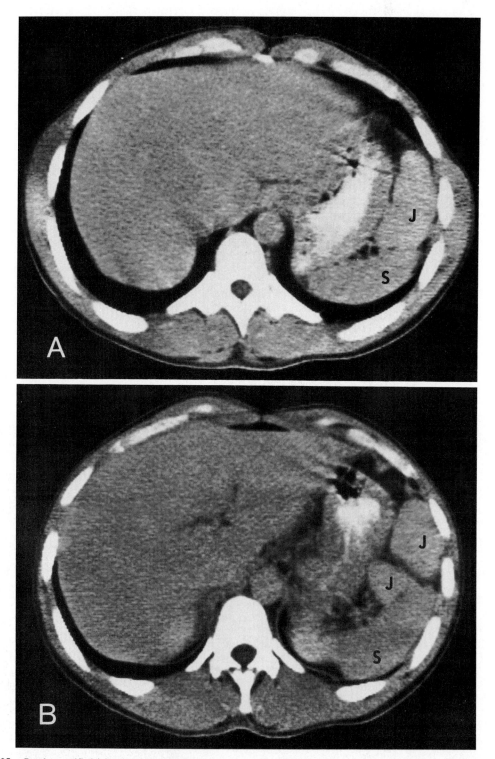

Figure 6.25. Poorly opacified jejunal segments (*J*) occupy an unusually high perisplenic position and simulate a fractured spleen or perisplenic clot. Delayed scans after additional oral contrast medium would help to distinguish these. In this patient, real-time sonography revealed bowel peristalsis. (*S*, spleen.)

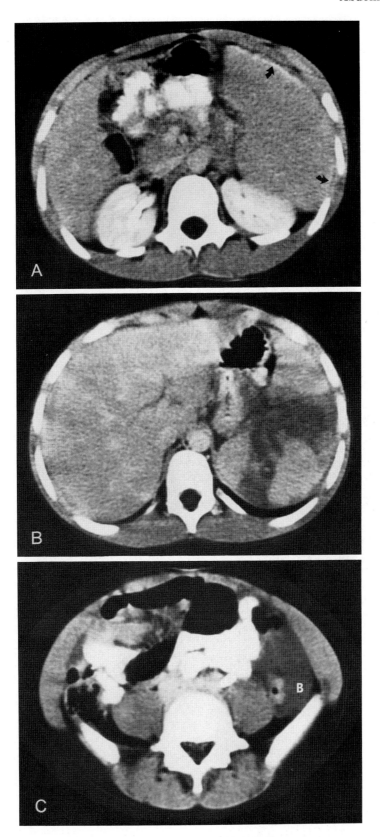

Figure 6.26.   Child with sickle-thalassemia and acute abdominal pain.
A. Splenomegaly and subcapsular calcification (*arrows*) due to chronic infarction.
B. Parenchyma is divided by heterogeneous low-density planes not typical for acute or chronic infarction.
C. Free blood in the paracolic gutters (*B*) helps to confirm diagnosis of splenic rupture.

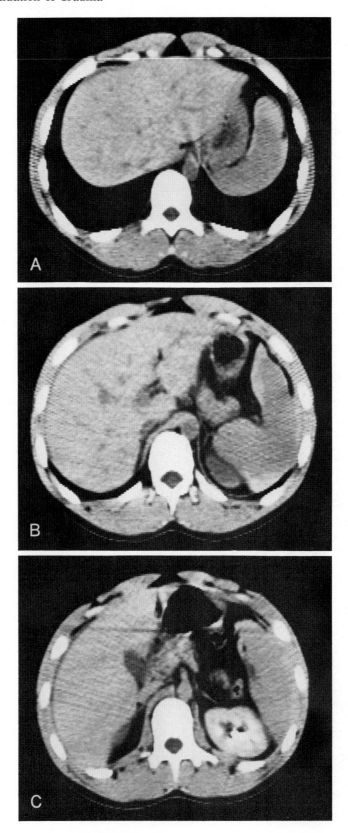

Figure 6.27.   Splenic laceration; "isodense" hematoma.
A, B. Scans performed before intravenous administration of contrast medium show perisplenic blood clot slightly more dense than the splenic parenchyma.
C. Scan repeated after infusion of only 50 ml of 60% contrast medium. The spleen and the hematoma are now almost isodense and difficult to distinguish. (Case courtesy of James E. Blackwell, M.D., Roanoke, VA.)

Liver Injuries

Injury to the liver is the second most common type of blunt intraperitoneal injury and causes a 15 to 45% mortality (27, 28). Injury to other abdominal organs is associated in many cases (45% had associated splenic lacerations in one report (29)), as are injuries to the head, chest, and limbs. The abdominal injury may be overlooked, although it carries the major significance for mortality. Morbidity and mortality increase when diagnosis and treatment are delayed or inadequate.

While many patients with blunt hepatic trauma are obvious candidates for urgent laparotomy (shock or peritonitis), those who are stable can definitely benefit from CT evaluation, which can help to determine optimal management of the hepatic lesion as well as any associated visceral injuries (30, 31).

Subcapsular Hepatic Hematoma

Collections of blood limited by the hepatic capsule may result from blunt or penetrating trauma, including iatrogenic injuries such as may occur during percutaneous liver biopsy (32). Subcapsular hematomas are difficult to diagnose on plain radiography. Arteriography and radionuclide scintigraphy may reveal at least the lateral component of a subcapsular hematoma, seen as an avascular or photopenic mass compressing liver parenchyma. Anatomic variants, such as abundant fat displacing liver from the lateral ab-

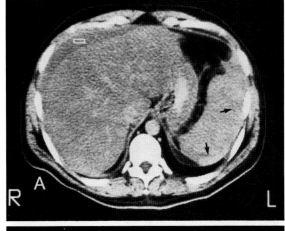

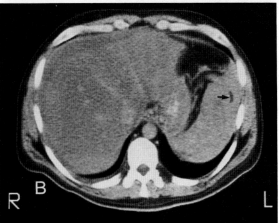

Figure 6.28. Splenic laceration; "isodense" hematoma.
A, B. Scans of a 17-year-old boy performed after administration of only 50 ml of contrast. Spleen and perisplenic hematoma are isodense, but small segments of perisplenic fat are interposed (*arrows*). Also note irregular "splenic contour" and less dense blood around the liver (*cursor*).

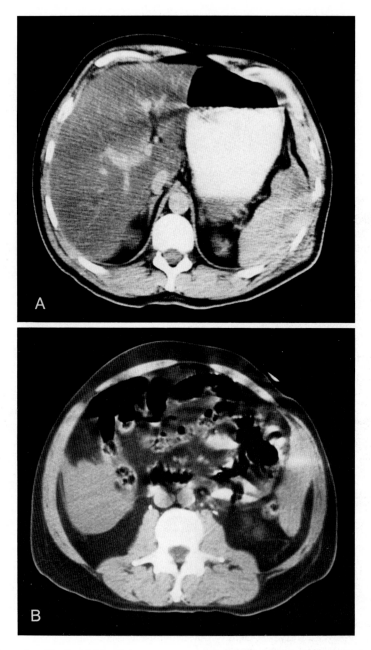

Figure 6.29.   Splenic laceration; "isodense" hematoma.
A. Subcapsular and perisplenic blood are nearly isodense with the spleen and obscure the parenchymal laceration. Incidental note of fatty liver.
B. Large volume of blood in the paracolic gutters is obvious.

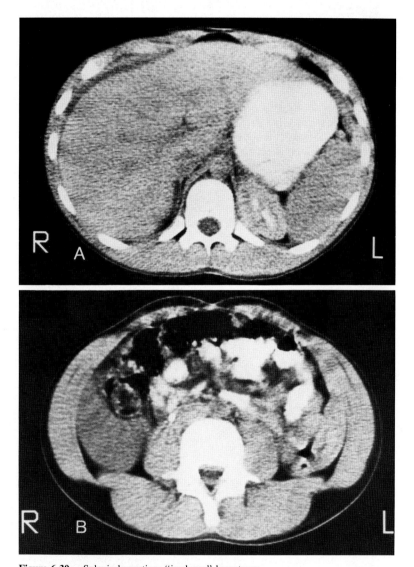

Figure 6.30.   Splenic laceration; "isodense" hematoma.
A. Parenchymal injury is obscured by isodense perisplenic clot.
B. Free peritoneal blood is obvious.

dominal wall, may cause errors in interpretation (Fig. 6.31), while CT clearly depicts the total extent of hematomas. Most hematomas are noted along the parietal surface of organs and appear as hypodense lenticular fluid collections that flatten or indent underlying hepatic tissue (33, 34) (Figs. 6.32–6.34).

Accurate assessment of the size and location of the hematoma and the presence or absence of associated parenchymal injuries is important, since limited injuries may be best managed nonoperatively. Percutaneous catheter drainage is another therapeutic option that can be aided by CT guidance (33).

Hepatic Laceration

Hepatic parenchymal lacerations vary from small lesions confined to the interior of the liver with no capsular disruption to large, complex lacerations with intrahepatic hematomas, extensive capsular disruption, and hemoperitoneum. The most commonly encountered pattern is an irregular fracture plane extending to the surface of the liver associated with a variable amount of free intraperitoneal blood. Limited bleeding is confined to the right subphrenic and subhepatic spaces (Morison's pouch) (Figs. 6.35 and 6.36). More extensive bleeding collects in the right paracolic gutter and pelvis (Fig. 6.37). Intrahepatic hematoma is commonly encountered as an inhomogeneous mass, with areas of high attenuation representing dense blood clot (Figs. 6.38 and 6.39).

Comprehensive injuries may cause stellate fractures of the liver, sometimes described as "bear claw" lacerations. On CT sections these may have an irregular branching pattern that superficially resembles the intrahepatic biliary or portal venous system (Figs. 6.40 and 6.41). Use of iodinated intravenous contrast enhancement and examination of contiguous CT sections allows differentiation.

Trauma to a fatty liver (hepatic steatosis) may be more difficult to assess. The attenuation of the liver may be uniformly or heterogeneously decreased as a result of fatty infiltration, making differentiation from hepatic parenchymal trauma more difficult (Fig. 6.42). Perihepatic blood may also be hypo-, hyper-, or isodense to the liver, depending upon the extent of fatty change and the physical state of the blood (clotted or lysed). However, hemoperitoneum can usually be diagnosed, and examination of liver sections with narrow window settings is useful. Focal fatty infiltration of the liver has been reported as a subacute (days to weeks) sequela of blunt trauma (35).

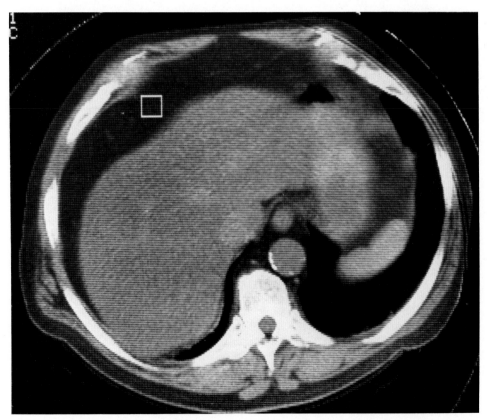

Figure 6.31.   Large amount of intraperitoneal fat (*cursor*) may flatten hepatic contour and displace liver from anterior and lateral abdominal wall. Such anatomic variants are easily recognized on CT but may cause diagnostic errors on radionuclide or angiographic studies.

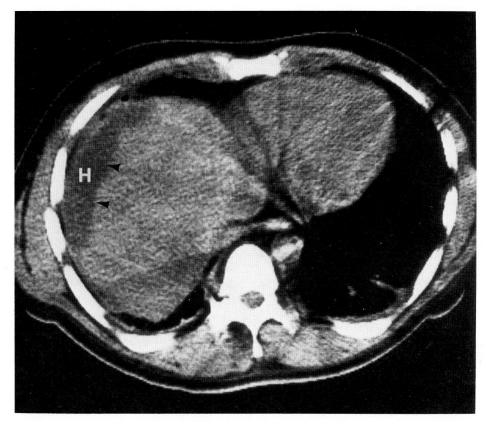

Figure 6.32.   Subcapsular hepatic hematoma. Lenticular low-density fluid collection (*H*) flattens underlying parenchyma (*arrowheads*).

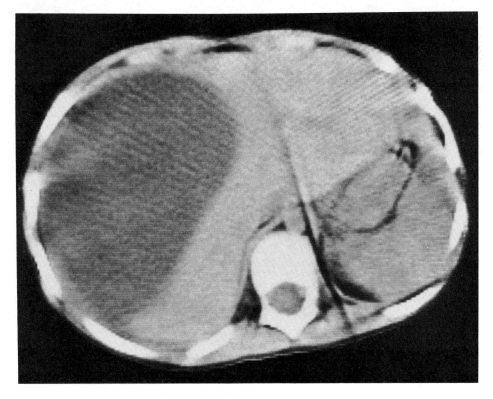

Figure 6.33.   Large subcapsular hepatic hematoma. An earlier CT had shown a much smaller lesion. The rapid increase in size led to surgical intervention for hemostasis.

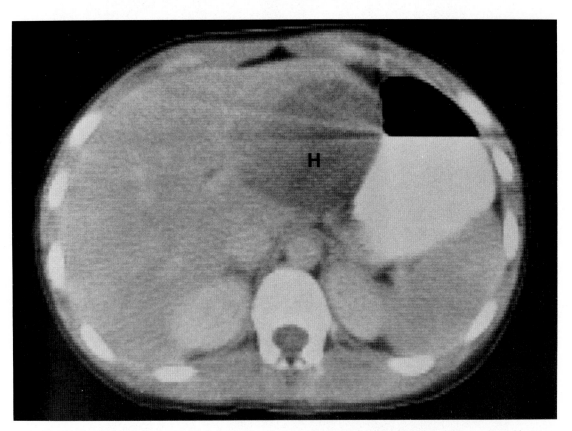

Figure 6.34.   Subcapsular hepatic hematoma (*H*) in unusual location, on posteromedial margin of left lobe of liver—due to blunt trauma.

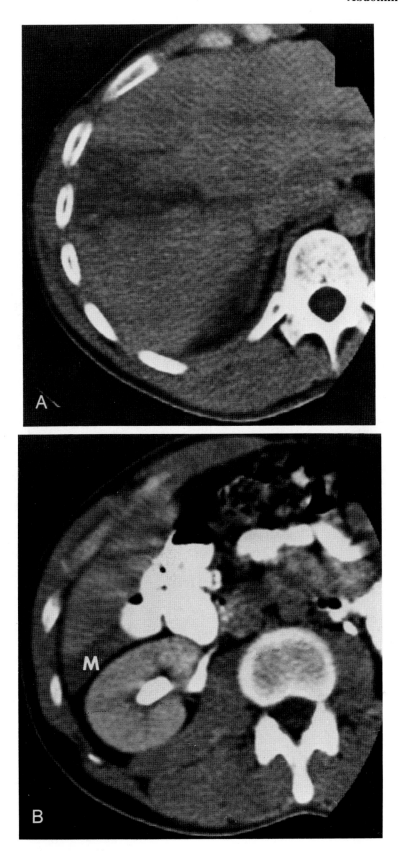

Figure 6.35.   Hepatic laceration; blunt trauma.
A. Irregular fracture plane in right lobe of liver.
B. Small amount of blood in Morison's pouch (*M*). The patient recovered uneventfully with conservative management.

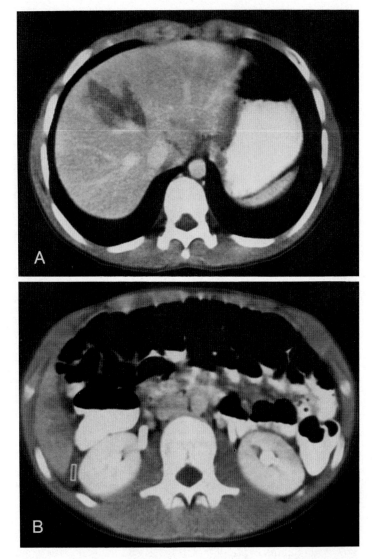

Figure 6.36.
A, B.   Irregular fracture plane in liver but small hemoperitoneum in Morison's pouch (*cursor*). Uneventful recovery without surgery.

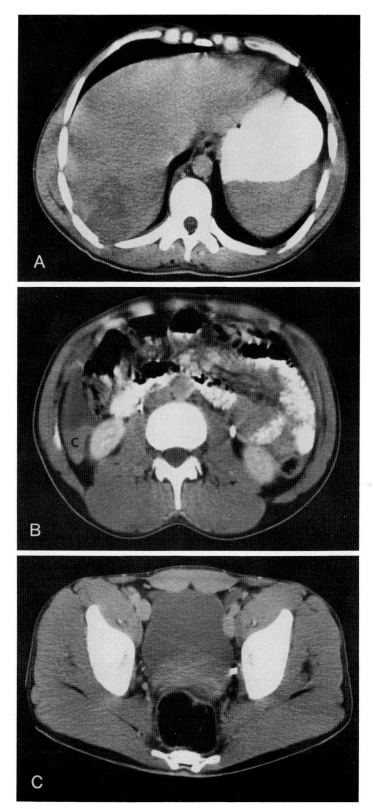

Figure 6.37.
A. Parenchymal hematoma/laceration in posterior right lobe.
B. Blood in right paracolic gutter with dependent clot (*C*).
C. Large collection of blood in the pelvis. Surgery was required because of extensive bleeding.

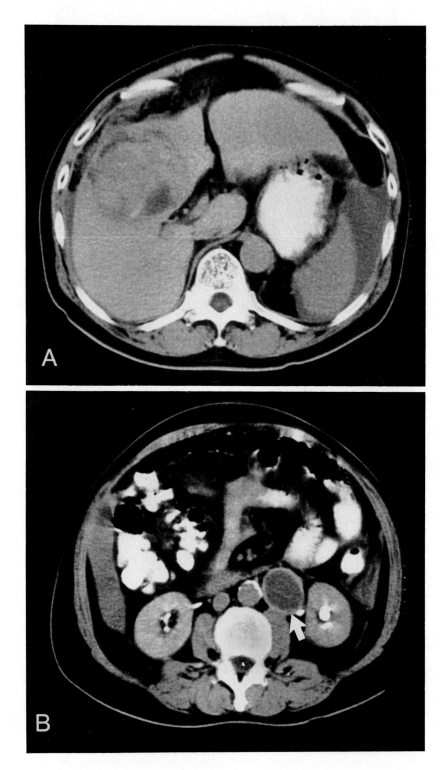

Figure 6.38.
A, B. Unusual round intrahepatic hematoma following minor trauma in a patient with a coagulopathy. Extensive hemoperitoneum. Incidental rounded left periureteral collection (*arrow*) was found to be an old organized hematoma.

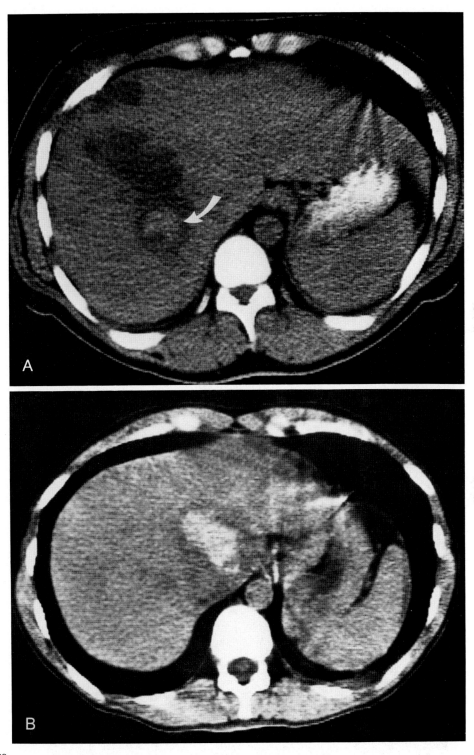

Figure 6.39.
A. Intrahepatic hematoma resulting from a gunshot wound. Irregular plane of low density representing damaged parenchyma and lysed hematoma. High-density focus (*arrow*) is freshly clotted blood. At laparotomy that preceded the CT scan, a small "nick" was seen on the surface of the liver and the extent of intrahepatic damage was not appreciated. (From Federle MP: Abdominal trauma: The role and impact of computed tomography. *Invest Radiol* 16:260, 1981.)
B. A different patient with a high-density intrahepatic hematoma.

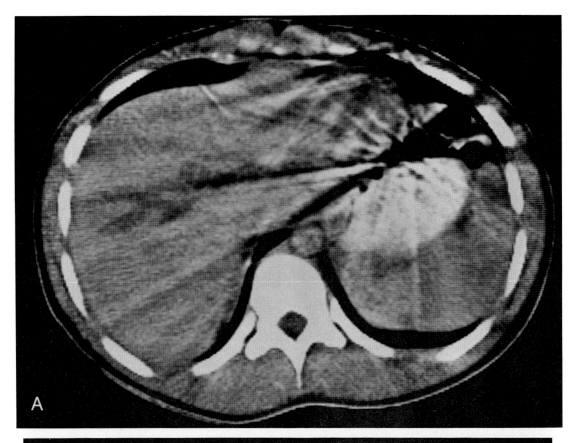

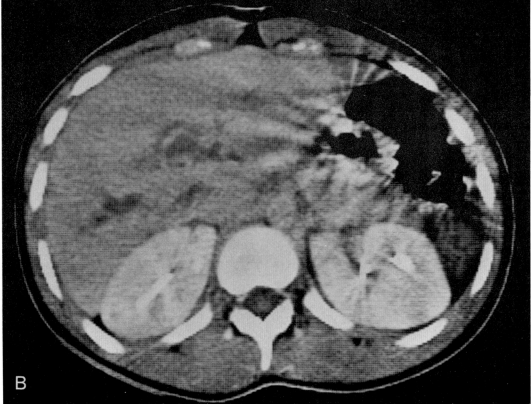

Figure 6.40. Hepatic laceration.

A, B. Branching linear lacerations (intrahepatic hematomas) simulate dilated bile ducts. Surgeons sometimes describe this type of injury as a "bear claw" laceration.

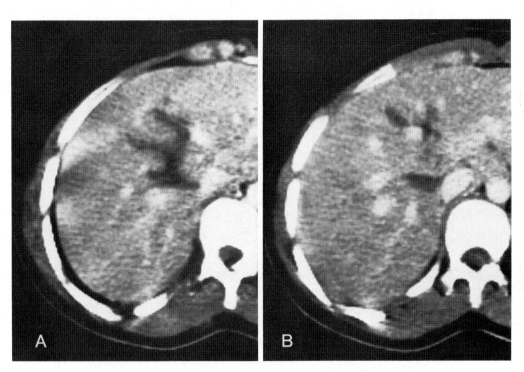

Figure 6.41.   Another patient with a "bear claw" laceration and a similar branching pattern.

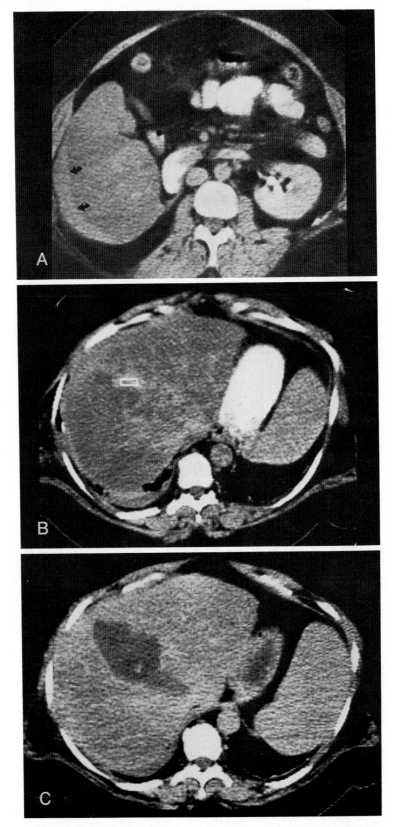

Figure 6.42. Trauma to a fatty liver.
A. Blood (50 H) lies lateral to the liver (*arrows*) and is more dense than the underlying liver parenchyma (40 H).
B. Liver parenchyma is heterogeneous. *Cursor* marks an area of mottled density that could represent intrahepatic hematoma or heterogeneous fatty infiltration.
C. A repeat CT scan 9 days later demonstrates an obvious parenchymal hematoma. The hematoma is low density (12 H) due to interval lysis of most of the clot.

Most hepatic lacerations occur in the right lobe, probably because of its larger size and its proximity to the lower ribs that are often fractured in blunt trauma. Laceration through the left lobe may be more difficult to identify, especially if the lobe extends unusually far across the midline and if the laceration divides the lobe in an anteroposterior plane (Figs. 6.43 and 6.44).

"Rib artifacts" and streak artifacts from gastric air-fluid levels can simulate parenchymal lesions or obscure parts of the liver. These can be minimized with careful technique and fast scan times, but they cannot be totally eliminated. Artifacts can often be differentiated from hepatic injuries by the regular linear appearance of the artifacts. While the accuracy of detecting small hepatic lacerations may be affected, the clinical impact may not be very important since the ability to diagnose hemoperitoneum is rarely affected by such artifacts and this is a major criterion for management.

Peripheral arterioportal fistulae are relatively frequent complications of hepatic biopsies and transhepatic catheterizations, though most resolve spontaneously. Dynamic CT is capable of diagnosing these lesions, showing a characteristic early opacification of portal vein branches and a triangular segment of hepatic parenchyma during the arterial phase of passage of the intravenous bolus of contrast medium (36, 37).

Accuracy and Effect on Management

In spite of the potential pitfalls described above, CT has proved to be a very accurate and useful tool in evaluating and managing hepatic trauma. The entire spectrum of hepatic trauma is detected, and injuries can be categorized by CT and clinical criteria as those likely to require surgical repair or those that can be managed nonoperatively. Clinical criteria for surgical intervention include hemodynamic instability, sepsis, or peritonitis. CT criteria are the extent of hepatic parenchymal injury, associated visceral injuries (especially splenic), and the presence and extent of hemoperitoneum (30).

The extent of hepatic parenchymal injury per se may influence outcome less than might be expected. If the hepatic capsule remains largely intact, and if extrahepatic bleeding is minimal, the hepatic injury may heal without sequelae, even if extensive (Fig. 6.45). More extensive hemoperitoneum and the presence of associated visceral injuries are more important criteria for surgery in our experience.

In the past several years we have diagnosed more than 30 cases of hepatic trauma that met our clinical and CT criteria for initial nonoperative therapy. Of these, only one patient subsequently required surgery, for a progressively enlarging subcapsular hematoma. Among the others, none subsequently had delayed bleeding requiring transfusion, nor developed evidence of biliary leakage or sepsis related to the hepatic injury.

With additional experience it is likely that cases of biloma or infected hematoma will be encountered, though these may occur regardless of initial operative or nonoperative management (38). CT has been demonstrated to be of value in detecting such complications and directing further therapy (3) (Figs. 6.46 and 6.47).

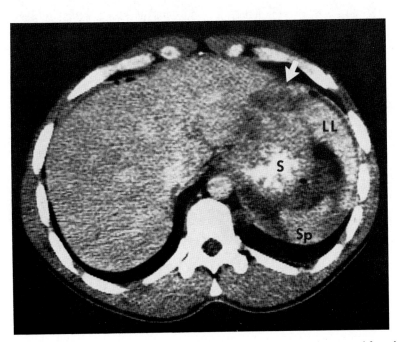

Figure 6.43.   Hepatic laceration, left lobe. The lateral segment of the left lobe (*LL*) is completely separated from the rest of the liver by a fracture plane (*arrow*). Close examination of contiguous sections may be necessary for confident detection of such lacerations and their relationship to nearby structures, such as stomach (*S*) and spleen (*Sp*).

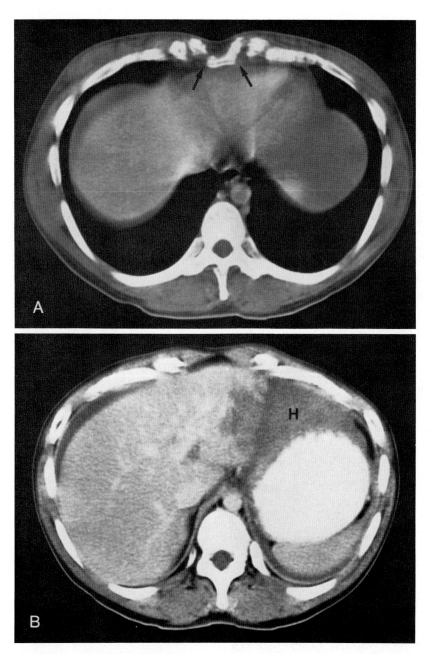

Figure 6.44.   Hepatic laceration, left lobe.
A. Depressed fracture of the sternum (*arrows*).
B. The left lobe of the liver is lacerated and a large adjacent hematoma (*H*) is noted.

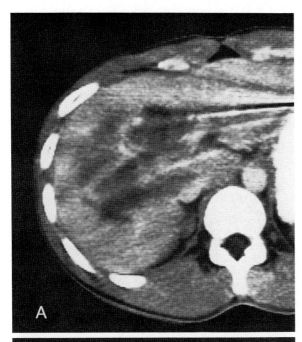

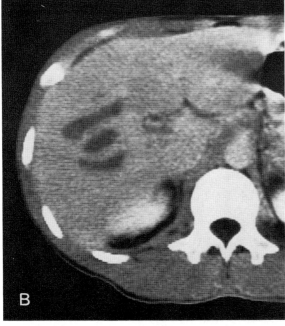

Figure 6.45.
A. Extensive intrahepatic hematoma/laceration in right lobe. Despite this extensive lesion, there was very little blood in the peritoneal cavity, and the patient was clinically stable.
B. Repeat CT scan after 8 days of bed rest shows substantial resolution of intrahepatic hematoma and no hemoperitoneum. Uneventful recovery without complications.

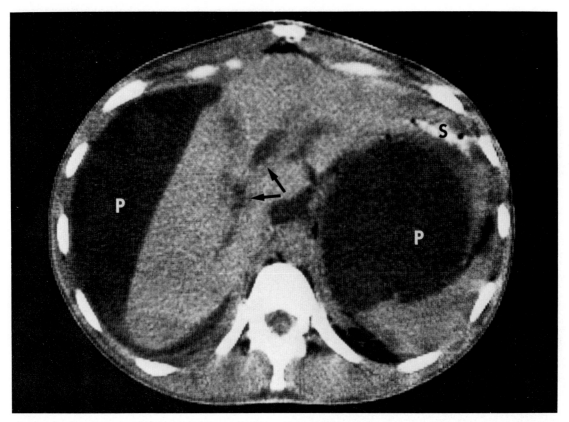

Figure 6.46. "Bile pseudocysts" (bilomas). Water density fluid collections (*P*) lateral to the liver and in the lesser sac, with forward displacement of the stomach (*S*). Dilated intrahepatic bile ducts (*arrows*). Patient had sustained a gunshot wound to the porta hepatis 2 weeks before CT. Damage to the bile duct was not appreciated at the time of initial surgery. (From Federle MP, Goldberg HI, Kaiser JA, et al: Evaluation of abdominal trauma by computed tomography. *Radiology* 138:637, 1981.)

Intestinal Injuries

Intestinal injuries may result from a direct blow or from sudden compression, as with an improperly positioned lap seat belt (39). The two segments of bowel most susceptible to blunt injury are the duodenum and proximal small bowel. The duodenum is fixed in a retroperitoneal position directly over the spine, and the proximal jejunum is relatively fixed by the ligament of Treitz. Injury may result in intramural hematoma, direct laceration, or "blowout" of the wall due to sudden increase in intraluminal pressure. Bowel perforation is considered a surgical emergency demanding early diagnosis and treatment. A 65% mortality rate for duodenal perforation due to blunt trauma has been reported when diagnosis was delayed for more than 24 hours (40).

Plain radiography is of limited value in diagnosing bowel injuries. The presence of free intraperitoneal or retroperitoneal gas should be carefully sought, and properly centered horizontal beam radiographs are essential. Nevertheless, Toxopeus et al. were able preoperatively to diagnose retroperitoneal duodenal rupture in only 33% of cases (41), and Kelly et al, failed to diagnose any of six patients with proven duodenal rupture by plain films (42).

Our experience suggests that CT scanning may be quite useful in the detection of retroperitoneal duodenal rupture and subsequent complications (43, 44). The gas and fluid liberated from retroperitoneal rupture are usually confined to the right anterior pararenal space, although trauma can result in violation of fascial planes, and thus gas may be found either intraperitoneally or in other retroperitoneal spaces. Because of its greater contrast resolution and tomographic nature, CT may demonstrate small amounts of retroperitoneal gas and extravasated contrast not evident on plain film examination (Fig. 6.48).

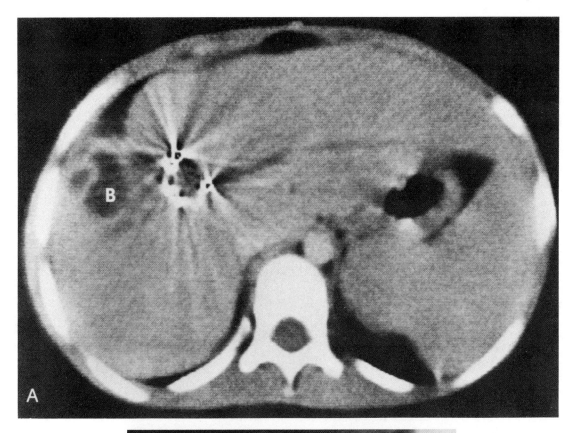

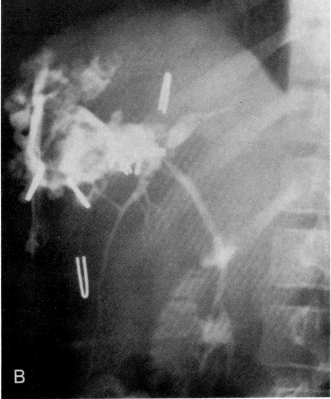

Figure 6.47.   Biliary-cutaneous fistula following blunt trauma.
A. CT demonstrates intrahepatic collection of bile (*B*) near site of prior hepatic laceration. Surgical clips cause artifacts.
B. Contrast injection of cutaneous fistula opacifies intrahepatic cavity and better defines the obstruction near the confluence of right and left hepatic ducts.

CT sections should be viewed with wide window widths so that extraluminal gas can be distinguished from fat or intraluminal gas. Small intestinal injuries are accurately diagnosed by CT, both only with careful attention to technique and close examination (7, 45). Oral contrast medium is essential and one must look carefully for extraluminal gas, contrast medium or blood (Figs. 6.49 and 6.50). Intramural hematoma is evident as diffuse fold thickening or a high-density (60 to 80 H) mass that narrows, distorts, or obliterates the bowel lumen. Children seem to be more susceptible to intramural hematoma, while adults more often suffer from bowel wall laceration.

Since the mechanism of injury is similar for duodenal and pancreatic trauma, CT scans obtained to evaluate possible pancreatic injury should be closely studied for evidence of duodenal laceration. We prefer CT examination as the initial study in such cases since the presence of barium or dense iodinated contrast material in the gut from a 0 preceding upper gastrointestinal examination seriously interferes with the quality of a subsequent CT study.

Small intestinal perforation may be difficult to diagnose specifically. We have studied 10 cases to date, and all have had signs of bowel injury, including intramural and mesenteric hematoma, and free per-

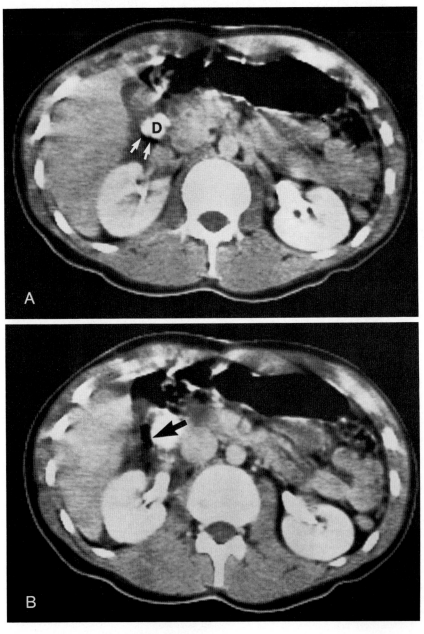

Figure 6.48.   Duodenal laceration; blunt trauma.
A, B. Extraluminal gas bubbles (*arrows*) are noted lateral and posterior to the contrast-opacified duodenal lumen (*D*).

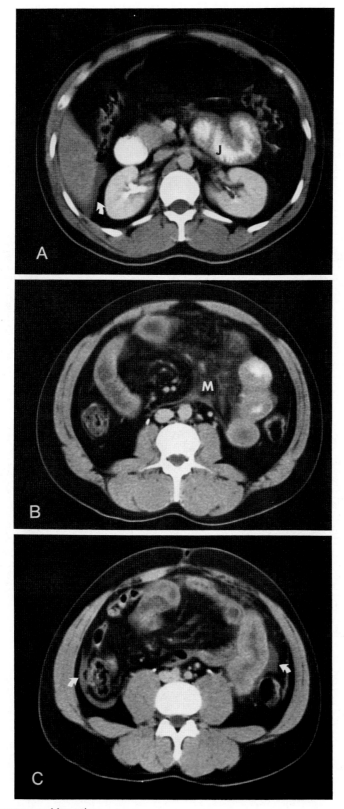

Figure 6.49.   Jejunal hematoma and laceration.
A–C. Several segments of proximal jejunum (*J*) have a thick wall, representing intramural hematoma. Mesenteric fat infiltration (*M*) and hemoperitoneum (*arrows*) are also noted. No extraluminal gas or Gastrografin is present, but jejunal hematoma with a small laceration was found at surgery.

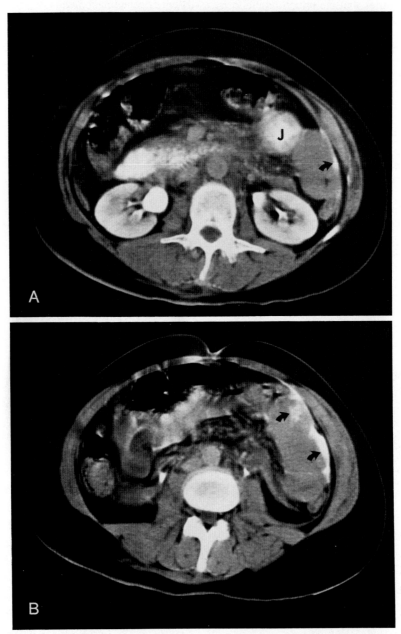

Figure 6.50.   Jejunal laceration.
A, B. The proximal jejunum (*J*) is thick walled, and there is a large adjacent amorphous collection of blood, bowel contents, and Gastrografin (*arrows*). In spite of this obvious laceration, no extraluminal gas is present, because the jejunum is usually fluid filled and almost gasless.

itoneal hemorrhage. Specific signs of laceration include extraluminal gas or Gastrografin, but these signs are not always present. Free intraperitoneal air can be detected by plain radiography in less than 30% of patients with small intestinal lacerations (46), probably because the small bowel is normally fluid filled and largely gasless.

Colonic injuries account for only 3 to 5% of all blunt abdominal injuries, but are important clinically because of potential life-threatening complications, such as peritonitis and hemorrhage (47). Clinical diagnosis is rarely made preoperatively, but can be apparent on CT. We have diagnosed several cases of intramural hematomas, depicted as distortion and narrowing of the colonic lumen by a high-density intramural mass (48) (Fig. 6.51). Colonic laceration is manifested by intra- or retroperitoneal spill of gas, stool, and blood (Fig. 6.52).

The omentum and mesentery are connecting folds of peritoneum enclosing a fatty areolar network of blood vessels, lymphatics, and nerves supplying the abdominal viscera. Because of their vascular nature, the omentum and mesentery are frequent sources of hemorrhage in abdominal trauma. The hemorrhage is often minor and self-limited (though detected as a "positive" peritoneal lavage), but more extensive hemorrhage may result and can be accurately diagnosed by CT (Figs. 6.53–6.55).

Pancreatic Injury

The most common etiology of pancreatic injuries in our experience has been blunt trauma, particularly from the impact of a steering wheel or a lap seat belt. Blunt or penetrating trauma may result in contusion of the pancreas, and the branches of the ductal system may be disrupted, leading to local hemorrhage and leakage of pancreatic enzymes. Pancreatic injuries are frequently associated with injuries to adjacent organs, and they result in a mortality rate of about 20% (49, 50). The difficulty in establishing a diagnosis of pancreatic injury has been stressed by various authors (49–51). Clinical, laboratory, and radiographic findings are highly variable and nonspecific. Even serum amylase levels are of little diagnostic value, particularly within the first 24 hours after injury.

CT is now well established as an accurate noninvasive means of detecting a wide variety of nontraumatic pancreatic lesions, including pancreatitis, pseudocysts, and abscess. Similar lesions are well-known sequelae of trauma, and CT has proved equally useful in this setting (52, 53).

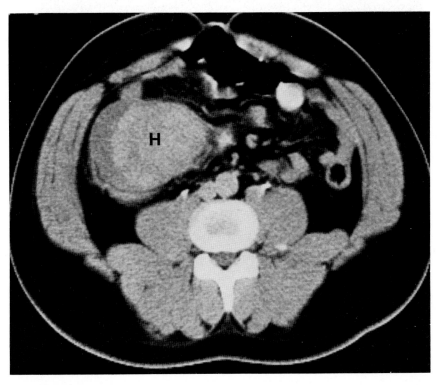

Figure 6.51. Hematoma of ascending colon following blunt trauma. On multiple CT sections a cylindrical high-density hematoma (*H*) was noted in the wall of the colon, distorting and narrowing the lumen. (From Jeffrey RB, Federle MP, Stein SM, Crass RA: Intramural hematoma of the cecum following blunt trauma *J Comput Assist Tomogr* 6:404, 1982.)

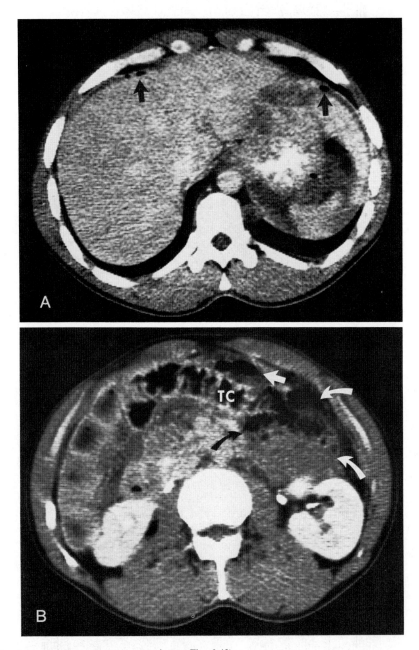

Figure 6.52.   Colon laceration; blunt trauma (same patient as Fig. 6.43).
A, B. Free extraluminal gas (*arrows*) is noted rising up under the diaphragm. The transverse colon (*TC*) is transected, leading to a collection of gas and bowel contents (*curved arrows*).

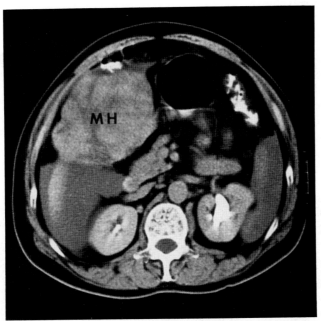

Figure 6.53.   Large, heterogeneous, high-density mesenteric hematoma (*MH*) following blunt trauma. Large hemoperitoneum is also noted.

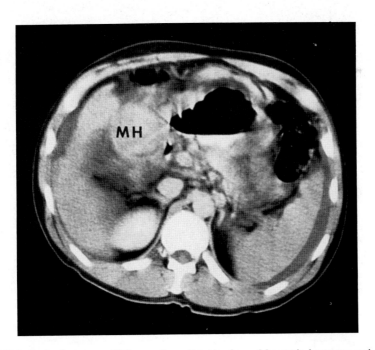

Figure 6.54.   Rounded high-density hematoma (*MH*) near the gallbladder fossa. Mesenteric hematoma and partial avulsion of the gallbladder were confirmed at surgery.

Mild traumatic pancreatitis generally appears as diffuse swelling of the gland (Fig. 6.56). More serious injuries generally result in a phlegmon, or large inflammatory mass, commonly extending into the mesentery ventral of the pancreas (Fig. 6.57). Spread of inflammation and blood throughout the anterior pararenal space is frequently noted (Figs. 6.58–6.60). These secondary signs of pancreatic injury are usually more evident than the primary parenchymal lesions and should be carefully sought in interpretation of the CT scan. If a pancreatic injury is not immediately recognized and treated, a pseudocyst may form within a week (Figs. 6.59 and 6.60). Pancreatic trauma accounts for about 5% of the pseudocysts encountered in the adult population, while virtually all pseudocysts in the pediatric population are the result of trauma (50).

Accuracy and Pitfalls

In our first 300 cases of blunt trauma CT scans, there were 13 surgically proved pancreatic injuries (52). Although CT correctly diagnosed 11 of the 13 injuries, there were four diagnostic errors, including two false positives. It is apparent that pancreatic injuries are more difficult to diagnose than other solid visceral injuries, but accuracy can improve with proper technique and attention to subtle findings.

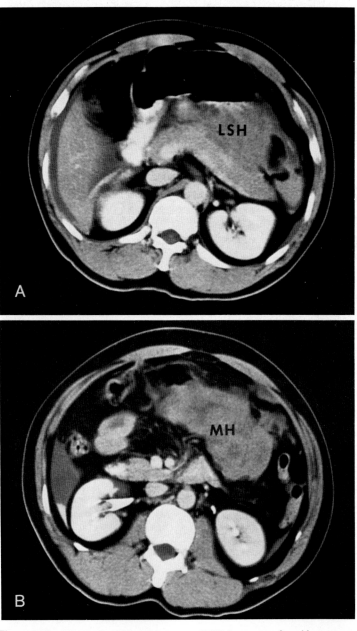

Figure 6.55.   Mesenteric (*MH*) and lesser sac (*LSH*) hematomas from blunt trauma.

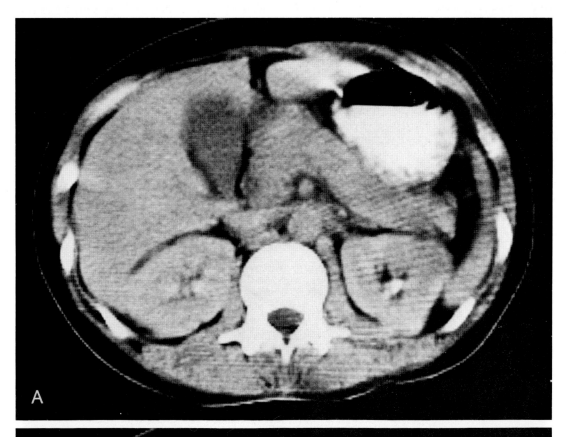

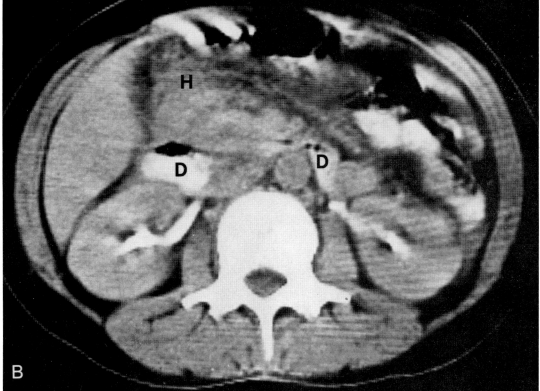

Figure 6.56.   Traumatic pancreatitis.
A. Mild diffuse swelling of pancreas.
B. On more caudal section, hematoma (*H*) and inflammation extend out into mesentery. (*D*, duodenum.)

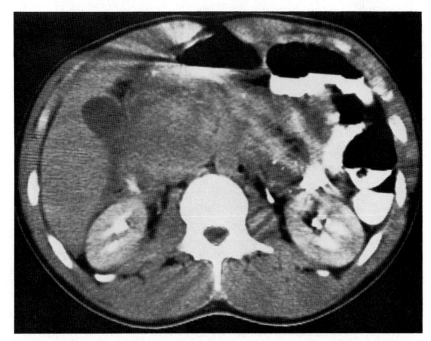

Figure 6.57. Traumatic pancreatic phlegmon; a large inflammatory mass envelopes the pancreas.

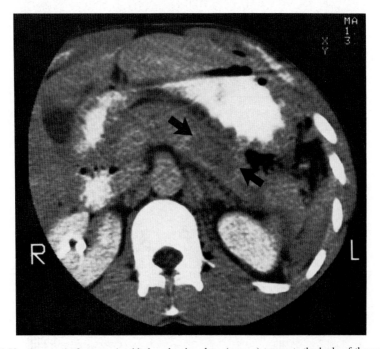

Figure 6.58. Pancreatic fracture. A wide low-density plane (*arrows*) transects the body of the pancreas.

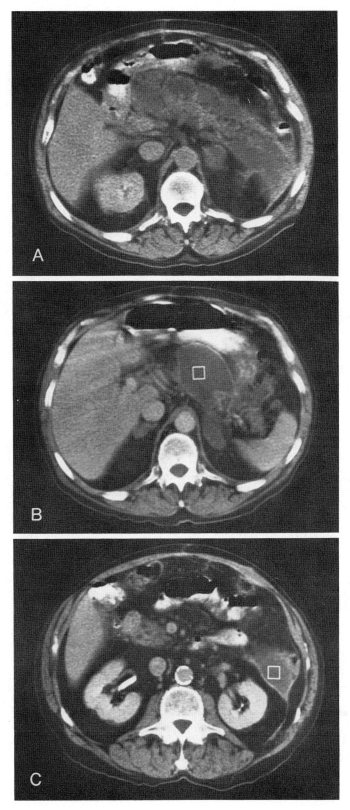

Figure 6.59. Evolution of post-traumatic pseudocyst.   A. Initial CT scan (12–29) demonstrated widespread infiltration of the peripancreatic fat planes.
B, C. Repeat CT (2–2) shows development of pseudocysts (*cursors*) in the lesser sac and left anterior pararenal space.

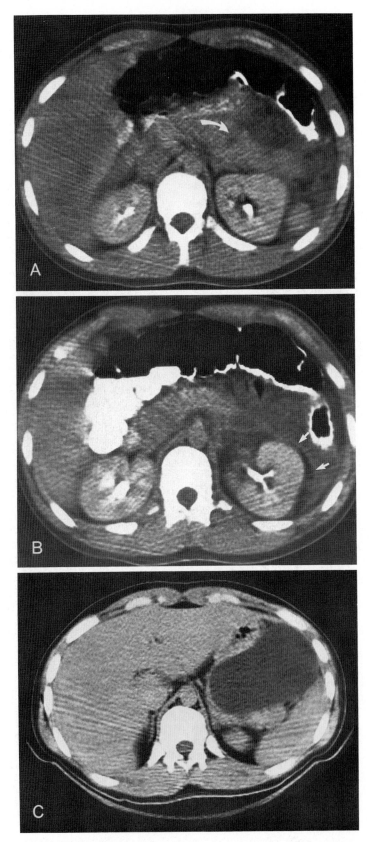

Figure 6.60.   Traumatic pancreatitis and pseudocyst.
A, B. Initial CT scan demonstrates a fracture plane through the body of the pancreas (**A**, *curved arrow*). Note widespread infiltration of anterior pararenal space limited posteriorly by the perirenal fascia (**B**, *arrows*).
C. Same patient after 9 days of conservative therapy. A post-traumatic pseudocyst is noted in the lesser sac.

Fracture or laceration of the pancreatic parenchyma is difficult to detect on CT for several reasons. The fracture plane may contain hemorrhagic or other exudate of density similar to pancreatic parenchyma, leading to a false negative diagnosis. Still, we have encountered no cases of pancreatic trauma with normal peripancreatic fat in the anterior pararenal spaces and mesentery.

False positive diagnoses can be described as "pseudofractures," attributable to streak artifacts and misinterpretation of normal anatomy. The latter situation is illustrated in Figure 6.61 and is due to misinterpretation of unopacified proximal jejunal loops as the pancreatic body, separated from the normal head-neck region by a fat plane around the mesenteric vessels. Streak artifacts must be minimized by gastric decompression, dilute oral contrast medium, and use of sedation if necessary. Scans obtained dynamically with table incrementation and bolus infusion of intravenous contrast medium can also be useful.

If doubt persists, repeating the CT scans the following day is often useful. Repeat scans are often unequivocally normal (usually due to fewer artifacts) or definitely abnormal, due to further peripancreatic inflammation and hemorrhage.

Renal Trauma

A major problem in the consideration of renal trauma has been proper assessment of the extent of injury, which determines the best therapeutic approach. Most investigations have attempted to divide injuries into three broad categories based on a combination of clinical and radiographic findings (Fig. 6.62) (54–57). Lesions in Category I are relatively minor, consisting of contusion and small cortical lacerations without disruption of the calyceal system. They account for 75 to 85% of cases in most series. Lesions in Category II are more serious, account for about 10% of cases, and include cortical lesions that

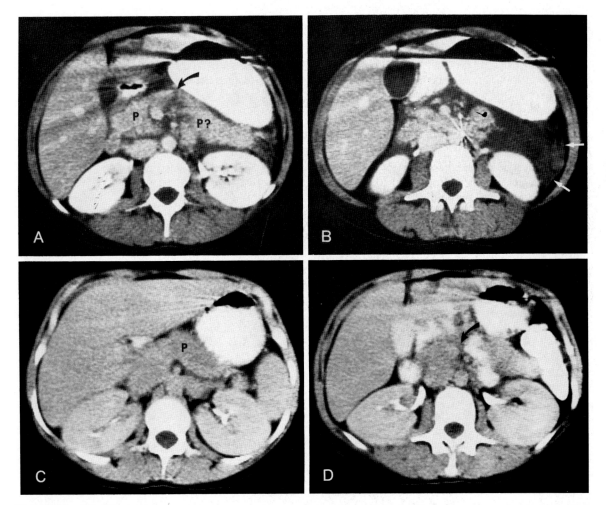

Figure 6.61. Pseudofracture.
A, B. Traumatic pancreatitis is suggested by infiltrated anterior pararenal space (**B**, *arrows*). A low-density plane (**A**, *curved arrow*) was interpreted as a fracture separating the pancreatic head (*P*) and body (*P?*).
C, D. Repeat CT scan 2 days later. Pancreas (*P*) is intact and peripancreatic edema has resolved. The "fracture" (**D**, *curved arrow*) was the normal plane between the head-neck of pancreas and proximal jejunal loops that were poorly opacified on the first study (due to ileus) and which had simulated the pancreatic body.

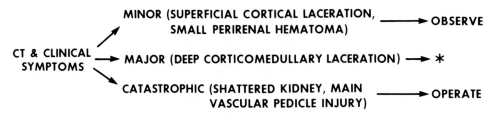

*Therapy depends on amount of nonviable tissue, extent of hemorrhage and extravasation of urine

Figure 6.62.   Classification and management of renal injuries.

communicate with the collecting system (complete laceration and renal fracture). Lesions in Category III are catastrophic, make up about 5% of the total, and consist of shattered kidneys and injuries to the renal vascular pedicle. There is general agreement among urologists that Category I (minor) injuries are best managed conservatively, while Category III lesions (catastrophic) require urgent surgery. Although opinion is divided over the proper management of Category II lesions, virtually all authors stress the need for accurate evaluation of the type and extent of injury so that therapy can be rationally planned (55, 58–61).

The four criteria that most influence therapy are the extent of parenchymal injury, presence of extravasated urine, extent of perirenal hemorrhage, and status of the renal vascular pedicle. Excretory urography may over- or underestimate the extent of injury. While a normal urogram generally indicates minor or no injury, the abnormal urogram is frequently nonspecific. In acute injury, excretory urography with nephrotomography accurately depicts the extent of renal injury in about 70 to 85% of cases (54–56), leaving a large number of patients (particularly those with more severe injuries) in whom the diagnosis is uncertain. Liberal use of angiography has been recommended by some authors to define such cases better (62–65).

Within the past 5 years, CT has replaced angiography in most medical centers as the procedure of choice in evaluating most types of major renal trauma (65–72). CT is capable of detecting virtually the entire spectrum of renal injury. Renal contusion is seen on conventional CT as delayed extravasation of contrast medium into the interstitial renal tissue. If a bolus of contrast medium is administered with rapid-sequence scanning, the contused area enhances during the capillary phase. Parenchymal tears and intrarenal hematomas appear as defects within a normally functioning kidney (Figs. 6.63 and 6.64). Complete lacerations, extending into the collecting system, dem-

onstrate a parenchymal tear with extravasation of contrast-opacified urine (Fig. 6.65). A renal fracture is a complete laceration extending through the kidney with separation of the renal poles (Figs. 6.66 and 6.67). Renal artery occlusion is diagnosed by failure of the kidney to enhance, as is discussed further below.

CT has clear advantages over excretory urography in assessing the extent of renal parenchymal damage and perirenal hemorrhage. A frequent urographic finding in trauma is a decreased unilateral nephrogram with evidence of perirenal mass effect. This is a nonspecific finding that may be encountered in relatively minor contusions and lacerations or severe renal disruptions. CT effectively distinguishes among these injuries and often demonstrates extravasation of urine not evident on urography, because of the improved contrast resolution and tomographic nature of CT.

The detection of renal vascular pedicle injuries remains a somewhat controversial topic. Renal arterial occlusion and, less commonly, avulsion may result from blunt trauma, with stretching of the vascular pedicle. Successful repair requires prompt diagnosis, and renal viability after 12 hours of ischemia is rare. Several reports have documented the ability of CT to diagnose global or segmental renal ischemia due to main or segmental renal arterial occlusion (72–75). The ischemic segment or kidney is near normal in size but fails to enhance with urographic contrast medium (Figs. 6.68 and 6.69). A "cortical rim" of enhancing peripheral tissue may be seen, presumably due to residual perfusion by capsular or collateral vessels.

Lang et al. have recently documented the ability of CT to diagnose renal injuries, including infarction, but still maintain a role for angiography when renovascular injury is strongly suspected (71). They point out that only angiography may diagnose certain vascular injuries, such as subintimal flaps, that may go on to occlusion.

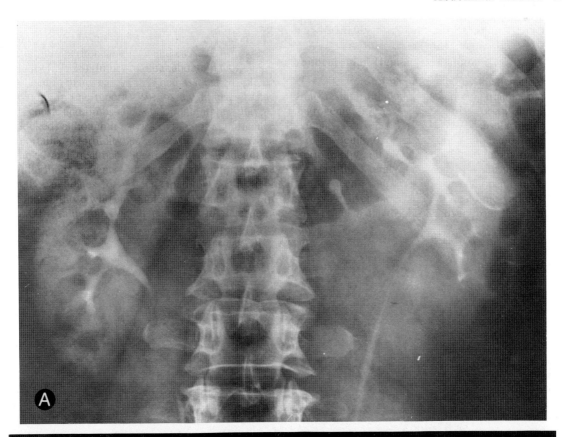

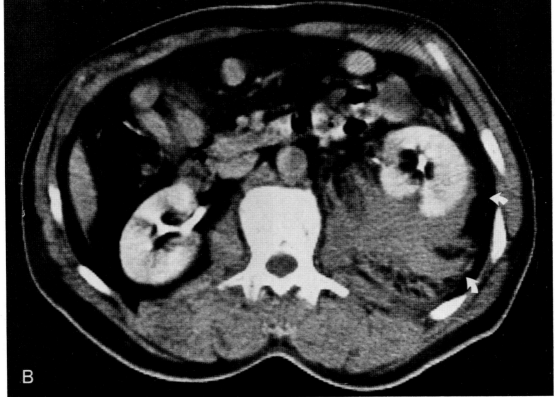

Figure 6.63.   Renal laceration.
A. Excretory urogram shows loss of left renal outline medially and mass effect with lateral displacement of the kidney.
B. CT demonstrates corticomedullary laceration and moderate perirenal hematoma extending to renal (Gerota's) fascia (*arrows*). Uneventful recovery on conservative management.

In our experience, subintimal flaps and arteriovenous fistulae are uncommon sequelae of blunt trauma, and fistulae that result from penetrating trauma usually close spontaneously. While angiography is undoubtedly more accurate than CT in diagnosing these specific injuries, we feel it is rarely indicated in evaluation of the acute blunt injury. Clinical and urographic criteria are poor predictors of renovascular injuries and many unnecessary angiograms would be performed before finding a surgically treatable lesion not already detected by CT. If a persistent arteriovenous fistula is suspected, angiography is optimal both to depict the lesion and for therapy, such as transcatheter embolization or balloon occlusion. Also, if massive hemorrhage results from acute penetrating injury, angiography should be performed for diagnosis and therapy of lacerated vessels (Fig. 6.70).

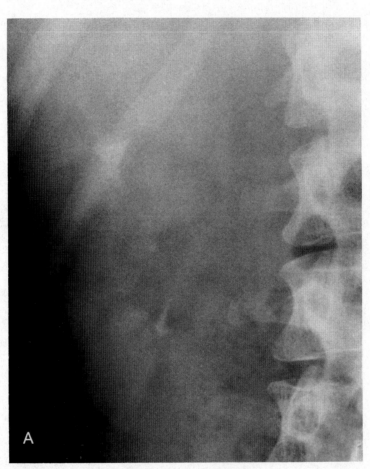

Figure 6.64. Major injury; deep corticomedullary laceration.
A. Excretory urogram shows diminished nephrogram and mass effect.

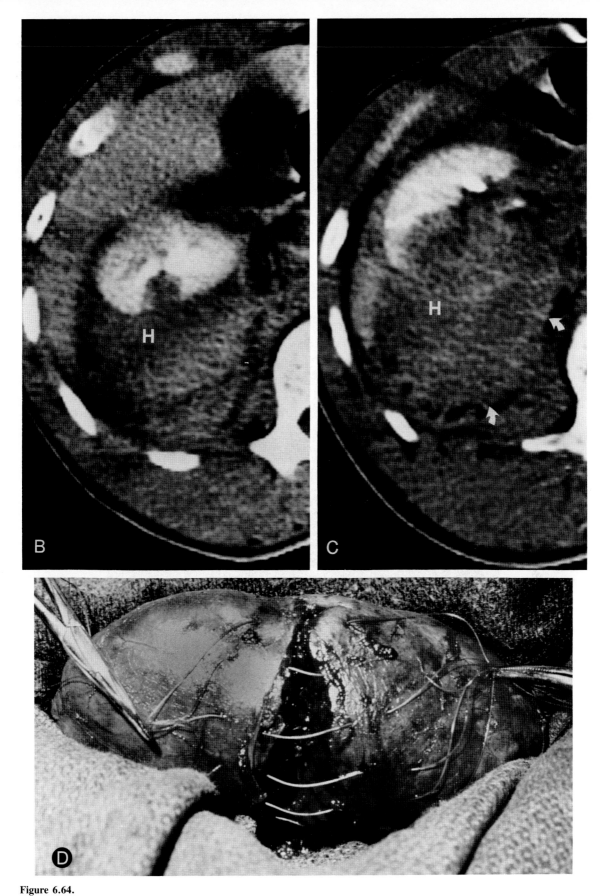

Figure 6.64.
B, C. CT shows deep corticomedullary laceration extending to renal hilus but no extravasation of opacified urine. Large perirenal hematoma (*H*) distends renal fascia (*arrows*). Sections above and below these showed normal renal parenchyma.
D. Surgical specimen with deep laceration not communicating with collecting system. Operation was required because of continued bleeding.

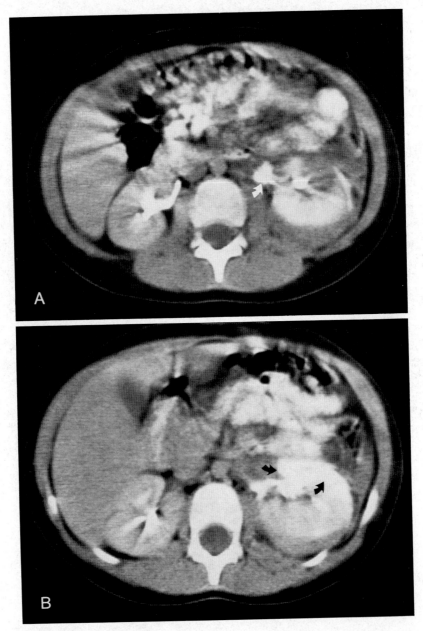

Figure 6.65.   Major injury; "complete" laceration.
A, B. Laceration through ventral half of kidney seen as absence of enhancing parenchyma. Extravasated opacified urine (*arrows*) indicates extension into the collecting system.

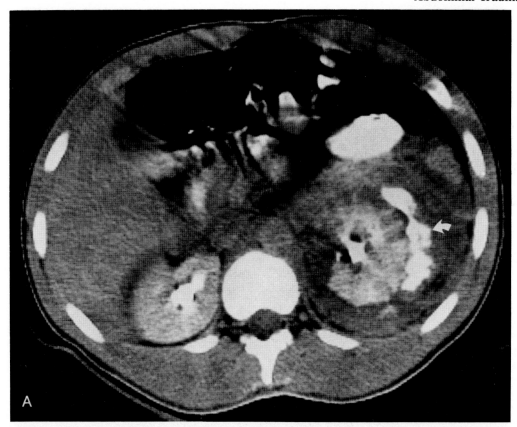

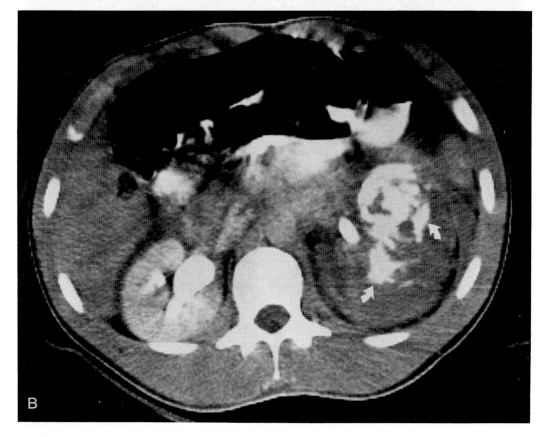

Figure 6.66.   Major injury; deep laceration with extravasation.
A, B. Midportion of kidney is shattered with marked extravasation of opacified urine (*arrows*) and large perirenal hematoma.

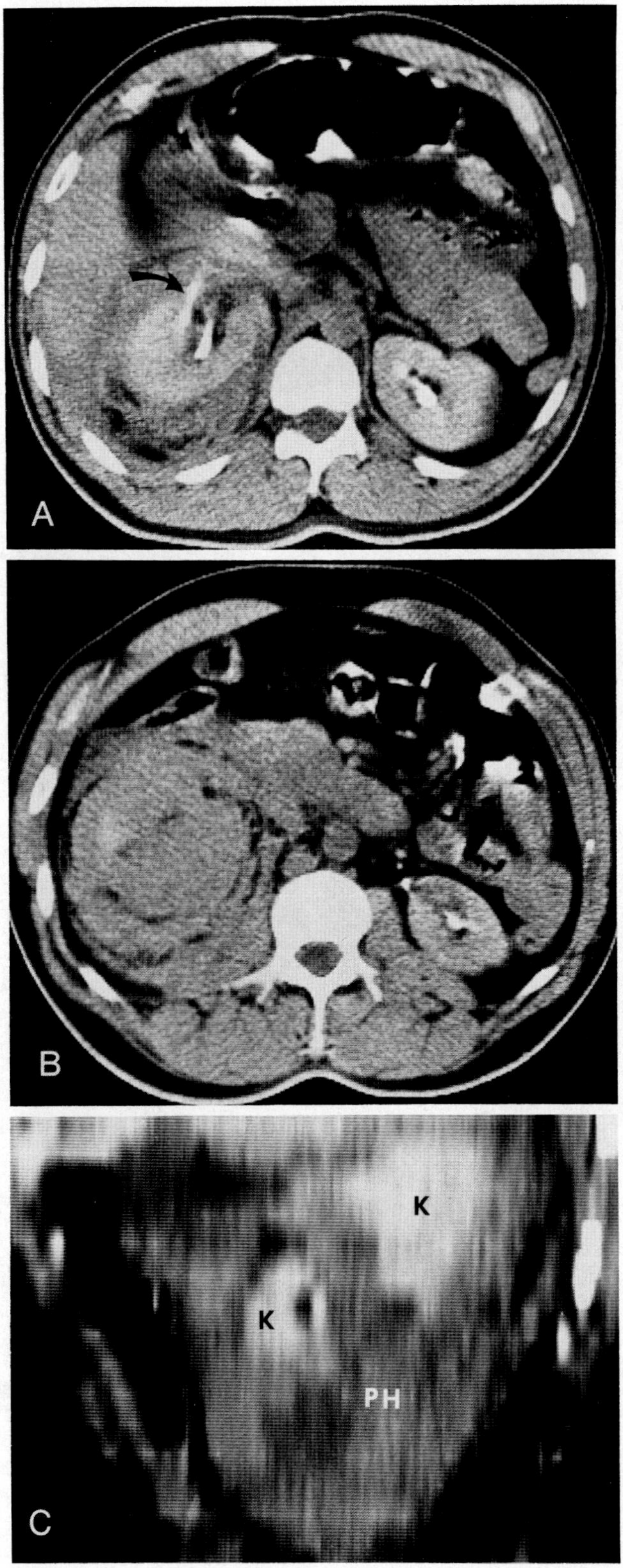

Figure 6.67.   Major injury; renal fracture.
A, B. Axial sections show absence of functioning parenchyma in midkidney with large perirenal hematoma and extravasation of opacified urine (*arrow*).
C. Sagittal reformation more clearly depicts the oblique fracture plane separating the upper and lower renal poles and the large perirenal hematoma (*PH*). (*K*, kidney.)

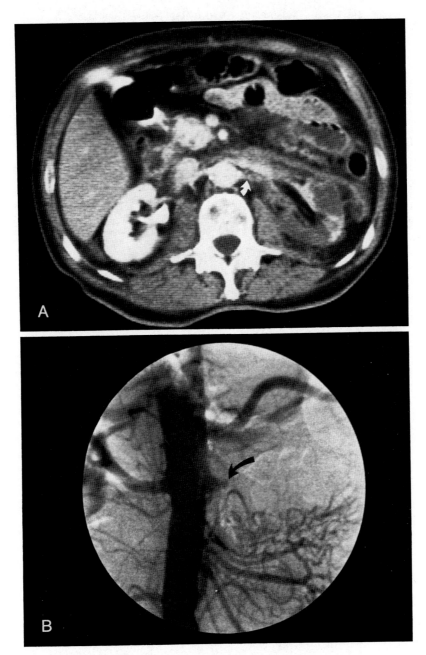

Figure 6.68. Vascular pedicle injury; blunt trauma.
A. CT shows normal size left kidney with minimal perirenal hemorrhage. Renal parenchyma fails to enhance except for small peripheral areas ("cortical rim sign"). Intact enhancing left renal vein and right renal artery are noted, while left renal artery fails to enhance (*arrow*).
B. Arteriogram confirms proximal left renal arterial occlusion (*arrow*).

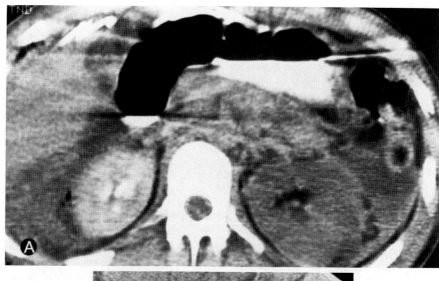

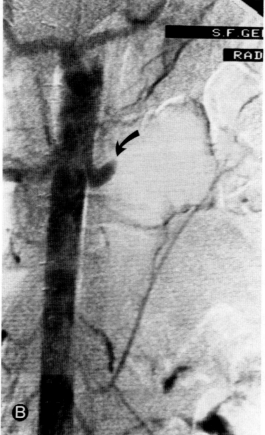

Figure 6.69.   Vascular pedicle injury; blunt trauma.
A. CT shows mildly swollen, nonenhancing left kidney. (Pancreatic and splenic lacerations, also diagnosed by CT, account for hemorrhage into pararenal space and Morison's pouch.)
B. Arteriogram confirms occluded left renal artery (*arrow*).

Penetrating Renal Trauma

In evaluation of acute penetrating renal trauma, CT can have a definite effect on management of selected patients. Patients who sustain gunshot wounds have a high incidence of associated intraperitoneal injuries and are *not* candidates for CT scanning. Those with stab wounds to the flank, however, can benefit from radiographic evaluation. Because urography correlates rather poorly with the extent of penetrating renal injury, most urologists have taken an aggressive surgical approach to such injuries. CT more accurately depicts the extent of parenchymal damage, perirenal hemorrhage, extravasation of urine, and the status of the vascular pedicle (Figs. 6.71–6.73). These objective criteria along with clinical assessment now allow confident nonoperative management in many cases of stab wounds to the flank.

Trauma to the Abnormal Kidney

It is particularly difficult to accurately define injuries to kidneys that have pre-existing congenital or acquired abnormalities. Renal neoplasms, simple cysts, and adult polycystic kidneys may bleed or rupture spontaneously or with relatively minor trauma. The urographic and clinical findings often seem out of proportion to the degree of trauma, and the underlying renal pathology is often masked by perirenal hemorrhage. Angiomyolipomas and hypernephromas have a particular tendency to hemorrhage. Angiography may be useful in diagnosing neoplasm in such cases, but CT has accurately detected three neoplasms in our experience (Fig. 6.74), including one that was not detectable by angiography (75). In none of the three cases of renal neoplasm was the tumor detected on excretory urography. Significant hemorrhage may occur in polycystic renal disease, either into the cystic

spaces or into the perirenal or retroperitoneal spaces (76, 77) (Fig. 6.75). Urography is of little diagnostic utility owing to renal insufficiency in most cases, while CT accurately and specifically detects hemorrhage due to its characteristically high attenuation value.

In similar fashion, CT may help to distinguish leaking or ruptured simple renal cysts from hemorrhage by the demonstration of near water density perirenal fluid (Fig. 6.76). Acute hemorrhage typically has an attenuation value in excess of 40 H.

Congenital renal anomalies may predispose to traumatic injury by virtue of size, shape, or location. An englarged kidney, like an enlarged spleen, is vulnerable to blunt or penetrating trauma. A horseshoe or pelvic kidney lies in an area unprotected by ribs and may be driven against the vertebral column by blunt trauma. CT makes it easier to distinguish traumatic lesions from congenital variations in such conditions (Fig. 6.77).

Extravasation of urine is considered by some urologists as a sign of major renal injury and an indication for operative repair of the lacerated collecting system. However, caliectasis and a dilated renal pelvis may predispose to laceration or forniceal rupture even without major renal parenchymal damage (Fig. 6.78). In these cases, extravasation may not have the same implication as if the kidney previously had been normal. Conversely, hydronephrosis accompanied by decreased renal function may cause a major renal injury to be missed at excretory urography, because extravasation of even large amounts of poorly opacified urine (and blood) may not be evident. Because of its greater low-contrast resolution and tomographic nature, CT may detect extravasation not seen on excretory urography, and CT better defines the extent of renal parenchymal damage (76).

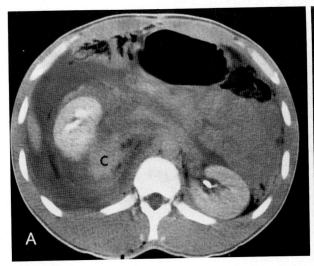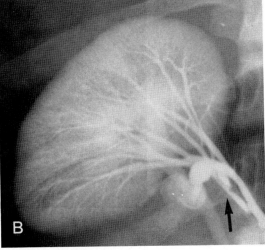

Figure 6.70.   Stab wound to back. Minimal hematuria and normal renal function on excretory urography.
A. CT shows massive perirenal hemorrhage including clotted blood (*C*) but no parenchymal injury.
B. Angiogram demonstrates partial transection of a major renal artery (*arrow*) with massive extravasation.

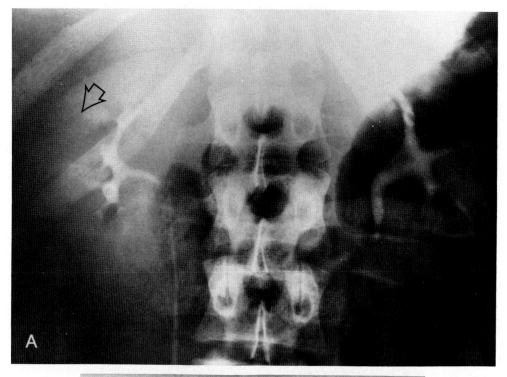

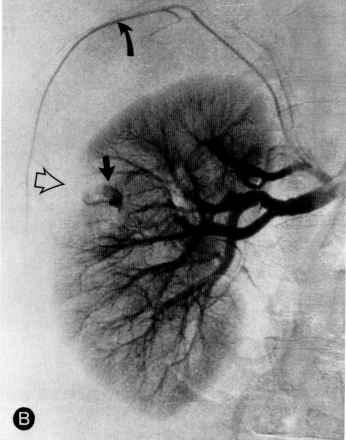

Figure 6.71. Major injury; deep laceration with extravasation (stab wound).
A. Excretory urogram demonstrates focal parenchymal defect (*arrow*) but no extravasation.
B. Arteriogram performed because of continuing hematuria and falling hematocrit. Stretched capsular artery (*curved arrow*) indicating extrarenal hematoma. Subtle parenchymal lesion (*open arrow*) and extravasation of opacified urine (*straight arrow*).

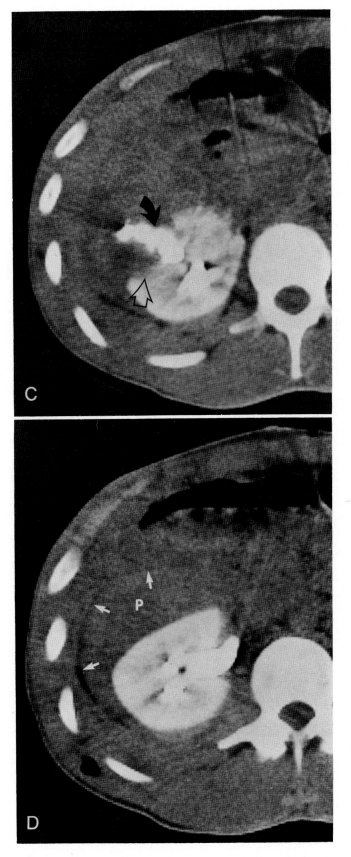

Figure 6.71.
C, D. CT scan followed arteriogram. Obvious corticomedullary laceration (*open arrow*) and extravasation of opacified urine (*curved arrow*). Large perirenal hematoma (*P*) extending to renal fascia (*white arrows*). (From Federle MP, Goldberg HI, Kaiser JA, et al: Evaluation of abdominal trauma by computed tomography. *Radiology* 138:637, 1981.)

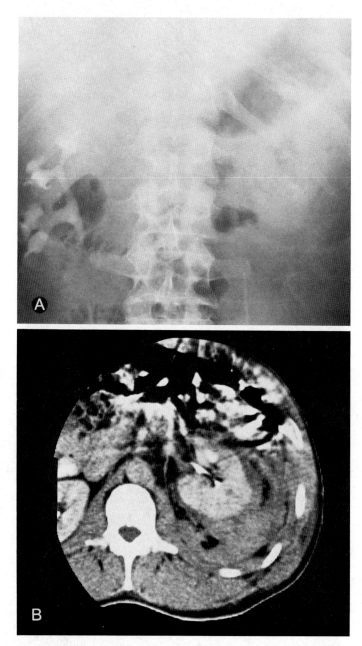

Figure 6.72. Stab wound to left kidney.
A. Urogram shows decreased nephrogram on left.
B. CT shows minimal parenchymal damage, no extravasation of urine, and a moderate subcapsular and perirenal hematoma. No surgery was required.

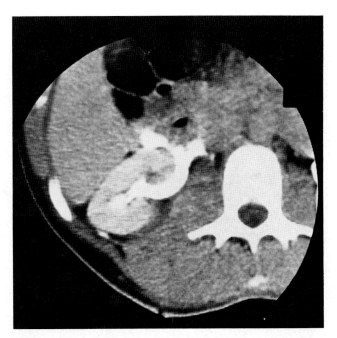

Figure 6.73.   Stab wound to right flank. CT shows no parenchymal damage or perirenal hemorrhage, but extravasation is noted surrounding the lacerated proximal ureter.

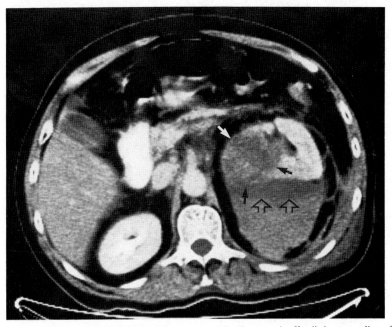

Figure 6.74.   Trauma to abnormal kidney. Fluid-fluid level (*open arrows*) is "hematocrit effect" due to settling of cellular elements of blood. Large rounded mass in kidney (*closed arrows*) of different attenuation is a renal cell carcinoma, actively bleeding from minor trauma.

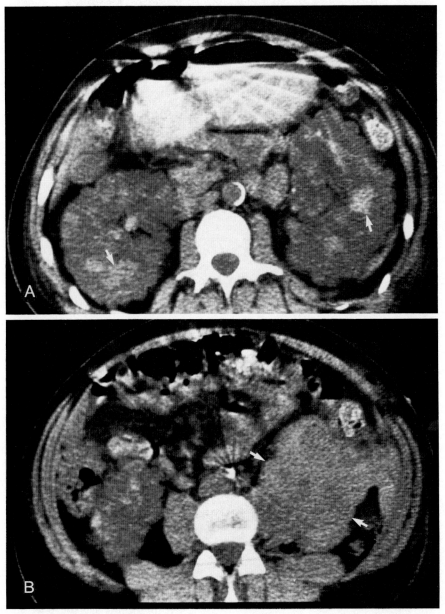

Figure 6.75. Hemorrhage with polycystic kidneys.
A. Both kidneys are grossly enlarged and deformed by cysts of varying attenuation. Recent hemorrhage into some cysts accounts for high-density areas (*arrows*).
B. Extrarenal hemorrhage distends the perirenal space below the left kidney (*arrows*).

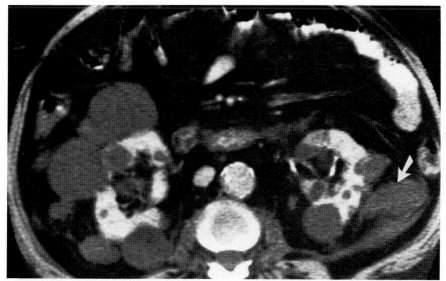

Figure 6.76. Ruptured simple cyst. Perirenal fluid (*arrow*) (10 H) is mostly cyst fluid with minimal hemorrhage. Urography was not helpful in assessing the extent of renal injury.

Imaging Approach to Renal Trauma

Because most renal injuries are minor and heal spontaneously, and because a normal urogram in a clinically stable patient practically excludes significant renal trauma, excretory urography (intravenous pyelography or IVP) remains a valuable screening procedure for patients suspected of having *isolated* renal trauma. If the urogram is abnormal or suggests major trauma, *or* if the patient seems to have major trauma in spite of a "normal" urogram (e.g., continuing gross hematuria, falling hematocrit) then CT should be performed (Fig. 6.79). For victims of major or multiple trauma for whom CT is to be performed, a preceding excretory urogram is a waste of time, and should not be performed. If urography has been performed in the usual and recommended manner (100 ml bolus of contrast material for adults) and CT is later requested, additional contrast media should be given in most cases. The delay between the urogram and CT diminishes renal parenchymal enhancement. An additional 50 ml bolus (for adults) provides optimal detection of renal and other solid visceral injuries. Angiography is almost never performed at our trauma center for evaluation of acute blunt renal trauma. It is useful for suspected arteriovenous fistulae and false aneurysms as discussed above. In our opinion, CT findings of traumatic renal arterial occlusion are specific and constitute an indication for urgent surgery. Angiography might provide a useful vascular "roadmap" in selected cases, but there is a danger of delaying surgery beyond the point of renal viability.

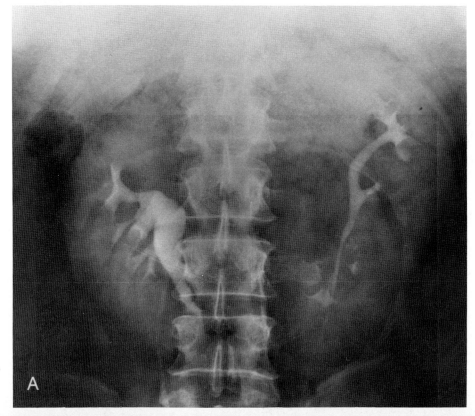

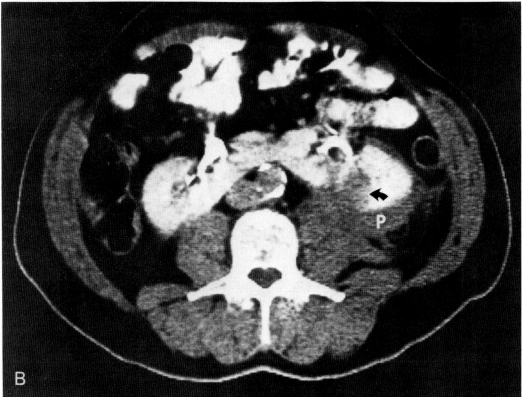

Figure 6.77.   Trauma to abnormal kidney.
A. Excretory urogram shows horseshoe kidney but no evidence of injury.
B. CT was performed because of continuing hematuria. Horseshoe kidney evident with functional tissue bridging the two sides. Deep corticmedullary laceration (*arrow*) and perirenal hematoma (*P*).

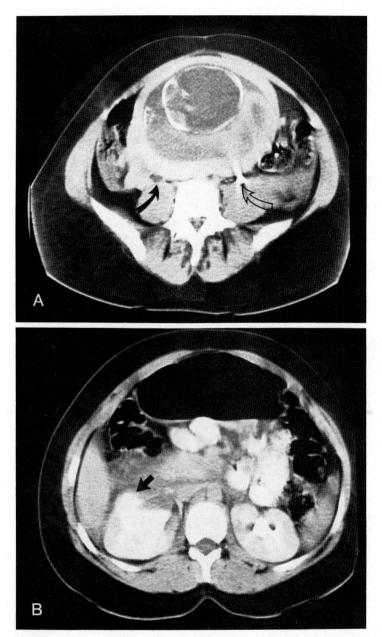

Figure 6.78.   Trauma to abnormal kidney; hydronephrosis of pregnancy. CT was performed after sonographic confirmation of fetal demise due to blunt abdominal trauma.
A. CT through uterus shows fetal head and high attenuation within the uterus that may represent hemorrhage into the amniotic fluid. Right ureter (*arrow*) is dilated and nonopacified, while the left ureter (*open arrow*) is densely opacified.
B. Right-sided hydronephrosis is present and extravasated urine (*arrow*) is present near the distended renal pelvis but the renal parenchyma is normal. At surgery, a minor forniceal rupture was found, not requiring repair. This is analogous to the forniceal rupture and extravasation that frequently accompany acute ureteral calculus obstruction.

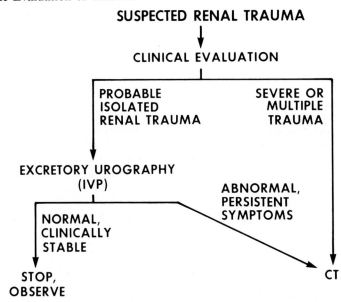

Figure 6.79.   Flow diagram with suggested role of excretory urography and CT in suspected renal trauma.

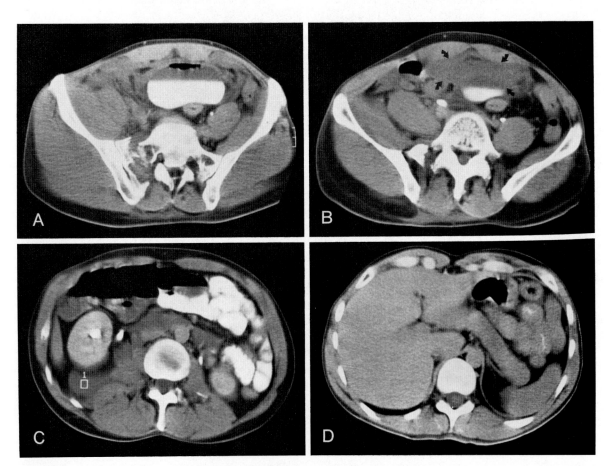

Figue 6.80.   Avoiding laparotomy for retroperitoneal hemorrhage.

A, B. Extensive pelvic fractures accompanied by bleeding into the right buttock, iliopsoas muscle, and retroperitoneum. A relatively small amount of blood is also present intraperitoneally in the anterior perivesicle space (*arrows*).

C, D. Retroperitoneal hemorrhage extends up behind the right kidney (*cursor*), but no intraperitoneal blood is present in the mid- or upper abdomen, and the abdominal viscera are intact. CT can help to avoid unnecessary laparotomy in such cases, even though peritoneal lavage would have been "positive" had it been done in this case.

COMPARISON WITH OTHER IMAGING MODALITIES

The choice of diagnostic imaging modalities for evaluation of abdominal trauma cannot, and should not, be legislated or relegated to algorithms or "decision trees" that are meant to apply to all patients at all hospitals. Rather the choice is influenced by many factors, including the results of clinical evaluation of the patient, the availability and quality of equipment and personnel, and the expertise and confidence of physicians interpreting the studies. It is useful to consider data comparing the accuracy and theoretical advantages of various imaging studies, but these must be interpreted in the context of one's own experience (78).

Radiography

Routine radiography (plain films and contrast studies) have a limited but important role in evaluation of blunt abdominal trauma. The initial assessment should include radiographs of the cervical spine, chest, and pelvis. As suggested by Ben-Menachem (79), the purpose of these films is not to screen the abdomen but rather to identify other potentially important injuries, such as cervical spine fracture, cardiopulmonary lesions, or extensive pelvic fractures. Abdominal films are rarely diagnostic of specific injuries and lack sensitivity (46, 80). While hemoperitoneum and free intraperitoneal or extraperitoneal gas might be considered diagnostic of an "operable" traumatic lesion, these findings are absent in the majority of patients, even those with proved solid or hollow visceral injuries. The normal abdominal film is, therefore, of little value.

Upper gastrointestinal or colonic contrast studies remain the procedures of choice when injury to the alimentary tube is specifically sought. Intramural hemorrhage and bowel wall laceration can be accurately diagnosed. We rarely perform gastrointestinal contrast studies as the initial imaging modality because the dense contrast material would produce artifacts limiting subsequent CT examination.

The role of excretory urography has been previously discussed, and it remains the initial procedure of choice when isolated renal trauma is suspected. In addition, we sometimes obtain an emergency "one-shot IVP" in the Emergency Department as part of the initial evaluation of a severely traumatized patient likely to be taken to laparotomy urgently. The study consists of a single supine abdominal film exposed after an intravenous bolus infusion of 50 to 100 ml of urographic contrast media, and is meant merely to confirm the presence of two functioning kidneys prior to abdominal exploration. Cystography and urethrography are valuable for diagnosing bladder and urethral injuries. We believe that bladder rupture can be accurately diagnosed by routine abdominopelvic CT as well, which might render subsequent cystography redundant, but must await the results of our prospective study.

Radionuclide Scintigraphy

Radionuclide scanning is a safe, noninvasive means of evaluating the liver, spleen, and kidneys (81–87). False negative results are very uncommon, and false positive results are reported as less than 10% in several series. Nonspecificity of "cold defects," including certain normal anatomic variants, such as splenic clefts and various hepatic lobulations, causes occasional diagnostic pitfalls. Exact accuracy figures and comparisons with other imaging studies, including CT, are difficult to evaluate because of a lack of surgical confirmation in all published series. The ability to evaluate parenchymal injuries, however, is not the limiting factor in scintigraphy. Rather, the inability to evaluate associated hemorrhage, extravasation of urine, and other visceral injuries makes radionuclide scanning less useful in the comprehensive evaluation of blunt abdominal trauma. While referring physicians frequently identify a specific abdominal organ as the one most likely injured, such organ-specific evaluation is often ill advised. In patients with splenic injuries, for instance, associated intra-abdominal injuries have been found in 18 to 48% of patients (88, 89). We have frequently identified solid or hollow visceral injuries in unsuspected sites while the "at risk" organ was normal.

When abdominal CT scans are obscured by artifacts (metallic clips, patient agitation, etc.) radionuclide scintigraphy may provide useful information.

Angiography

Angiograhy is of limited value in blunt abdominal trauma because it is invasive, time consuming, and relatively insensitive and nonspecific (90). In splenic trauma, poor correlation of angiographic and pathologic findings has been reported (91). Angiography cannot comprehensively evaluate all abdominal and retroperitoneal viscera and cannot evaluate associated hemoperitoneum. Angiography does remain the most accurate way of evaluating vascular injuries, and it is essential in the early evaluation of suspected blunt thoracic aortic injury (see Chapter 5). We rarely utilize angiography in the initial evaluation of blunt abdominal trauma, but find it useful in the subsequent evaluation of patients with blunt or penetrating trauma and occult bleeding, who are considered at risk for vascular injuries. Suspected traumatic pseudoaneurysms and arteriovenous fistulae are best evaluated by selective angiography, which may also lead to therapeutic embolization (92–94). Pelvic fractures with associated hemorrhage are also best evaluated and treated by angiographic techniques.

Ultrasonography

Ultrasonography in trauma has not been extensively studied, but certain limitations have been noted in several reports (7, 95–97). Comprehensive evaluation of the abdomen is extremely difficult due to a lack of "acoustic windows" imposed by open wounds, broken ribs, intestinal gas, and inability to reposition the patient. In one prospective study of liver and spleen injuries, ultrasound could not be adequately performed in 19% of patients because of superficial injuries or pain (98). In several reports, almost 50% of splenic injuries have been missed on ultrasonography due to the similar low-level echogenicity of splenic parenchyma and blood clot (7, 97). Renal parenchymal injuries and perirenal fluid can be detected by ultrasound, but sonography provides only morphologic, not functional, information, unlike CT and urography. Because it is noninvasive and accurately identifies fluid collections, sonography may find its greatest utility in the follow-up of patients with known abdominal injuries, to document progressive resolution of parenchymal laceration and hemorrhage.

COMPARISON WITH PERITONEAL LAVAGE

Many patients with abdominal injuries have either equivocal or absent physical and laboratory findings, and initial assessment has been found accurate in only 55 to 84% of patients (80, 99, 100). Diagnostic peritoneal lavage has been extensively studied as a supplement to clinical evaluation (101, 102). Peritoneal lavage entails installation and subsequent recovery of sterile saline solution in the peritoneal cavity. The recovered lavage fluid can be examined for blood and other contaminants such as bowel contents and amylase concentration.

Peritoneal lavage is very sensitive in detecting intraperitoneal hemorrhage. Various criteria for a "positive" result have been proposed, but many regard *any* evidence of blood as an indication for laparotomy. Such an approach results in many nontherapeutic laparotomies, with reports of 6 to 25% of patients with trivial injuries and positive results of lavage (red blood cell count of greater than 100,000) not requiring laparotomy (101–103). False positive lavage can also result from traumatic insertion of the trocar, or retroperitoneal or pelvic hematomas with blood entering the peritoneal cavity through torn fascial planes or by diapedesis of red cells across an intact peritoneal membrane. Extraperitoneal injuries can give rise to both false positive and false negative results, because the extraperitoneal location of the urinary bladder, pancreas, kidneys, and other structures precludes evaluation by peritoneal lavage. Peritoneal lavage is also less accurate and more dangerous in patients with a prior laparotomy or other cause of peritoneal adhesions.

We have evaluated more than 50 cases of retroperitoneal or extraperitoneal pelvic hemorrhage without intraperitoneal visceral injury (18). None of these had laparotomy except for six patients with pancreatic lacerations and one patient with intraperitoneal rupture of the bladder. Three other patients with blood in both the retroperitoneal and intraperitoneal spaces were spared surgery, partly based on the absence of parenchymal laceration as demonstrated by CT (Fig. 6.80).

CT has certain advantages over peritoneal lavage in evaluation of intraperitoneal injuries as well. The sensitivity and specificity of CT for visceral lacerations are very high. Absence of a parenchymal laceration on CT is strong evidence that laparotomy is unnecessary even if a small hemoperitoneum is demonstrated. CT may reveal the source of bleeding, such as pelvic fractures or a mesenteric hematoma. CT may also demonstrate relatively minor parenchymal lesions such as superficial liver lacerations with a small hemoperitoneum. In our experience, about 60% of patients with hepatic lacerations detected by CT have been spared surgery based on the CT findings and a stable clinical course (104). Presumably, all of the patients with hemoperitoneum would have had a positive peritoneal lavage and would have gone to surgery had this been a major criterion. Kuhn and Berger (105) reported a similar experience in their study of pediatric patients in which 79% of those with CT-demonstrated splenic injuries were managed nonoperatively. CT demonstration of a limited hepatic or splenic laceration with little or no hemoperitoneum correlated well with a stable clinical course.

Because CT scan detects any significant amount of hemorrhage, usually detects the specific source, and evaluates all of the intraperitoneal and extraperitoneal structures in a quick noninvasive study, it has largely replaced peritoneal lavage in the evaluation of blunt trauma at San Francisco General Hospital. The remaining role for lavage is in the evaluation of patients requiring urgent extra-abdominal surgery. For example, a patient requiring emergency craniotomy or operative fixation of extremity injuries might have peritoneal lavage while being anesthetized in the operating room, if the urgency of the situation precluded abdominal CT examination. Peritoneal lavage should *not* precede abdominal CT because the retained intraperitoneal gas and fluid may simulate traumatic lesions on CT.

CLINICAL IMPACT OF ABDOMINAL CT IN TRAUMA

San Francisco General Hospital (SFGH) is the only designated major trauma center servicing a population of over 700,000. This setting has allowed us to study large groups of unselected patients representative of the entire spectrum of urban trauma in both the pre-CT and CT eras.

In a 2-year period (1975–1976) prior to installation of a CT scanner at SFGH, the negative laparotomy rate following blunt trauma was 18.2% (42 negative; 231 total) (106). An additional uncalculated percentage of patients had nontherapeutic laparotomies, during which minor traumatic injuries (e.g., superficial hepatic and mesenteric lacerations) were discovered that had spontaneously stopped bleeding and required no other intervention. These figures are similar to the nontherapeutic laparotomy rate of 25% cited for the Maryland Institution for Emergency Medical Services Systems (29). Peritoneal lavage was in common use at

SFGH, and angiography, radionuclide scintigraphy, and conventional radiography provided additional diagnostic information in many cases.

In a recent 1-year period (1983) during which abdominal trauma CT was commonly employed at our trauma center, the nontherapeutic laparotomy rate was 12.3% (9 "negative"; 73 total). Seven of the 9 negative laparotomies were performed on patients in shock on the basis of massive head trauma and in whom an abdominal source of hypotension had to be excluded. In another patient with closed head injury, a trivial liver laceration was discovered at laparotomy. Importantly, only 1 of the 9 patients who underwent nontherapeutic laparotomy had had a preoperative CT scan, and it correctly indicated absence of trauma, although it had been initially misinterpreted by the on-call residents as abnormal. The negative laparotomy rate, therefore, of those who had a CT scan prior to surgery was 2% (1 of 73). There was one false positive CT interpretation. Of the 125 patients who underwent abdominal CT scans, 50% showed significant trauma (thoracic, abdominal, or pelvic) and 50% were negative for trauma. Using findings at surgery, clinical follow-up, and repeat radiographic studies (including CT) as proof, our data indicate an overall accuracy of 97.6% with 98.3% sensitivity and 96.8% specificity (107).

It is apparent that CT can substantially reduce the rate of nontherapeutic laparotomy in patients who are stable enough to undergo CT evaluation safely. It must be emphasized that patients who do not respond to initial resuscitation are not candidates for CT or other diagnostic modalities that may delay operative therapy. Thus, we can never expect to eliminate nontherapeutic laparotomies completely in the critically injured group of patients. Nevertheless, assuming proper patient selection, avoiding unnecessary laparotomy has several obvious benefits, including reduced medical costs and reduced perioperative morbidity and mortality.

CT has also substantially decreased the use of other imaging modalities and peritoneal lavage. Radionuclide scintigraphy and angiography are rarely performed for initial evaluation of blunt trauma at this institution, and peritoneal lavage is used primarily in the operating room for emergency evaluation of patients undergoing extra-abdominal surgery, as previously discussed.

REFERENCES

1. Freeark RF: Abdominal trauma. In Hardy JE (ed): *Rhoad's Textbook of Surgery*, ed 5. Philadelphia, JB Lippincott, 1977, pp 239–250.
2. Trunkey DD: Trauma. *Sci Am* 249:28, 1983.
3. Federle MP, Goldberg HI, Kaiser JA, et al; Evaluation of abdominal trauma by computed tomography. *Radiology* 138:637, 1981.
4. Toombs BD, Lester RG, Ben-Menachem Y, Sandler CM: Computed tomography in blunt trauma. *Radiol Clin North Am* 19:17, 1981.
5. Druy EM, Rubin BC: Computed tomography in the evaluation of abdominal trauma. *J Comput Assist Tomogr* 3:40, 1979.
6. Berger PE, Kuhn JP: CT of blunt abdominal trauma in childhood. *AJR* 136:105, 1981.
7. Kaufman RD, Towbin R, Babcock DS, et al; Upper abdominal trauma in children: Imaging evaluation. *AJR* 142:449, 1984.
8. Federle MP: Computed tomography of blunt abdominal trauma. *Radiol Clin North Am* 21:461, 1983.
9. Nelson EW, Holliman CJ, Juell BE, Mintz S: Computerized tomography in the evaluation of blunt abdominal trauma. *Am J Surg* 146:751, 1983.
10. Federle MP, Crass RA, Jeffrey RB, Trunkey DD: Computed tomography in blunt abdominal trauma. *Arch Surg* 117:645, 1982.
11. Wall SD, Federle MP, Jeffrey RB, Brett CM: CT diagnosis of unsuspected pneumothorax after blunt abdominal trauma. *AJR* 141:919, 1983.
12. Meyers MA: *Dynamic Radiology of the Abdomen*. New York, Springer-Verlag, 1976.
13. Bergstrom M, Ericson K, Levander B, et al: Variation with time of the attenuation values of intracranial hematomas. *J Comput Assist Tomogr* 1:57, 1977.
14. New PF, Aranow S: Attenuation measurements of whole blood and blood fractions in computed tomography. *Radiology* 121:635, 1976.
15. Norman D, Price D, Boyd D, et al: Quantitative aspects of computed tomography of blood and cerebrospinal fluid. *Radiology* 123:335, 1977.
16. Wolverson MK, Crepps LF, Sundaram M, et al: Hyperdensity of recent hemorrhage at body computed tomography: Incidence and morphologic variation. *Radiology* 148:779, 1983.
17. Swenson SJ, McLeod RA, Stephens DH: CT of extracranial hemorrhage and hematomas. *AJR* 143:907, 1984.
18. Federle MP, Jeffrey RB: Hemoperitoneum studied by computed tomography. *Radiology* 148:187, 1983.
19. Mall JC, Kaiser JA: CT diagnosis of splenic laceration. *AJR* 134:263, 1980.
20. Korobkin M, Moss AA, Callen PW, et al: Computed tomography of subcapsular splenic hematoma—clinical and experimental studies. *Radiology* 129:441, 1978.
21. Gruenberg JC, Horan DP: Delayed splenic rupture: The phoenix, *J Trauma* 23:159, 1983.
22. Taylor CR, Rosenfield AT: Limitations of computed tomography in the recognition of delayed splenic rupture. *J Comput Assist Tomogr* 8:1205, 1984.
23. Wright FW, Williams EW: Large post-traumatic splenic cyst diagnosed by radiology, isotope scintigraphy and ultrasound. *Br J Radiol* 47:454, 1974.
24. Jeffrey RB, Laing FC, Federle MP, Goodman PC: Computed tomography of splenic trauma. *Radiology* 131:719, 1981.
25. Glazer GM, Axel L, Goldberg HI, Moss AA: Dynamic CT of the normal spleen. *AJR* 137:343, 1981.
26. Federle MP: CT of upper abdominal trauma. *Semin Roentgenol* 19:269, 1984.
27. Defoe WW, Mattox LK, Jordan GL, Beall AC: Management of 1590 consecutive cases of liver trauma. *Arch Surg* 111:495, 1976.
28. Patcher HL, Spencer FC: Recent concepts in the treatment of hepatic trauma. *Ann Surg* 190:423, 1979.
29. Haney PJ, Whitley NO, Brotman S, et al: Liver injury and complications in the postoperative trauma patient: CT evaluation. *AJR* 139:271, 1982.
30. Moon KL Jr, Federle MP: Computed tomography in hepatic trauma. *AJR* 141:309, 1983.
31. Toombs BD, Sandler CM, Rauschkolb EN, et al: Assessment of hepatic injuries with computed tomography. *J Comput Assist Tomogr* 6:72, 1982.
32. Tyler U, Hoevels J, Nilsson U: Computed tomography of iatrogenic hepatic lesions following percutaneous transhepatic cholangiography and portography. *J Comput Assist Tomogr* 5:15, 1981.
33. Bhatt GM, Jason RS, Delaney HM, Rudavsky AZ: Hepatic hematomas: Percutaneous drainage. *AJR* 135:1287, 1980.
34. Iino S, Sawada T, Kusunoki T: Computed tomography in neonatal subcapsular hemorrhage of the liver. *J Comput Assist Tomogr* 5:416, 1981.

35. Pardes JG, Haaga JR, Borkowski G: Focal hepatic fatty metamorphosis secondary to trauma. *J Comput Assist Tomogr* 6:769, 1982.

36. Axel L, Moss AA, Berninger W: Dynamic computed tomography demonstration of hepatic arteriovenous fistula. *J Comput Assist Tomogr* 5:95, 1981.

37. Mathien D, Larde D, Vasile N: CT features of iatrogenic hepatic arterioportal fistulae. *J Comput Assist Tomogr* 7:810, 1983.

38. Esensten M, Ralls PW, Colleth P, Halls J: Posttraumatic intrahepatic biloma: Sonographic diagnosis. *AJR* 140:303, 1982.

39. Orloff MJ, Charters AC: Injuries of the small bowel and mesentery and retroperitoneal hematoma. *Surg Clin North Am* 52:729, 1972.

40. Roman E, Silva Y, Lucas C: Management of blunt duodenal injury. *Surg Gynecol Obstet* 132:7, 1971.

41. Toxopeus MD, Lucas CE, Krabbenhoft KL: Roentgenographic diagnosis in blunt retroperitoneal duodenal rupture. *Radiology* 115:281, 1972.

42. Kelley G, Norton L, Moore G, Eiseman B: The continuing challenge of duodenal injuries. *J Trauma* 18:160, 1978.

43. Glazer GM, Berg JN, Moss AA, et al: CT detection of duodenal perforation. *AJR* 137:333, 1981.

44. Karnayl GC, Sheedy PF, Stephens DH, McLeod RA: Computed tomography in duodenal rupture due to blunt abdominal trauma. *J Comput Assist Tomogr* 5:267, 1981.

45. Plojoux O, Hauser H, Wettstein P: Computed tomography of intramural hematoma of the small intestine. *Radiology* 144:559, 1982.

46. Love L: Radiology of abdominal trauma. *JAMA* 23:1377, 1975.

47. McKenzie AD, Bell BA: Nonpenetrating injuries of the colon and rectum. *Surg Clin North Am* 52:735, 1972.

48. Jeffrey RB, Federle MP, Stein SM, Crass RA: Intramural hematoma of the cecum following blunt trauma. *J Comput Assist Tomogr* 6:404, 1982.

49. Donovan AJ, Turrill F, Berne CJ: Injuries of the pancreas from blunt trauma. *Surg Clin North Am* 52:649, 1972.

50. Waugh JM, Lynn TE: Clinical and surgical aspects of pancreatic pseudocysts: Analysis of fifty-eight cases. *Arch Surg* 77:47, 1985.

51. Bach R, Frey CF: Diagnosis and treatment of pancreatic trauma. *Am J Surg* 121:20, 1971.

52. Jeffrey RB, Federle MP, Crass RA: Computed tomography of pancreatic trauma. *Radiology* 147:491, 1983.

53. Ivancev K, Kullendorff CM: Value of computed tomography in traumatic pancreatitis in children. *Acta Radiol (Diagn)* 24:441, 1983.

54. Richter MW, Lytten B, Myerson D, et al: Radiology of genitourinary trauma. *Radiol Clin North Am* 11:593, 1973.

55. Cass AS: Immediate radiological evaluation and early surgical management of genitourinary injuries from external trauma. *J Urol* 122:771, 1979.

56. Mahoney SA, Perskey L: Intravenous drip nephrotomography as an adjunct in the evaluation of renal injury. *J Urol* 99:513, 1968.

57. Morrow JW, Mendez R: Renal trauma. *J Urol* 104:649, 1970.

58. Kazmin MH, Brosman SA, Crockett ATK: Diagnosis and early management of renal trauma: A study of 120 patients. *J Urol* 101:783, 1969.

59. Evins SC, Thomason B, Rosenblum R: Nonoperative management of severe renal lacerations. *J Urol* 123:247, 1980.

60. Mendez R: Renal Trauma. *J Urol* 118:698, 1977.

61. Thompson IM, Latourette H, Montie JE, et al: Results of nonoperative management of blunt renal trauma. *J Urol* 118:522, 1977.

62. Halpern M: Angiography in renal trauma. *Surg Clin North Am* 48:1221, 1968.

63. Lang EK, Trichel BE, Turner RW, et al: Renal arteriography in the assessment of renal trauma. *Radiology* 98:103, 1971.

64. Elkin M, Meng C-H, de Paredes RG: Roentgenologic evaluation of renal trauma with emphasis on renal angiography. *AJR* 98:1, 1966.

65. Federle MP, Kaiser JA, McAninch JW, et al: The role of computed tomography in renal trauma. *Radiology* 141:455, 1981.

66. McAninch JW, Federle MP: Evaluation of renal injuries with computerized tomography. *J Urol* 128:456, 1982.

67. Kuhn JP, Berger PE: Computed tomography in the evaluation of blunt abdominal trauma in children. *Radiol Clin North Am* 19:503, 1981.

68. Sandler CM, Toombs BD: Computed tomographic evaluation of blunt renal injuries. *Radiology* 141:461, 1981.

69. Schaner EG, Balow JE, Doppman JL: Computed tomography in the diagnosis of subcapsular and perirenal hematoma. *AJR* 129:83, 1977.

70. Rosenbaum R, Hoffsten PE, Stanley RJ, Klahr S: Use of computerized tomography to diagnose complications of percutaneous renal biopsy. *Kidney Int* 14:87, 1978.

71. Lang EK, Sullivan J, Frenty G: Renal trauma: Radiological studies. Comparison of urography, computed tomography, angiography and radionuclide studies. *Radiology* 154:1, 1985.

72. Lang EK: Assessment of renal trauma by dynamic computed tomography. *Radio-Graphics* 3:566, 1981.

73. Ishikawa I, Matsuura H, Onouchi Z, Suzuki M: CT appearance of the kidney in traumatic renal artery occlusion. *J Comput Assist Tomogr* 6:1021, 1982.

74. Haynes JW, Walsh JW, Brewer WH, et al: Traumatic renal artery occlusion: CT diagnosis with angiographic correlation. *J Comput Assist Tomogr* 8:731, 1984.

75. Steinberg DL, Jeffrey RB, Federle MP, McAninch JW: The computerized tomography appearance of renal pedicle injury. *J Urol* 132:1163, 1984.

76. Rhyner P, Federle MP, Jeffrey RB: CT of trauma to the abnormal kidney. *AJR* 142:747, 1983.

77. Bush WH, Orme BM: CT diagnosis of symptomatic cystic hemorrhage in polycystic renal disease. *J Comput Assist Tomogr* 7:1115, 1983.

78. Jones TK, Walsh JW, Maull KI: Diagnostic imaging in blunt trauma of the abdomen. *Surg Gynecol Obstet* 157:389, 1983.

79. Ben-Menachem Y: Logic and logistics of radiography, angiography, and angiographic intervention in massive blunt trauma. *Radiol Clin North Am* 19:9, 1981.

80. Fitzgerald JB, Crawford ES, deBakey ME: Surgical considerations of nonpenetrating abdominal injuries. *Am J Surg* 100:22, 1960.

81. McConnell BJ, McConnell RW, Guibertean MJ: Radionuclide imaging in blunt trauma. *Radiol Clin North Am* 19:37, 1981.

82. Freedman GS: Radionuclide imaging of the injured patient. *Radiol Clin North Am* 11:461, 1973.

83. Nebesar RA, Rabinov KR, Potsaid MS: Radionuclide imaging of the spleen in suspected splenic injury. *Radiology* 110:609, 1974.

84. Chopp RT, Hekmat-Ravan H, Mendez R: Technetium-99 in glucoheptonate renal scan in diagnosis of acute renal injury. *Urology* 15:201, 1980.

85. Lutzler LG, Chun KJ: Radionuclide imaging in the nonsurgical treatment of liver and spleen trauma. *J Trauma* 21:382, 1981.

86. Gelfand MJ: Scintigraphy in upper abdominal trauma. *Semin Roentgenol* 19:296, 1984.

87. Utkoff LB, Wyffels PL, Adams CS, et al: A prospective study comparing nuclear scintigraphy and computerized axial tomography in the initial evaluation of the trauma patient. *Ann Surg* 198:611, 1983.

88. Stevelman RL, Glaubitz JP, Crampton RS: Laceration of the spleen due to nonpenetrating trauma: One hundred cases. *Am J Surg* 106:888, 1963.

89. Livingston CD, Sirinek KR, Levine BA, et al: Traumatic splenic injury; its management in a patient population with a high incidence of associated injury. *Arch Surg* 117:670, 1982.

90. Casarella WJ, Martin EC: Angiography in the management of abdominal trauma. *Semin Roentgenol* 19:321, 1984.

91. Fisher RG, Foucar K, Estrada R, et al: Splenic rupture in blunt trauma: Correlation of angiographic and pathologic records. *Radiol Clin North Am* 19:141, 1981.

92. Chuang VP, Reuter SR: Selective arterial embolization for the

control of traumatic splenic bleeding. *Invest Radiol* 10:18, 1975.

93. Rubin BE, Katzen BT: Selective hepatic artery embolization to control massive hepatic hemorrhage after trauma. *AJR* 129:253, 1977.

94. Lang EK: The role of arteriography in trauma. *Radiol Clin North Am* 14:353, 1976.

95. Kuligowska E, Mueller PR, Simeone JF, Fine C: Ultrasound in upper abdominal trauma. *Semin Roentgenol* 19:281, 1984.

96. Kay CJ, Rosenfield AT, Armm M: Gray-scale ultrasonography in the evaluation of renal trauma. *Radiology* 134:461, 1980.

97. Asher WM, Parvin S, Virgilio RW, et al: Echographic evaluation of splenic injury after blunt trauma. *Radiology* 118:411, 1976.

98. Froelich JW, Simeone JF, McKusick KA, et al: Radionuclide imaging and ultrasound in liver/spleen trauma: A prospective comparison. *Radiology* 145:457, 1982.

99. Strauch GO: Major abdominal trauma in 1971. *Am J Surg* 125:413, 1973.

100. Jordan GL, Beall AC: Diagnosis and management of abdominal trauma. *Curr Probl Surg* 3:5, 1971.

101. Powell DC, Bivens BA, Bell RM: Diagnostic peritoneal lavage. *Surg Gynecol Obstet* 155:257, 1982.

102. Fisher RP, Beverlin BC, Engrav LH, et al: Diagnostic peritoneal lavage. *Am J Surg* 136:701, 1978.

103. Soderstrom CA, DuPriest RW Jr, Cowley RA: Pitfalls of peritoneal lavage in blunt abdominal trauma. *Surg Gynecol Obstet* 151:513, 1980.

104. Meyer AA, Crass RA, Lim RC, et al: Selective non-operative management of blunt liver injury using abdominal CT guidance. *Arch Surg* 120:550, 1985.

105. Kuhn JP, Berger PE: Computed tomography in the evaluation of blunt abdominal trauma in children. *Radiol Clin North Am* 19:503, 1981.

106. Petersen SR, Sheldon GF: Morbidity of a negative finding at laparotomy in abdominal trauma. *Surgery* 148:23, 1979.

107. Wing VW, Federle MP, Morris JA Jr, et al: The clinical impact of computed tomography for blunt abdominal trauma. *Radiology* in press.

Chapter 7

CT in the Evaluation of Pelvic Trauma

MICHAEL P. FEDERLE, M.D.

Pelvic fractures from motor vehicle accidents are a cause of substantial morbidity and permanent disability, and are the third leading cause of death following blunt trauma (1–3). Associated extremity fractures are common (4), and injury to abdominal and pelvic viscera may occur. Difficulty in establishing the source of hemorrhage may be encountered, especially since pelvic fractures with extraperitoneal bleeding may result in intraperitoneal bleeding through torn fascial planes (5).

The difficulty in properly diagnosing and managing complex fractures of the pelvis and acetabulum is well documented (6, 7). Prognosis is influenced by the type and extent of pelvic fracture and associated soft tissue injuries. Computed tomography (CT) has proved to be a valuable tool in evaluation of these complex and life-threatening injuries.

INDICATIONS AND TECHNIQUE

Virtually all patients with complex acetabular or pelvic fractures are studied by CT at this institution. Simple or isolated fractures of the pubic rami or ilium are excluded unless there are other clinical concerns, such as unexplained blood loss or evidence of hip joint problems (e.g., decreased motion, instability).

In some cases of blunt trauma to the pelvis and abdomen, CT sections of the acetabulum and pelvis are obtained while evaluating the abdomen for visceral injury. In such cases we generally obtain 10 mm sections at intervals of 10 or 20 mm through the pelvis and abdomen to determine the type of fracture and the extent of hemorrhage and abdominal injury, if any.

If pelvic fracture is the only injury, initial radiographic evaluation consists of anteroposterior and bilateral 45° oblique films whenever possible. Inlet and outlet views of the pelvis are also obtained when disruptions of the pelvic ring are suspected. Fracture-dislocations of the hip are reduced, spontaneously or by manipulation, prior to other radiographic studies. Most patients are first studied by CT after a period of bed rest, clinical evaluation, and traction. Patients may remain in traction while the CT scan is performed (8). The CT examination begins with a digital radio-graph (Scoutview) of the pelvis in the anteroposterior projection (Fig. 7.1). Transaxial sections are obtained through the region of suspected fractures. Contiguous 5 mm sections are obtained through the acetabulum and femoral head, while 10-mm sections may be obtained for more extensive fractures of the upper sacrum or iliac wings. The axial or transverse plane is optimal for evaluation of the femoral head and major part of the acetabulum, while coronal and sagittal reformations are utilized to best demonstrate fractures of the acetabular dome and their relationship to the femoral head. These reformations are easily and quickly obtained by computer programs available as standard features on most modern CT scanners, and they entail no additional radiation to the patient. Some authors have advocated direct coronal CT sections of the pelvis, using angulation of the CT gantry and tilting the patient on a specially constructed board. Experience to date is limited, and the potential value of this technique has yet to be proved.

ANATOMY

The pelvis is an osseous ring composed of the following major components: the pubic rami and ischium, ilium, sacrum, and the pubic symphysis and sacroiliac joints. Because it is a ring, disruption of any point in the ring is almost always associated with a break through some other osseous or cartilaginous component of the ring.

The acetabulum is a complex structure, basically consisting of a concavity located at the apex of arch formed by two columns of bone (Fig. 7.2). The strong posterior or ilioischial column extends from the central portion of the obturator foramen through the middle of the acetabulum and then obliquely and posteriorly to the greater sciatic notch. This segment includes the ischial tuberosity. The anterior column extends forward from the same point on the obturator foramen through the acetabulum and then anteriorly to the anteroinferior iliac spine. Fractures may occur in either of the two columns, independently or together, and with or without involvement of the dome fragment or the adjacent ilium. The dome segment is

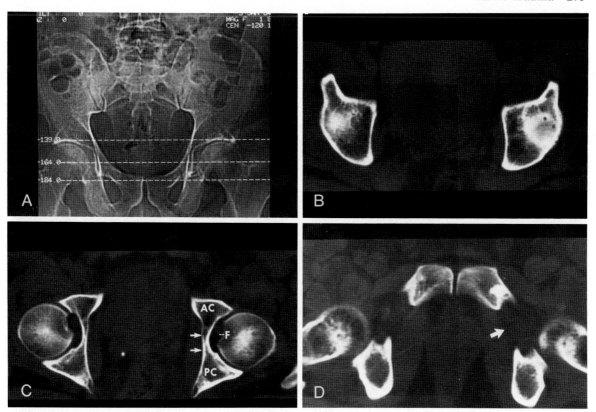

Figure 7.1.
A. Digital radiograph (Scoutview), *Labeled dashed lines* indicate level of axial sections (**B–D**).
B. Roof (dome segment) of acetabulum.
C. Midacetabulum. (*F*, fovea of femoral head, seen as a small concavity; *AC*, anterior column; *PC*, posterior column.) *Arrows* denote quadrilateral surface connecting the anterior and posterior columns.
D. Level of symphysis pubis and acetabular notch, seen as a discontinuity (*arrow*) in the anteroinferior portion of the acetabulum.

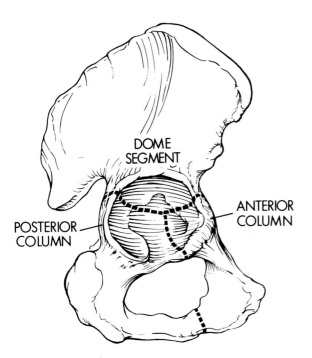

Figure 7.2.   Drawing of the acetabulum viewed from the lateral side. The *dashed line* indicates the divisions into anterior and posterior columns. The dome segment is the very strong and important superior aspect of the acetabulum, extending from the anterior-inferior iliac spine toward the greater sciatic notch.

the extremely strong bone extending from the posterior column to the anterior-inferior iliac spine. The acetabulum is rimmed by a thick ledge of bone called the conduit labrum, which forms a 320° arch and is complete except for the anterior and inferior segments (acetabular notch). On axial sections, the acetabulum is semicircular and partially surrounds the femoral head (Fig. 7.1).

MECHANISM AND CLASSIFICATION OF FRACTURES

In a simple classification of pelvic injuries there are two major types: stable and unstable (Fig. 7.3). Stable fractures consist of single breaks in the pelvic ring or fractures of the peripheral margins that do not disrupt the ring. Unstable fractures are those that disrupt the pelvic ring in two or more places and usually consist of fractures in both the posterior and anterior arches. Stable fractures account for two-thirds of all pelvic fractures and are usually the result of moderate trauma, such as a fall. Unstable fractures constitute one-third of pelvic fractures and are usually the result of severe trauma such as sustained in a motor vehicle or auto-pedestrian accident.

In blunt pelvic trauma, three types of disruptive forces are recognized: anterior compression, lateral compression, and vertical shear injuries (9, 10). All three types of forces may result in an unstable pelvis in which fractures through two portions of the pelvic ring cause separation of an unstable fragment from the rest of the pelvis.

Anterior injuries are caused by direct pressure on the anterior-superior iliac spines causing disruption of the symphysis pubis, but not resulting in an unstable fracture unless the ilium is involved posteriorly.

Lateral compression injuries cause a variety of fracture patterns and are responsible for the majority of pelvic fractures. When a lateral force is applied anteriorly on one side of the hemipelvis, that side is rotated inwardly causing a fracture pattern through the superior and inferior pubic rami in the posterior entry through the ipsilateral sacrum, sacroiliac joint, or ilium (Fig. 7.4). If the rotation is even more severe, disruption of the posterior ligaments occurs, and an unstable hemipelvis is the result. Such injuries resulting from violent lateral forces have the highest association with soft tissue injuries and the highest degree of mortality among all pelvic fractures.

Vertical shear injuries are all unstable fractures and constitute the most common form of unstable fracture, accounting for 14% of all pelvic fractures. The classical fracture pattern described by Malgaigne consists of a fracture through the pubic rami or pubic symphysis associated with a posterior disruption either through the sacrum, sacroiliac joint, or ilium (Figs. 7.4 and 7.5). The ipsilateral hemipelvis is unstable, and actual cranial displacement is not uncommon (Fig. 7.5).

STABLE

SINGLE BREAK IN PELVIC RING

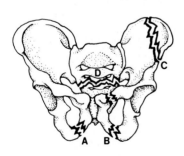

A. SINGLE PUBIC RAMUS

B. UNILATERAL PUBIC RAMI

C. ILIAC (DUVERNEY)

D. SACRUM OR COCCYX

UNSTABLE

DOUBLE BREAKS IN PELVIC RING

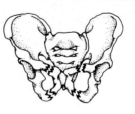

STRADDLE

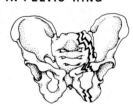

MALGAIGNE

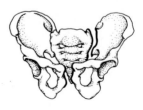

DISLOCATION

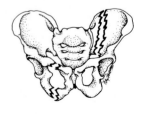

BUCKET HANDLE

Figure 7.3.   Typical patterns of stable and unstable pelvic fractures.

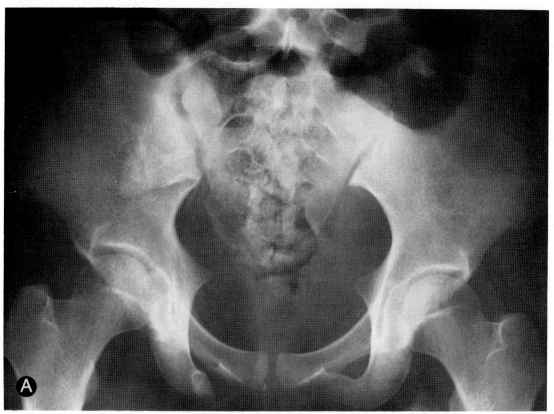

Figure 7.4.
A. Undisplaced Malgaigne fracture, plain radiograph.

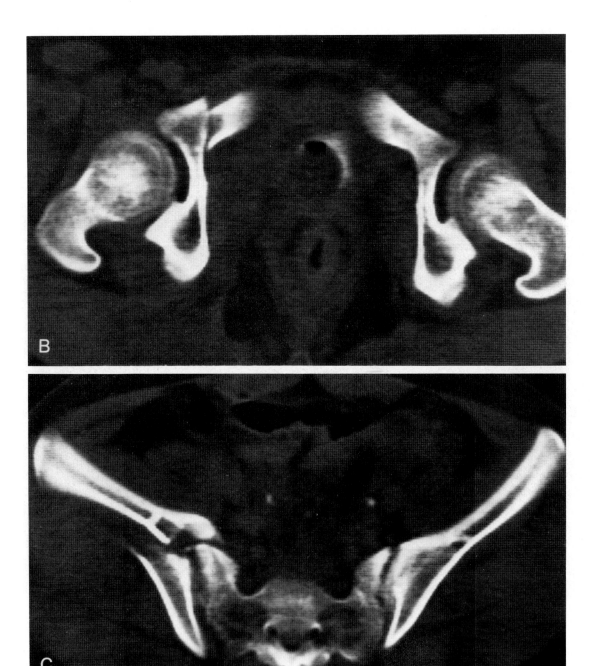

Figure 7.4.
B. Axial CT section demonstrating right superior pubic ramus fracture.
C. Iliac fracture with diastasis of the sacroiliac joint. This is an unstable pelvis.

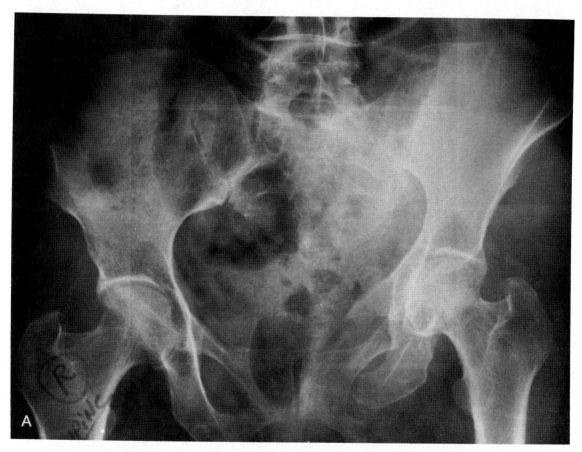

Figure 7.5.
A. Displaced Malgaigne fracture showing cephalic displacement of left hemipelvis.

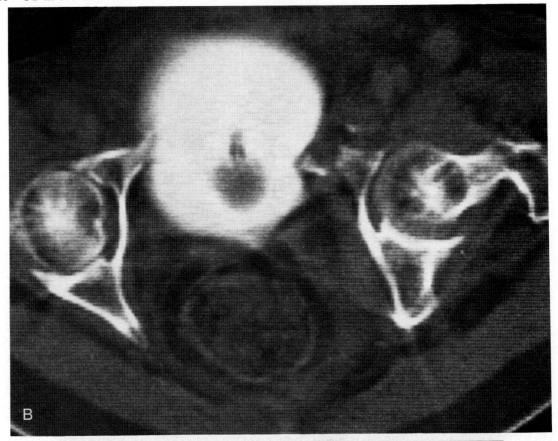

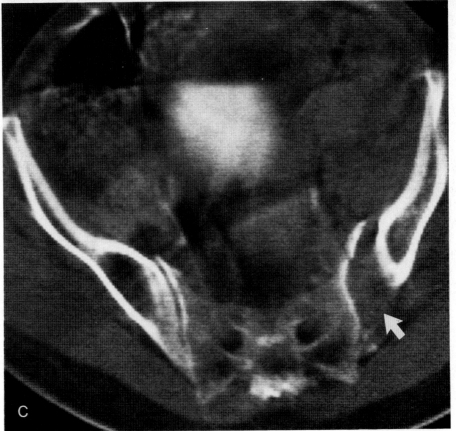

Figure 7.5.
B, C. CT sections demonstrate wide diastasis of the sacroiliac joint and fracture of the pubic rami.

Isolated fractures or fracture-dislocations of the acetabulum most often affect automobile passengers. With sudden deceleration (and failure to wear seat belts), the passenger is typically thrown forward, striking his knee on the dashboard, and driving the femoral head posteriorly out of the acetabulum. Acetabular fractures are discussed in detail below.

Trunkey et al. (1) have reviewed a large series of patients from this institution with pelvic fractures and noted a high morbidity and mortality due to uncontrolled bleeding and later complications, such as sepsis, thromboembolism, and the respiratory distress syndrome. They classified the types of pelvic injury and found this correlated with morbidity and mortality. Comminuted or crush fractures of the pelvis are the most serious type of injury and have the highest mortality. These injuries involve fractures or disruptions of three or more of the osseous or cartilaginous components of the pelvic ring and are often associated with massive hemorrhage and intra-abdominal injuries (Figs. 7.6 and 7.7).

Unstable pelvic fractures comprise Trunkey's second category and include acetabular fractures and vertical shear fractures (also known as double vertical

or Malgaigne fractures). These are important to recognize because they require immobilization or traction to reduce hemorrhage and to maintain the position of weight-bearing portions of the pelvis (Figs. 7.4 and 7.5).

The third category of injury includes stable fractures such as isolated pelvic fractures and fractures of the pubic rami. Immobilization in these cases is usually unnecessary except for symptomatic relief, and serious hemorrhage and other complications are uncommon, although they may occur (Fig. 7.8).

ROLE OF COMPUTED TOMOGRAPHY

Pelvic Fractures

The basic components of most pelvic fractures can be demonstrated by routine radiography. The proper role of CT in such injuries is still under evaluation, but we have found it to be most useful in selected cases. In evaluating the osseous component of pelvic injuries, CT is an important adjunct to plain radiography. CT may demonstrate fractures that are not visible on plain radiographs, particularly sacral fractures and diastasis of the sacroiliac joint (11, 12).

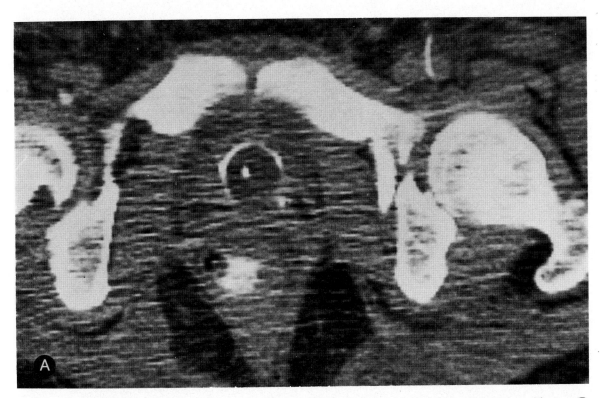

Figure 7.6.   Crush fracture of pelvis. Components of the injury include bilateral pubic rami fracture (**A**), acetabular and sacral fractures (**B, C**). Note extensive hemorrhage into soft tissues over the sacrum. The patient nearly exsanguinated from this injury but was stabilized following transcatheter Gelfoam embolization of pelvic bleeding vessels preceding the CT scan.

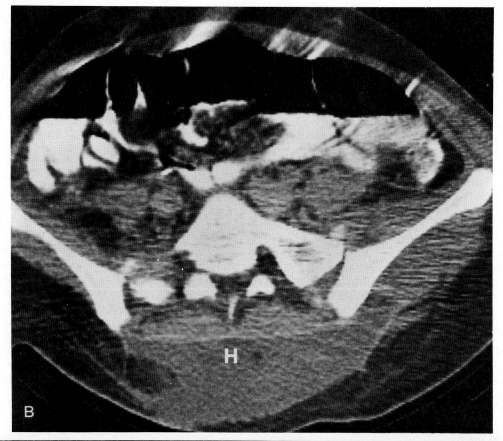

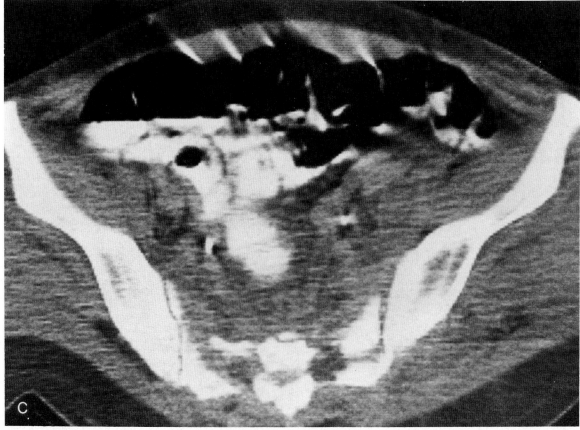

Figure 7.6.   B, C.

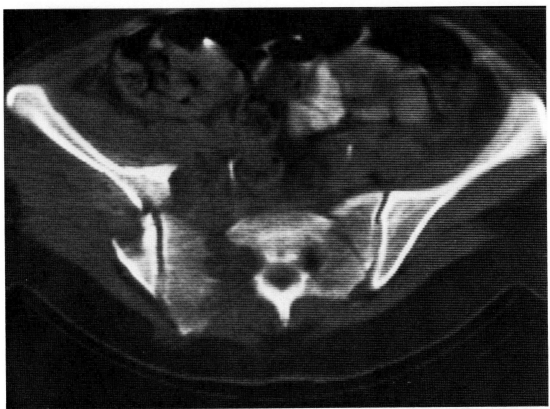

Figure 7.7. Crush fracture. Comminuted and displaced fractures of the sacrum and iliac wing are seen. Also present were acetabular and pubic rami fractures.

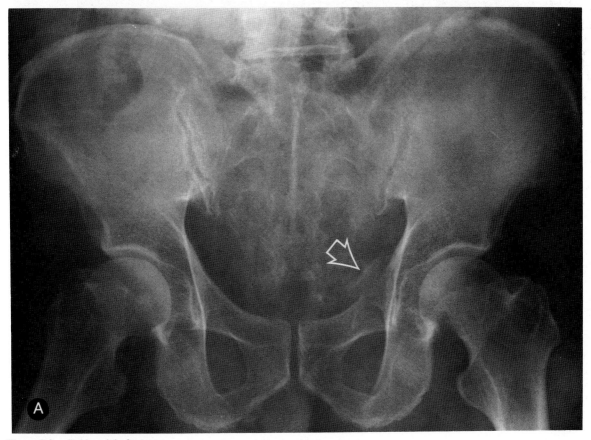

Figure 7.8. Stable pelvic fracture.
A. Plain radiograph shows displaced fracture of superior pubic ramus (*open arrow*).

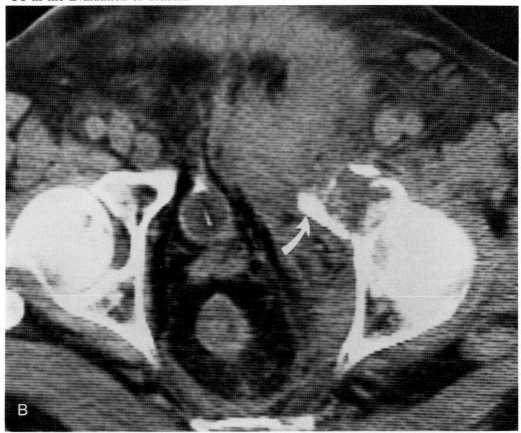

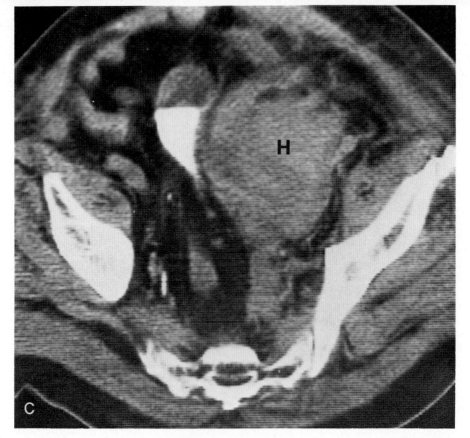

Figure 7.8.
B, C. CT sections demonstrate displaced comminuted fracture of superior pubic ramus and a large intrapelvic hematoma (*H*). CT was obtained because of continued blood loss which seemed out of proportion to the extent of pelvic fracture. Hemorrhage may have resulted from a spicule of bone (*solid arrow*) lacerating an artery.

These structures are frequently obscured by overlying bowel gas and stool. The tomographic nature of CT and the potential for multiplanar reformations of the axial sections also provide an inherently more complete understanding of the complex nature of pelvic fractures. In particular, CT may better depict stable and unstable fracture components (13–17). In one recent report (12) comparing CT and plain radiography for pelvic fractures, CT was judged to be "useful" or "extremely helpful" in 85% of cases by demonstrating additional fractures and better delineation of fracture fragment size, configuration, and displacement.

Since pelvic fractures usually result from blunt trauma, possible damage to abdominal and retroperitoneal structures is of great clinical concern. As noted above, peritoneal lavage is of limited value in this setting and may be misleading, since intraperitoneal blood may result from large pelvic hematomas with torn fascial planes in the absence of abdominal injury. In our experience, CT has been of value in excluding intra- or retroperitoneal visceral trauma while demonstrating the osseous and soft tissue components of the pelvic injury, including some estimation of the amount of hemorrhage (Fig. 7.9). In most cases, therapy can properly be directed toward the orthopaedic injuries without incurring the delay and additional morbidity of abdominal exploration. Extensive surgical exploration of pelvic hematomas is contraindicated since interruption of the tamponading effect of the peritoneum and fascia may cause exsanguination. CT demonstration of a large extraperitoneal hematoma and absence of intra-abdominal injury may lead to angiography as the next diagnostic procedure, should continued bleeding be clinically suspected. Angiography may demonstrate the source of hemorrhage, and provides a route for transcatheter occlusion of bleeding vessels, which is the most effective therapy (18). The incidence of severe hemorrhage and thus the need for embolic therapy has decreased due to the early use of external fixation of pelvic fractures by adjustable metallic frames (Hoffmann frame) that are fixed to the pelvic ring by metallic screws in the bone (Fig. 7.10).

Acetabular Fractures

Several methods of describing or classifying acetabular fractures are in use, and some terminology from each will be incorporated into this discussion (10, 19–21). Simple or partial fractures are those involving only the anterior or posterior column or noncomminuted transverse fractures. Isolated fractures of the anterior column are uncommon and generally carry a good prognosis, since the anterior column has less of a weight-bearing function and the anterior lip provides little stability for the hip joint (Figs. 7.11 and 7.12). Fractures of the strong posterior (ilioischial) column are more common and are usually associated with posterior dislocation of the hip. Fractures of the posterior lip of the acetabulum often result in intra-articular fragments and other complications to be discussed later (Fig. 7.13).

Falls from a height may drive the femoral head into the dome of the acetabulum, often resulting in complex or stellate fractures. In T-shaped fractures, the acetabulum is split, separating the anterior and posterior columns (Fig. 7.14). This feature has considerable prognostic and surgical importance, since operative fixation of both columns may be required. CT can accurately depict the stable and unstable components (13, 16, 17).

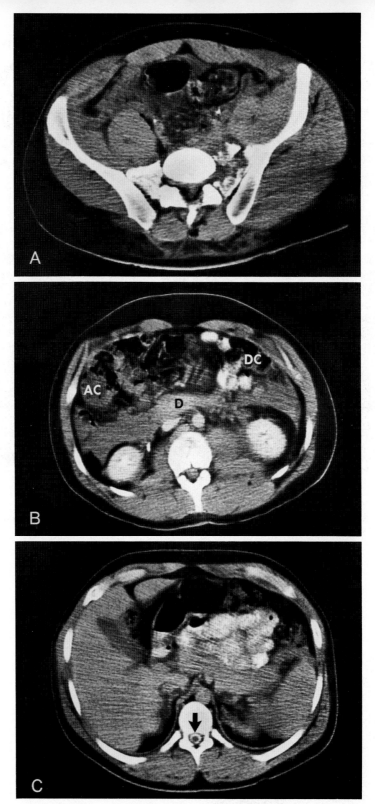

Figure 7.9. Complex pelvic and spine fractures. A 25-year-old man jumped 40 feet from a freeway overpass, suffering vertebral and pelvic fractures. A falling hematocrit caused concern for abdominal visceral injuries. An abdominal-pelvic CT scan was requested to evaluate fracture extent, the source of hemorrhage, and coexisting abdominal visceral injury or hemoperitoneum. It was performed after administration of oral, intravenous, and intrathecal contrast. The latter was administered via a C1-C2 puncture to evaluate the extent of compromise of the spinal canal by the lumbar fracture.
A. Extensive pelvic fractures including comminuted fractures of both sacral ala. Fractures of the pubic rami were present on caudad sections, constituting an unstable double vertical fracture. Note the soft tissue swelling (hemorrhage) into the left buttock and iliopsoas muscles.
B. Fracture through L1 with an absence of intrathecal metrizamide at this and lower levels due to block by fracture fragments. Note extensive hemorrhage into the anterior pararenal spaces bilaterally surrounding the third portion of duodenum (*D*) and displacing ascending (*AC*) and descending colon (*DC*) anteriorly. Note the absence of blood in the paracolic gutters lateral to the vertical colon segments.
C. Normal spleen, liver, and pancreas with no hemoperitoneum. Note metrizamide surrounding the thoracic spinal cord (*arrow*). CT thus excluded intraperitoneal hemorrhage, and when continued hemorrhage was clinically suspected, diagnostic angiography was performed next. Bleeding vessels were occluded with Gelfoam emboli and hemostasis was achieved without laparotomy.

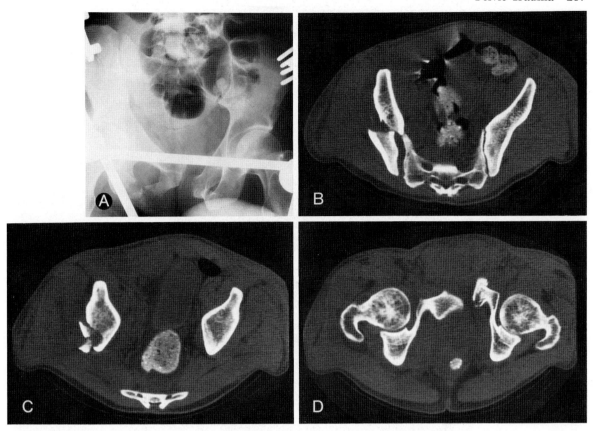

Figure 7.10.   Displaced Malgaigne fracture in external fixation frame.
A. Plain radiograph with stabilizing frame fixed to pelvis.
B, C. Axial CT sections demonstrate diastasis of sacroiliac joint with a fracture of the ilium extending into the dome fragment.
D. Axial CT section demonstrates diastasis of pubic symphysis and internal rotation of the right hemipelvis.

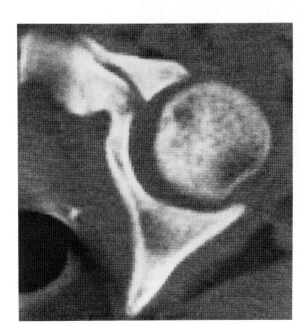

Figure 7.11.   Fracture of anterior column. As an isolated injury, these fractures generally carry a good prognosis.

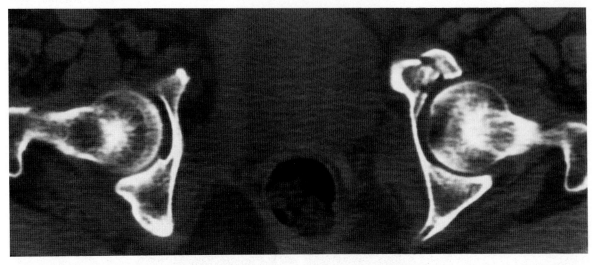

Figure 7.12. Comminuted fracture of anterior column.

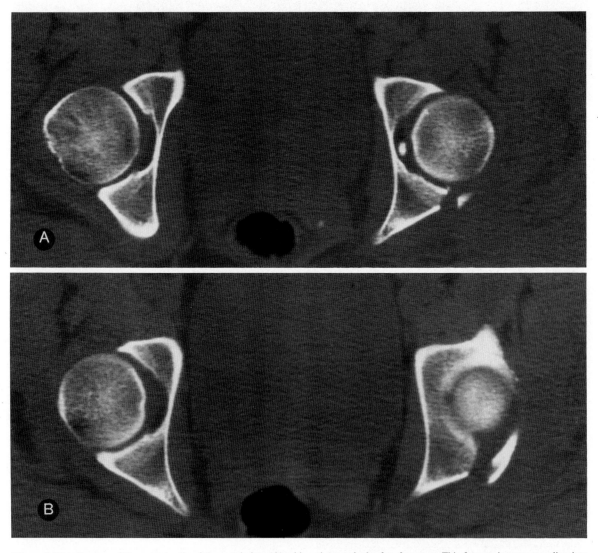

Figure 7.13. Fracture of the posterior lip of the acetabulum (**A**) with an intra-articular free fragment. This fracture is seen extending into the dome fragment (**B**).

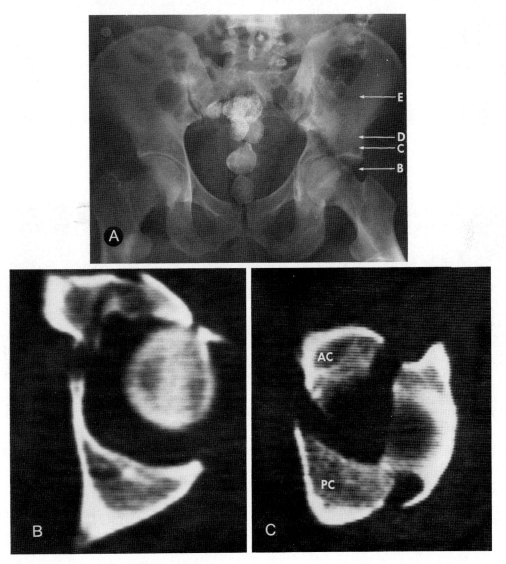

Figure 7.14.   Complex T-shaped fracture of acetabulum.
A. Anteroposterior radiograph shows complex acetabular fracture and probable diastasis of the left sacroiliac joint. *Arrows* and *letters* indicate corresponding axial sections.
B–E. Axial sections through acetabulum demonstrate fractures separating anterior (*AC*) and posterior columns (*PC*) (**B, C**), extending into iliac wing (**D**) and causing diastasis of the sacroiliac joint (**E,** *arrow*).
F, G. Coronal (**F**) and sagittal (**G**) reformations further demonstrate the complex nature of this fracture and best depict the relationship of the femoral head (*F*) to the dome fragment (*DF*). *Solid line* (*) indicates location and plane of reformation.

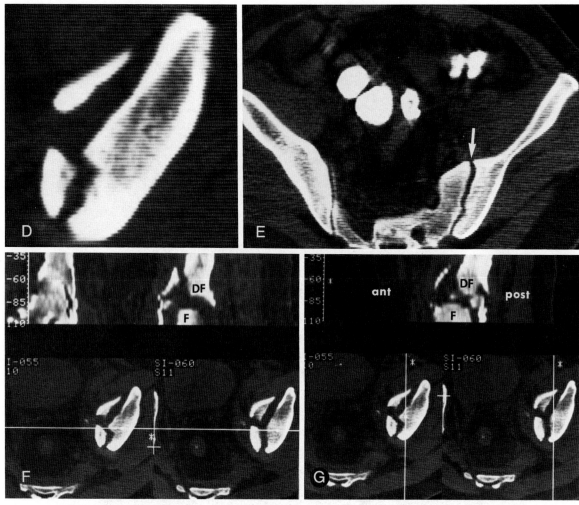

Figure 7.14.   D–G.

Complex fractures of the dome always have important implications, since the dome fragment is the major superior weight-bearing portion of the acetabulum. Some authors consider a displaced dome fragment the single most important indication for surgery in acetabular fractures (Fig. 7.15) (20, 22).

Complex fractures that involve the iliac wing carry a worse prognosis than those that do not. The wing fragment is often displaced and externally rotated, and failure to reduce this component prevents surgical reduction of the acetabular fracture (Fig. 7.16). If an iliac wing fracture is not found, sacroiliac disruption is often present with a similar external rotation of the hemipelvis and difficulty in reduction. Proper demonstration of all components of complex fractures, including the degree of comminution and displacement, is important in determining if open reduction is warranted and in planning the surgical approach (20, 22). The combination of plain radiographs and CT has proved optimal in this regard.

Beyond the anatomic classification of acetabular fractures, orthopaedic surgeons recognize several important considerations that may influence the choice of open surgical therapy or nonoperative management. Judet and colleagues (19) have described four complications of fracture-dislocation of the hip that often require open reduction. It was these authors' attempts to better define these abnormalities that led them to devise the oblique radiographs of the pelvis commonly known as the Judet views. It appears that the unique properties of CT are even better able to detect these complications, and these four criteria should be carefully evaluated on every CT examination.

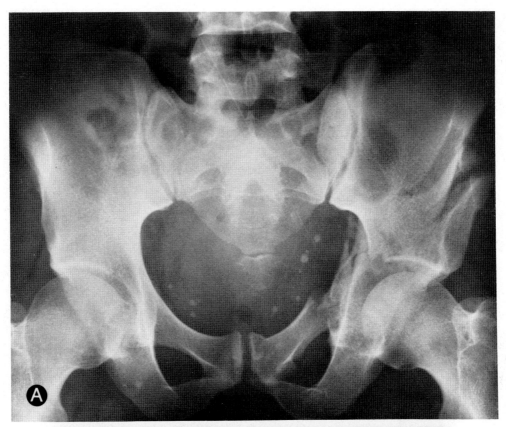

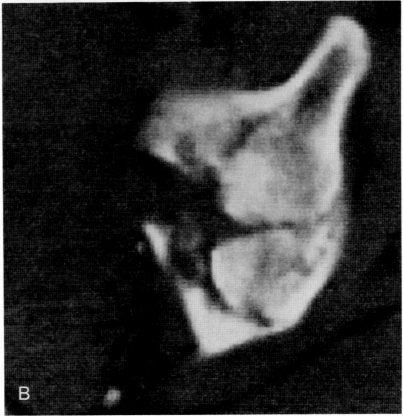

Figure 7.15.   Complex fracture of the dome fragment.
A. Plain radiograph shows complex comminuted fracture.
B. Axial CT section shows comminuted fracture of dome segment.

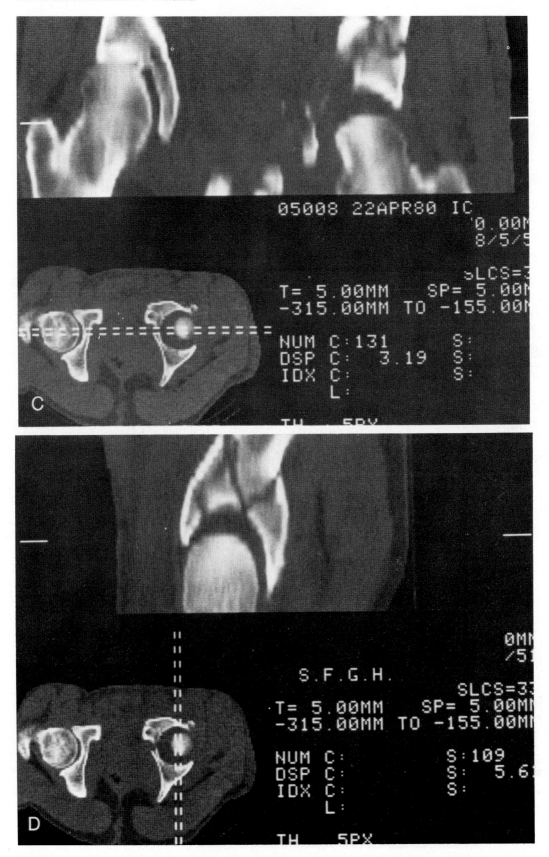

Figure 7.15.
C, D. Coronal (**C**) and sagittal (**D**) reformations better demonstrate the components of the dome fracture and the relationship of the femoral head to the dome. *Dashed lines* through axial image show plane of reformation.

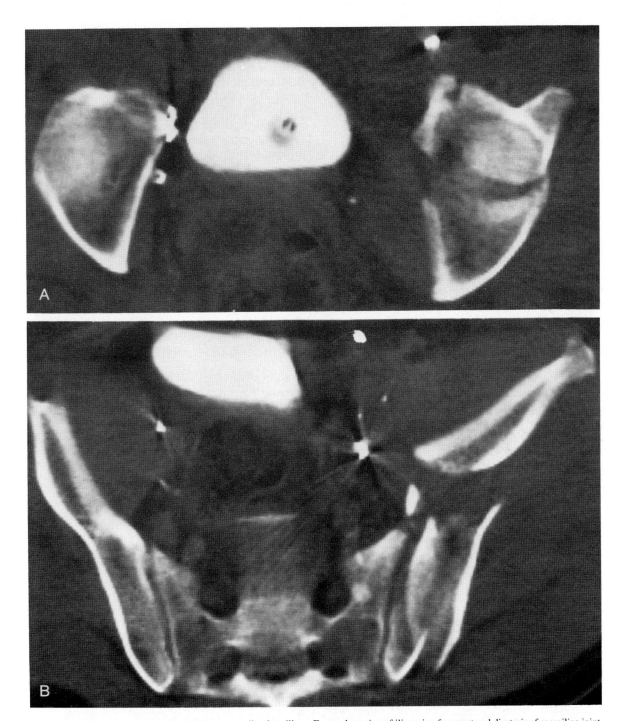

Figure 7.16.   Complex fracture of acetabulum extending into ilium. External rotation of iliac wing fragment and diastasis of sacroiliac joint imply a less favorable prognosis and must be reduced for proper surgical reduction of the acetabular fracture.

1. Stability of the hip joint

The two major osseous structures that stabilize the femoral head within the joint are the dome segment and the posterior lip of the acetabulum. Axial CT sections clearly demonstrate fractures of the posterior lip along with the degree of rotation, comminution, and displacement (Fig. 7.17). While fractures of the dome are easily detected on axial sections, the important relationship of the dome fragment to the femoral head is best depicted by coronal and sagittal reformations of the CT scans in planes passing through the femoral head (Fig. 7.18).

2. Intra-articular fragments

Osseous or cartilaginous fragments from the acetabulum or femoral head are frequently displaced into the hip joint following fracture-dislocation. Such debris may limit joint mobility or lead to degenerative changes, and demonstration of such fragments is important even if surgical reduction is planned (20). Plain radiographs often fail to demonstrate loose bodies. CT is more sensitive in determining their presence, size, and site of origin (Figs. 7.13 and 7.19) (13, 23–25). One limitation of CT, however, is its inability to demonstrate small cartilaginous fragments (21).

3. Fractures of the femoral head

Posterior fracture-dislocations may result in a "shear" fracture of the femoral head as it is driven past the irregular fractured surface of the posterior lip of the acetabulum (Fig. 7.19). Occasionally, impacted fractures of the femoral head result from trauma (Figs. 7.20 and 7.21) even in the absence of acetabular fracture or dislocation. CT appears to be more sensitive in demonstrating the size and location of femoral fragments than routine radiographs or conventional tomography (13, 23–25).

4. Congruity of fracture fragments

Complex fractures of the medial wall or dome of the acetabulum can lead to severe degenerative changes and long-term disability, as the femoral head articulates with an irregular acetabular surface. Precise definition of the position and alignment of fragments is necessary to guide the orthopaedic surgeon in the formidable task of reconstructing this complex anatomic unit (22). In addition to defining complex acetabular fractures more completely, CT may detect central acetabular fractures that cannot be visualized on routine radiographs (26). Fractures through the superior-medial portion of the dome may be particularly difficult to demonstrate on plain radiographs, and these may clinically simulate hip fractures.

Future Developments

New computer software programs are being evaluated by several manufacturers of CT equipment that allow three-dimensional reconstructions from standard axial sections through major anatomic units (Fig. 7.22). These images can be manipulated to show bone or soft tissue detail optimally and can be rotated in space in real time. Such precise and detailed information has already been demonstrated to be of value to plastic surgeons in reconstructing complex maxillofacial deformities that have resulted from trauma or congenital anomaly. We will soon begin prospectively studying complex pelvic and acetabular fractures using a similar program, and we anticipate that the improved preoperative understanding of the pathologic anatomy will faciliate surgical reconstruction with decreased long-term morbidity.

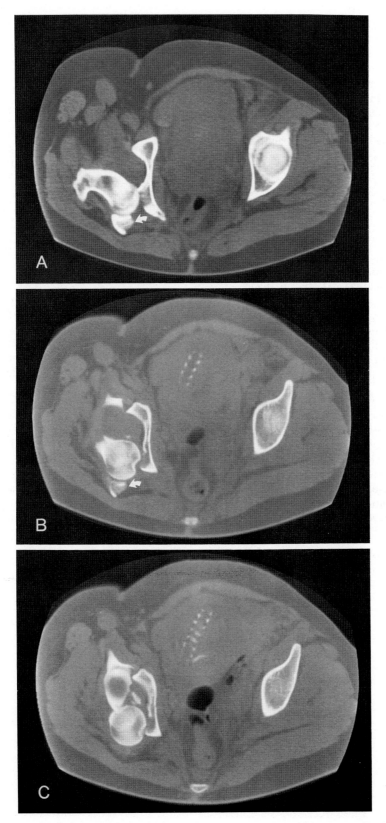

Figure 7.17. Unstable acetabular fracture-dislocation. Young pregnant woman in motor vehicle accident suffered abdominal and pelvic trauma causing fetal demise. Axial sections (**A–C**) show posterior dislocation of femoral head and intra-articular debris. The two most important elements for hip stability, the posterior lip and dome segment, have been fractured and displaced (*arrows*). Surgical fixation was required.

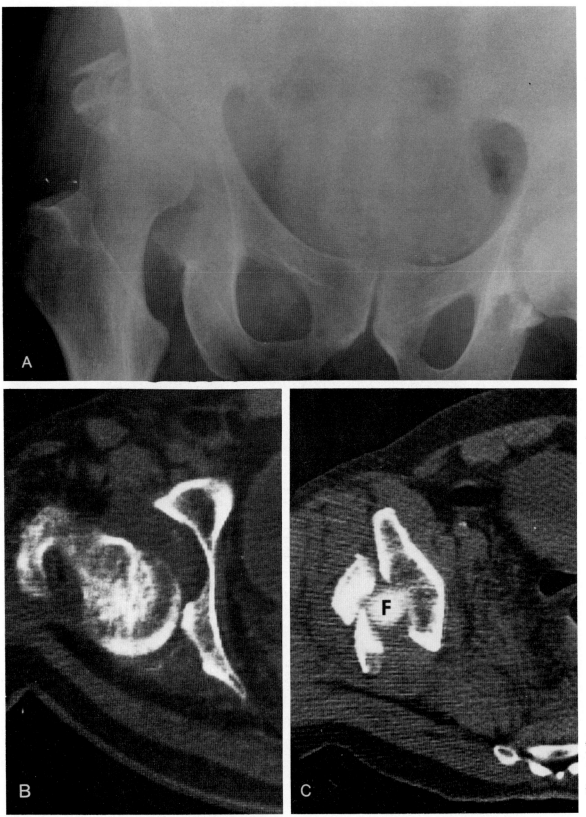

Figure 7.18. Unstable acetabular fracture-dislocation.
A. Plain radiograph demonstrates comminuted fracture and superolateral displacement of femoral head.
B, C. Axial sections following traction show displacement of femoral head (*F*) which lies lateral to the iliac wing. Femoral head is also displaced posteriorly due to fracture of posterior lip of acetabulum.

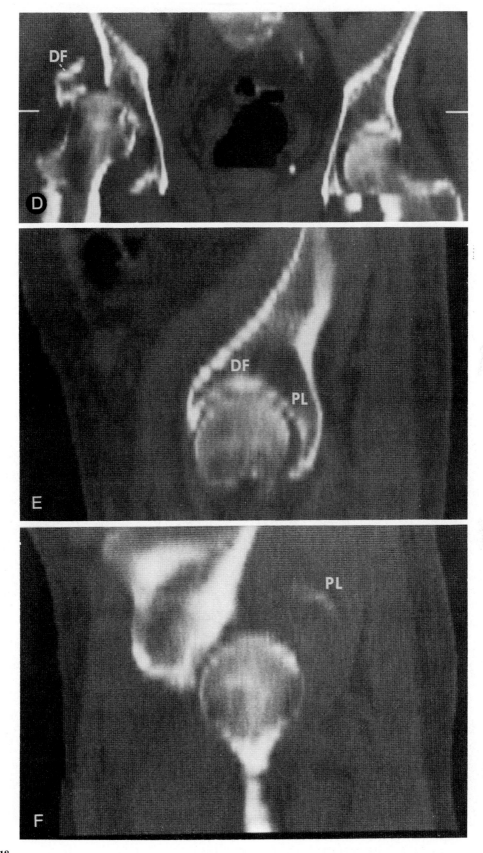

Figure 7.18.
D. Coronal reformation shows displaced dome fragment (*DF*), allowing superior subluxation of femoral head.
E, F. Sagittal reformation of normal (**E**) and abnormal (**F**) hip in this patient. Note the complete displacement of the posterior lip (*PL*) of the acetabulum.

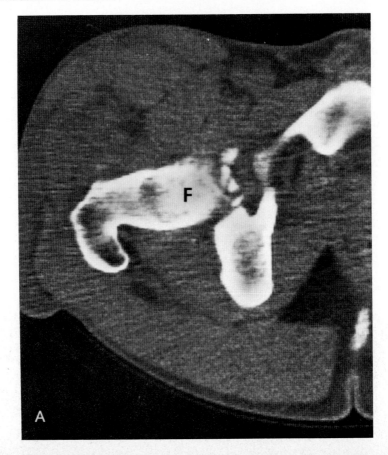

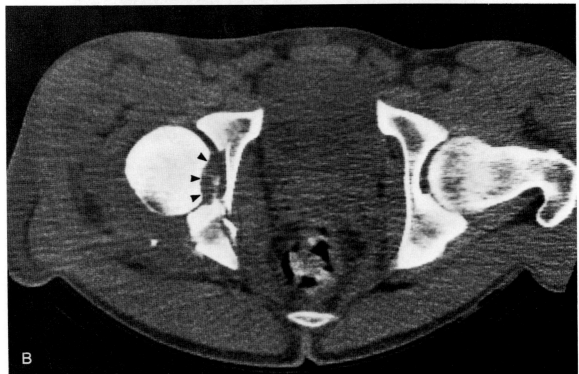

Figure 7.19.   Intra-articular fragments and femoral head fracture.
A. Multiple bony fragments interposed between femoral head (*F*) and acetabulum.
B. "Shear" fracture of femoral head. The scooped-out defect (*arrows*) is larger than the normal indentation at the fovea. Note fracture of the posterior lip of the acetabulum, which occurred at the time of dislocation.

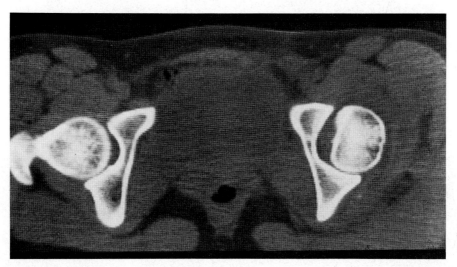

Figure 7.20.   Impacted femoral head fracture. This appears similar to a shear fracture and also resulted from posterior dislocation of the hip. However, no fracture fragments or intra-articular debris are noted.

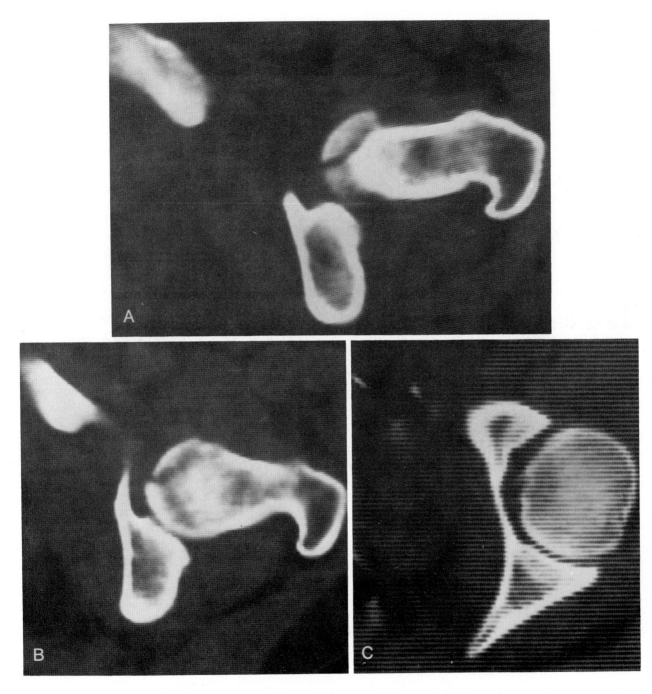

Figure 7.21.   Impacted fracture of femoral head without acetabular fracture.

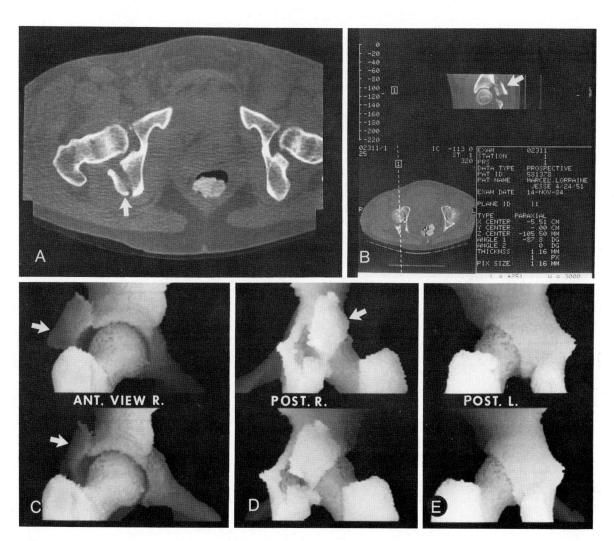

Figure 7.22. Three-dimensional reconstruction of acetabular fracture. Axial section (**A**) and sagittal reformation (**B**) demonstrate a displaced fragment (*arrows*) from the posterior lip of the acetabulum. Three-dimensional reconstructions can be rotated in any plane for viewing. Anterior (**C**) and posterior (**D**) views graphically demonstrate the large displaced fragment and its relationship to the rest of the pelvis and the femoral head. Posterior views of the normal left acetabulum (**E**) are shown for comparison.

REFERENCES

1. Trunkey DD, Chapman MW, Lim RC Jr, Dunphy JE: Management of pelvic fractures in blunt trauma injury. *J Trauma* 14:912, 1974.
2. Naam NH, Brown WH, Hurd R, et al: Major pelvic fractures. *Arch Surg* 118:610, 1983.
3. Melton LJ III, Sampson JM, Morrey BF, Ilstrup DM: Epidemiologic features of pelvic fractures. *Clin Orthop* 155:43, 1981.
4. Ward RE, Clark DG: Management of pelvic fractures. *Radiol Clin North Am* 19:167, 1981.
5. Hubbard SG, Bivens BA, Sachatello CR, Griffen WO Jr: Diagnostic errors with peritoneal lavage in patients with pelvic fractures. *Arch Surg* 114:844, 1979.
6. Epstein HC: Posterior fracture-dislocations of the hip. *J Bone Joint Surg* 56A:1003, 1974.
7. Baines SN, Stewart MJ: Central fractures of the acetabulum: A critical analysis and review of literature. *Clin Orthop* 114:276, 1976.
8. Robertson J, Federle MP: Simple traction-immobilization device for CT scanners. *AJR* 141:1331, 1983.
9. Tile M: Pelvic fractures: Operative versus nonoperative treatment. *Orthop Clin North Am* 11:423, 1980.
10. Pennal GF, Tile M, Waddell JP, Garside H: Pelvic disruption: Assessment and classification. *Clin Orthop* 151:12, 1980.
11. Gilula LA, Murphy WA, Tailor CC, Patel RB: Computed tomography of the osseous pelvis. *Radiology* 132:107, 1979.
12. Dunn EL, Berry PH, Connally JD: Computed tomography of the pelvis in patients with multiple injuries. *J Trauma* 23:378, 1983.
13. Sauser DD, Billimoria PE, Rouse GA, Mudge K: CT evaluation of hip trauma. *AJR* 135:269, 1980.
14. Hubbard LF, McDermott JH, Garrett G: Computed axial tomography in musculoskeletal trauma. *J Trauma* 22:388, 1982.
15. Whelan MA, Gold RP: Computed tomography of the sacrum: 1. Normal anatomy. 2. Pathology. *AJR* 139:1183, 1982.
16. Harley JD, Mack LA, Winquist RA: CT of acetabular fractures: Comparison with conventional radiography. *AJR* 138:413, 1982.
17. Mack LA, Harley JD, Winquist RA: CT of acetabular fractures: Analysis of fracture patterns. *AJR* 138:407, 1982.
18. Kam J, Jackson H, Ben-Menachem Y: Vascular injuries in blunt pelvic trauma. *Radiol Clin North Am* 19:171, 1981.
19. Judet R, Judet J, Letournel E: Fractures of the acetabulum: Classification and surgical approaches for open reduction. Preliminary report. *J Bone Joint Surg* 46A:1615, 1964.
20. Letournel E: Acetabulum fractures: Classification and management. *Clin Orthop* 252:81, 1980.
21. Senegas J, Liorzou G, Yates M: Complex acetabular fractures. *Clin Orthop* 151:107, 1980.
22. Tile M: Fractures of the acetabulum. *Orthop Clin North Am* 11:481, 1980.
23. Lange TA, Alter AJ Jr: Evaluation of complex acetabular fractures by computed tomography. *J Comput Assist Tomogr* 4:849, 1980.
24. Shirkhoda A, Brashear HR, Staab EV: Computed tomography of acetabular fractures. *Radiology* 134:683, 1980.
25. Blumberg ML: Computed tomography and acetabular trauma. *Comput Tomogr* 4:47, 1980.
26. Rogers LF, Novy SB, Harris NF: Occult central fractures of the acetabulum. *AJR* 124:96, 1975.

Index